ETHICAL DIMENSIONS in the HEALTH PROFESSIONS

Fourth Edition

Ruth B. Purtilo, PhD

Professor and Director of Ethics Initiative
MGH Institute of Health Professions
Boston, MA

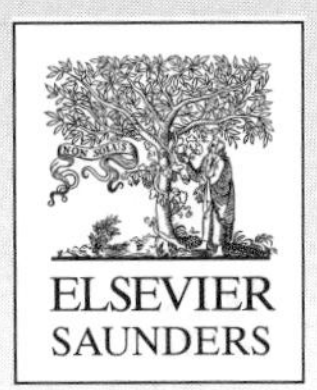

ELSEVIER
SAUNDERS

The Curtis Center
170 S Independence Mall W 300E
Philadelphia, Pennsylvania 19106

ETHICAL DIMENSIONS IN THE HEALTH PROFESSIONS, EDITION FOUR

NOTICE

Physical Therapy and other health professions are ever-changing. Standard safety precautions must be followed, but as new research and clinical experience broaden our knowledge, changes in treatment and drug therapy may become necessary or appropriate. Readers are advised to check the most current product information provided by the manufacturer of each drug to be administered to verify the recommended dose, the method and duration of administration, and contraindications. It is the responsibility of the licensed prescriber, relying on experience and knowledge of the patient, to determine dosages and the best treatment for each individual patient. Neither the publisher nor the author assumes any liability for any injury and/or damage to persons or property arising from this publication.

Previous editions copyrighted 1999, 1993, 1981

ISBN-13: 978-0-7216-0243-1
ISBN-10: 0-7216-0243-6

Acquisitions Editor: Marion Waldman
Developmental Editor: Jacqui Merrell
Publishing Services Manager: Melissa Lastarria
Senior Designer: Julia Dummitt

Printed in the United States of America

Last digit is the print number: 9 8 7 6 5 4 3

With gratitude to my colleagues
at the Creighton University Center for Health Policy and Ethics
for their ongoing support and generosity of ideas
and for their daily reminder that work can be both meaningful
and fun.

Preface

There has never been a more challenging or generative time to enter the health professions. As this fourth edition goes to press, the news is filled with discussion of life-prolonging technologies, including artificial or animal organs for transplantation, and with talk of a "post human era" populated with cyborgs, robots, and other fusions of computer technology with biological entities. Embryonic and other stem cell research and the promises and cautions of genomic medicine are also being debated. Healthfulness and health maintenance programs have adherents in all parts of the globe. Worldwide, the population is growing older and with it is the unintended side effect of an unprecedented number of persons with chronic impairment, including Alzheimer's disease and other dementias. Smaller and smaller newborns are taking up residence in larger and larger newborn intensive care units. The AIDS epidemic is into its third decade while the age-old ravages of war and other violence persist. In addition, the organizational and institutional dimensions of health care are changing locally and worldwide. For example, partial or total privatization of health care systems is emerging in many nations, raising serious questions about who will gain access to services and on what conditions. At the same time, specialized information technology and improved transportation have brought with it new opportunities for effective clinical interventions to reach people in the most remote communities.

Everyday health professionals confront the ethical issues raised by the above issues and more. This textbook is expressly for health professions students–those members of society who are prepared to gain the appropriate skills for leadership as professionals. The text gives these students the ethical tools to use for recognizing ethical issues, building understanding, and working toward the resolution of ethical problems. The goal is to improve the lives of patients, the community, and themselves. In the course of their professional education, practitioners in the health professions are members of society who are transformed from simply caring to learn to also learning to care. The tone is practical throughout—this is not a book for philosophers or distant observers of the health care enterprise, but for people on the front lines of health care decision making.

The fourth edition stands on the shoulders of the previous three, grounded securely in those enduring concerns that have supported the need for professional ethics and ethical professionals since the beginnings of health care. The current edition also builds on my abiding conviction that health professionals can and should assume a strategic position to help shape the contours of today's health care environment so that it embraces and protects cherished social values. The weight of responsibility for constructing or reinforcing high ethical standards must be shouldered by all health professionals, not just by doctors or nurses and not turned over to philosophers, theologians, administrators, or policy makers.

This new edition also reflects educators' increased awareness that ethics has to be taught, and taught well, so that students will be well prepared for their role. Society expects its health professionals to be informed about current ethical issues and be moral agents in helping to address them. In response, administrators and teachers in professional education continue to work toward offering more and better professional ethics courses, ethics seminars, and continuing education opportunities. Furthermore, in many educational programs educators skillfully have woven ethics theory and practice into the very fabric of the student's educational experience. With these changes, it is not surprising that there has been a proliferation of written and online resources for new students and lifelong learners alike. In short, I have observed a promising increase in sophistication and interest in professional ethics and in a commitment to providing educational experiences geared to improving knowledge and skills in this area. My goal in preparing this updated and expanded edition has been to reflect these positive changes by offering an instrument that educators can use to meet the changing needs of the classroom, seminar, and self-learning settings while maintaining the no-frills approach that has helped assure the book's utility during the past decade.

What's New in this Edition

With these encouraging considerations as guideposts, the fourth edition of *Ethical Dimensions in the Health Professions* introduces *an explicit focus throughout on the overarching goal of professional practice,* namely *the search for a caring response.* Chapter 1 introduces the idea, and at the beginning of Chapter 2 I delineate the specific characteristics of "care" that are relevant to professional ethics, setting the groundwork for how "care" figures into professionals' relationships with patients, their colleagues, health care institutions, and society. Care for oneself, sometimes missing in ethics discussions, is included. In every chapter the goal of a caring response helps to orient the reader, providing the basic reason for his or her ethical concern and attempt to solve ethical problems in everyday practice.

In Chapter 2, immediately following the description of "care" and what, exactly, is entailed in "a caring response," I introduce the four basic prototypes of ethical problems, highlighting how each one challenges the professional who is in search of a caring response in a particular situation. Readers of the previous editions will recognize that *the prototypes of problems are introduced earlier* than in previous editions, my intent being to help students think, at the beginning of their study in ethics, about their role as moral agents.

In the previous editions two chapters were devoted to ethical theories and approaches. In this edition *the description of ethical theories and approaches have been summarized into one chapter* (Chapter 3), the organization flowing from those that emphasize character and virtue to those more designed to aid action. In other words, the professional (i.e., moral agent) who has a disposition to care also needs ethical tools to discern the direction a caring response will take when action is required.

The six-step problem-solving method is retained and further refined. In concert with the goal of a caring response, *this six step process serves much more of an organizing function in the subsequent chapters than in previous editions.* I use Chapter 4 to incorporate the welcome input from readers of the previous edition regarding use of the method and to tie each step of the process to the material introduced in the earlier chapters.

The fourth edition again takes both traditional and emerging roles of health professionals seriously: *Updated cases and other examples pay special attention to societal trends or concerns* (e.g., bioterrorism, genetic conditions, the need for competence related to ethnic and cultural diversity, new members of the health care team and sites where care is provided). There is added attention *to dealing ethically with mistakes.* New population trends are taken into account for their ethical implications; for example there is *a new chapter on chronic conditions and long-term care.* The book addresses the health professional as an individual moral agent (including one's moral agency as a student) and as a moral participant in team decisions. The reader also has an opportunity to learn about how he or she is shaped by organizational structures and can be effective as a framer of ethical policies and practices in the institutions of health care.

As in previous editions, the textbook does not assume that the reader has engaged in any previous formal study of ethics. For those who have, parts should provide a quick and helpful review. The scope is broad and the focus multidisciplinary. Those wanting more rigorous study in a particular topic or discipline fortunately will find ample materials available, both on-line and in hard copy. For those wishing additional work in basic philosophical, theological, or other theories and approaches to ethical issues, there are excellent texts and courses, including an increasing number of short-term intensive courses offered.

Ethical Dimensions in the Health Professions is a basic map, backpack, and fresh water supply for what I trust will be a lifelong and generative journey of professional ethics exploration, reflection, and effective professional judgment and action. This journey is, I believe, the key to finding self-fulfillment in professional life. Once begun, the reader will find many other trekkers to walk and talk with along the way, each compelled and all connected by wanting to help foster the best type of health care possible.

Ruth Purtilo

Acknowledgments

Edition Four

The first edition of this book was coauthored with my respected colleague and friend, Dr. Christine Cassel. Readers familiar with her outstanding work will recognize her ideas and insights again woven into the very warp and woof of the text.

I owe a debt of gratitude, too, to the health professions students I have had the opportunity to teach and learn from during the life of this book: at the University of Nebraska Medical Center, the Karolinska Institute, the MGH Institute of Health Professions, Harvard Medical School, and Creighton University.

As for the current edition, I am especially grateful to Ms. Helen Shew my colleague at the Creighton University Center for Health Policy and Ethics. Her skill in helping to prepare the manuscript, then review, proof, and prod it into its final form was a great gift. Ms. Gina Svendsen worked diligently and skillfully with publishers and authors to secure permission to reprint material, and I am grateful for her help as well. Ms. Rita Nutty and Ms. Marybeth Goddard provided important back-up support. As the reader can conclude, the book was a team effort.

During 2003-2004 I was invited to be a Sherrill Visiting Professor in Ethics at the MGH Institute of Health Professions, Boston, Massachusetts during which time considerable work on this edition took place. Their support of this project, as well as the opportunity to discuss many ideas with colleagues, enhanced my own thinking and is reflected in the quality of this product.

Thanks, too, to my husband Vard Johnson. His deep support for the highest ideals of who I want to be as a person and deep respect for what I want to do in my professional life bring joy to the tasks of both.

Notes to Instructors on Using This Edition

The core purpose of this book is to provide the tools for addressing common, everyday ethical issues in the health professions. I hope you will find it student *and* instructor user-friendly!

The goal of a caring response (Chapter 2), combined with *the six-step process of ethical decision-making* (Chapter 4) is your organizing framework. A quick look through the table of contents will highlight that they appear throughout almost every chapter in the book. In addition, each chapter includes a story to help focus the student's thinking.

The Six Steps	Building Blocks	Chapter(s)
Step 1: Gather relevant information	One must pay attention to the details of the narrative for its ethical content.	1, 3, examples in later chapters
Step 2: Identify the type of ethical problem	The *three prototypes* of problems will organize the details of the narrative into categories for further analysis.	2, examples in later chapters
Step 3: Analyze the problem using ethics theories or approaches	One must attend to methods and concepts that take means and ends into account, as well as use principles as guides towards appropriate action. Virtue helps position one for appropriate moral action.	3, examples in later chapters
Steps 4: Explore the practical alternatives	This step requires life experience and creativity.	Examples are provided throughout the book

Step 5: Act	Resolve to proceed is needed. Courage helps.	Examples are provided throughout the book
Step 6: Evaluate the process and outcome	Ethics require self-reflection on moral situations and decisions. Each act must be evaluated for how it might have been better and what can be learned for next time.	4, find sections and examples throughout

Other Instructional Tools

At the beginning of each chapter are

- Educational objectives for the chapter
- New terms introduced in the chapter
- A quick cross reference of key concepts used in the chapter and where each first appeared in the book

At the end of each chapter are questions for thought and discussion.

Objectives

Through reading this book and discussing the Questions for Thought and Discussion, students will be able to

1. Increase their sensitivity to the influence of ethics in professional practice.
2. Identify how the need to find a caring response factors into a wide range of ethical issues in their practice.
3. Competently apply a straightforward problem-solving method to ethical decision making.
4. Become familiar with basic ethics approaches and concepts widely used today in addressing ethical dimensions of professional practice and policy.
5. Recognize current and longstanding themes in professional ethics and cite examples of concrete ethical situations reflecting them.
6. Gain insight into ethical situations and problems that are unique to their own profession, in contrast to those shared by a wide range of health professionals.
7. Find resources useful for more in-depth study of professional ethics.

Contents

Guide to Cases and Stories in Text

Section I

Introduction to Ethical Dimensions in the Health Professions

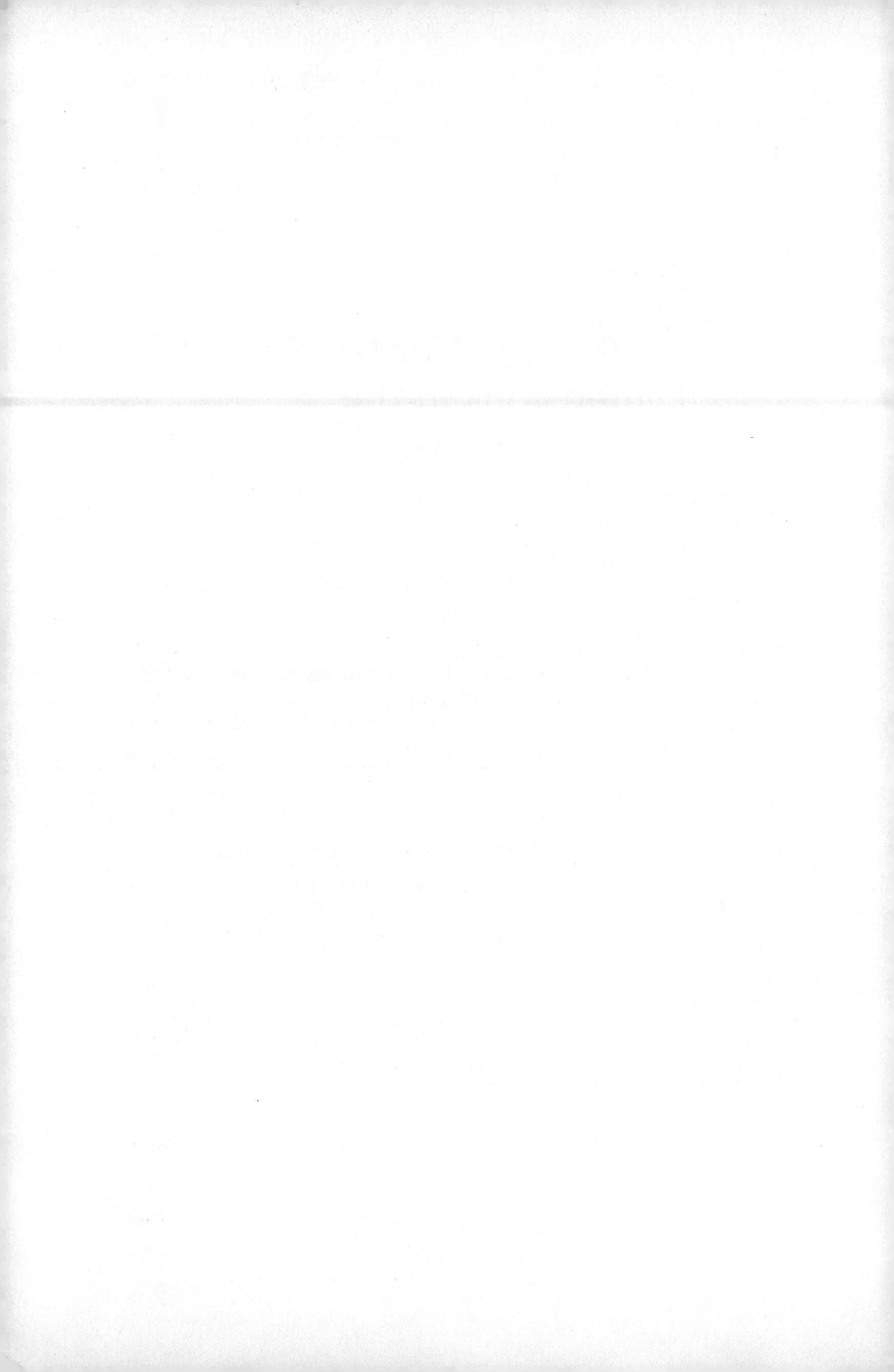

1

Morality and Ethics:
What Are They and Why Do They Matter?

Objectives

The student should be able to:

- Define morality and ethics and distinguish between the two.
- Describe three moralities that health professionals must integrate into their own moral life.
- Identify some major sources of moral beliefs in Western societies.
- Distinguish between an ethical issue and ethical problem.
- List three ways that ethics is useful in everyday professional practice.
- Describe what material cooperation entails.
- Identify some mechanisms available to protect the personal moral convictions of health professionals.

New terms and ideas you will encounter in this chapter

morality	values	duties
moral character/virtue	personal morality	societal morality
group morality	ethics	ethicists
ethics committees	ethical issue	ethical problem
conscience	material cooperation	state interest
licensing laws	moral repugnance	deductive theories
inductive theories	individualistic theory	common good theories
role of reason	role of emotion	the Hippocratic Oath

Introduction

Your adventure into the world of health care ethics begins with a story. Throughout this textbook you will meet patients, health professionals, families, and others who are facing challenges posed by their situations and the health care environment. Their stories illustrate the types of ethical issues you yourself may face as a caregiver, a patient, or a family member. The underlying ethical themes in the stories are woven into the very fabric of health care. This book attempts to pull out the threads, examine them for their unique or interesting characteristics, and assess the role each plays in the overall scheme of good professional practice.

The following story is about the Harvey family and the health care system into which they are catapulted after the tragic events of a beautiful late spring day.

The Story of the Harvey Family

Drew Harvey was undoubtedly one of the most popular students at Mountmore College. Now, in his senior year, he was captain of the college basketball team which had had its best season ever, going to regional competition, and had his own band that played every Saturday night at the most popular local pub, the Mole Hole. He had played more than studied during his first 2 years of college, having never had to "crack the books" in high school. But after his sophomore year he worked as an assistant in a local law firm. When he returned in his junior year he announced that he was going to become a lawyer. He buckled down, gaining an almost straight "A" record, never having to give up basketball or the band.

May 20

And so the violent incident that occurred during the weekend before commencement rocked the entire community. Drew's band was playing at the Mole Hole at an event reserved for the college seniors and their friends. At the end of the first set, just as Drew was acknowledging the band members to the applause and howls of the audience, he suddenly staggered backward and blood appeared on his forehead as he fell forward off the platform. After a moment of stunned silence someone screamed, "He's been shot!" Pandemonium broke out. Someone must have called 911. Drew mumbled, a confused and frightened look on his face, "What's going on?" Then he lost consciousness. He was taken to the emergency department of a hospital, where it was determined that a bullet had lodged in his skull, penetrating it above his left temple.

The physician assistant and nurses on duty administered first aid trauma measures. By now his parents had arrived. The physician on call asked Drew's mother, Alice, to sign informed consent, insurance, and other forms and began to prepare Drew for immediate surgery to remove the bullet and for subsequent admission to the hospital.

Mrs. Harvey wept. When a nurse put an arm across Alice's shoulder and said, "I'm sorry," Alice began to cry inconsolably. Alfonso Harvey, Drew's father, stood off to one side, staring straight ahead as if in shock. The nurse offered to get Alice a drink of water and guided them to a private waiting room while explaining what would happen next. Police were everywhere.

June 11

After 2 weeks in the intensive care unit, Drew regained consciousness. The shunt that had been placed in his skull to relieve the swelling of his brain was working well. He was beginning to focus his gaze, and the nurses believed he was trying to say something, though no one else saw this gesture yet. On the 18th day, the physician reported that Drew would be transferred to the medical unit. This morning, 22 days after the shooting, the physician told Alice that Drew was "stabilized" and would be going home soon. "Home!" Alice gasped. "How can we possibly manage at home? He can barely talk, can't walk, can't go to the bathroom alone!" The social worker who was standing at the foot of the bed explained that the Harveys would be visited by a home care nurse and for some time (depending on his progress) by a physical therapist, speech therapist, and others. The physician reminded the Harveys that Drew's progress exceeded their expectations, likely a reflection of the excellent physical shape he was in before his trauma. The social worker added that a home health aide also would visit periodically. The physician did caution that although Drew was improving, it was impossible to predict how much he would finally improve. However, she said the entire team was hopeful.

July 11

At home Drew's right arm and hand regained function so that he could almost dress himself. He couldn't walk because of spasticity of the right leg, although the spasticity seemed at times to be subsiding. He suffered from a limited vocabulary but increasingly caught himself when he used a wrong word. Because of this progress the case manager authorized another 6 weeks of physical therapy, speech therapy, and other interventions.

Mr. and Mrs. Harvey were understandably anxious but very supportive throughout the entire ordeal, encouraging their son toward as much independence as possible and offering support when needed. Drew's older brother made some adjustments in the Harveys' home to accommodate Drew's impaired state.

Today (April 1)

The several health professionals working with Drew have grown attached to him and his family. They have rejoiced with every sign of progress and have struggled with him through the frustration and depression that accompany such a catastrophe. But the health professionals are now faced with a difficult situation. Another treatment review is due. Understandably, when no further progress can be shown, authorization for his treatments (and therefore the reimbursements for them) will be discontinued. At the moment his progress seems to have stopped.

Anyone who works with patients who experience brain trauma knows that the team faces a critical and delicate situation. The rate of "progress" is not always constant. It may be marked by periods of rapid improvement interspersed with other periods of almost no perceptible change (plateaus). If the patient ceases to receive maintenance treatments during these plateau periods, a dramatic loss in functioning may occur. Yet, many insurance plans or other reimbursement mechanisms make little or no allowance for these plateau periods, and treatment usually is discontinued. The patient must regress to the point at which a symptom becomes acute again before treatment can be reinstituted. In summary, although progress eventually does end, the failure to allow for a plateau period often results in the patient being prematurely discontinued from treatment altogether. This is precisely the ambiguity facing the health professionals who have been treating Drew Harvey.

The Story of the Harvey Family (continued)

Drew's speech and progress in being able to walk have reached a plateau. Yet, the health professionals have not reached an agreement regarding whether more improvement may be on the way if he is not allowed to slip back. Maybe he will be able to avoid lifelong use of a wheelchair if his treatment is not discontinued at this critical juncture. But his university's health plan insurers use success ("outcomes") measures that make it unlikely he will continue to be reimbursed for therapy costs. The health professionals know that continued payments for treatment depend on their report of his progress. What should they do?

- Should they "bend the truth a little," reporting that Drew continues to make daily progress, so that he will be less likely to lose an opportunity for possible further progress?
- Should they tell the truth and let Drew be discontinued from treatment at this time?
- Are there alternatives to an either/or solution to this perplexing problem?

- Should they get involved in trying to change the insurance company policies that put them in this difficult situation in the first place?

Reflection

Suppose *you* are treating Drew and feel like you are the one who has to be an advocate for him and his family. You probably will try to figure out some way to report on his condition that gets him a chance at a few more treatment sessions. Questions with a broader outlook might occur as well. For instance, is it fair to continue treating him if you are not prepared to make a similar defense for all patients in a comparable situation? Or, an even broader scope may be encompassed: Are you as a health professional responsible for trying to change the system so that such situations do not occur and you can more easily give patients what you think they need? Take a minute to jot down what you think are the most important challenges facing health professionals involved with Drew Harvey's situation, regardless of whether they are suggested in the above text:

1. ____________________

2. ____________________

3. ____________________

4. ____________________

Responses to these challenges are not to be found in the textbooks that deal with the technical skills of your chosen field. You are beginning to use your understanding of morality and how ethics figures into your professional life if you are thinking about what would be *right* or *wrong* conduct for you in this situation and *why*; what your *duties* are to everyone involved, and what your (and everyone else's) *rights* are; the type of *character traits* you want to preserve; or what constitutes *fairness* for all patients in similar situations. In a word, what is involved in showing Drew and his family that you *care*?

> **SUMMARY**
>
> Facing difficult human questions about right and wrong conduct, duties, rights, character traits, and fair treatment are part and parcel of your professional challenges.

These considerations may even make you think about what type of society you want to help build in your professional career. In all of these areas of your professional life you are dealing with morality and moral values.

Morality and Moral Values

When "the moral life" or "morality" is mentioned, you might think of what you were told to do or not to do as a child. That *is* a part of morality. But morality is a much richer idea than that. From the earliest societies onward people have established guidelines designed to preserve the very fabric of their society. Taken collectively, these guidelines are a society's morality.

Morality, then, is concerned with relationships between people and how, ultimately, they can best live in peace and harmony. The goal of morality is to protect a high quality of life for an individual or for the community as a whole. Most people recognize this and try to act in accordance with morality in their everyday activity. They know that "certain things ought or ought not to be done because of their deep social importance in the ways they affect the interests of other people."[1] It makes things go better and gives more meaning to life. Morality is made up of a lot of values and duties and character traits based on beliefs that people take for granted most of the time.

Values is the language that has evolved to talk about objects or things a person holds dear. An apt example is life itself. Without it you cannot do anything else. Many moral values build on this basic value of life and describe certain qualities that constitute "a good life" from the perspective of how individuals can live full lives, finding support for their basic interests and providing it to others.

Duties is a language that has evolved to describe actions in response to claims on you that are either self-imposed or imposed by others. Moral duties describe certain *actions* required of you if you are to play your part in preventing harm and building a society in which individuals can thrive. *Moral character* or *virtue* is a language used to describe *traits* and *dispositions* or attitudes that are needed to be able to trust each other and to provide for human flourishing in times of stress, such as compassion, courage, honesty, faithfulness, respectfulness, humility, and other ways of being in the world that we want to be able to count on. These traits taken together and exercised regularly make up what we mean when we say a person is "of high moral character."

As a child you acquired parts of your morality from parents and friends, from reading and television, from your religious teaching, and in school. Behavior was modified when knowingly or unknowingly you did something outside of what you had been taught is right, and you were punished or shamed by others for what you did (or failed to do). One of the primary tasks of growing up is to internalize or personalize aspects of the morality that have come from various sources in your life. In fact, there is a whole area of study in psychology called "moral development" that deals with theories of how and why individuals become the types of moral beings they are.

Reflection

Consider some sources that have informed your own moral beliefs. Your answers can be personal reference points as you read on about morality.

1. Who or what have been five important influences on your understanding of right and wrong?

a. ____________________

b. ____________________

c. ____________________

d. ____________________

e. ____________________

2. Name three people whom you admire. They can be people you know personally or only by reputation. What makes them admirable?

a. ____________________

b. ____________________

c. ____________________

Morality informs many decisions in your everyday experience, but usually you are so accustomed to moving through your life in accordance with its values and duties that you have little conscious awareness of it. In short, it is safe to say that morality is habitual, shaping the character of individuals and communities, the majority of the time without them even realizing it.

As a student entering the health professions you must reckon with at least three subgroups of morality: your personal morality, societal morality, and the morality of the health professions and its institutions. Fortunately, there are large areas of overlap. Whether as an individual among family members or friends, as a citizen, or as a professional, the sources of moral belief usually derive from similar understandings of value, of right and wrong, of virtues and vices, and large groups of society interpret their dictates similarly.

Personal Morality

Personal morality is made up of the virtues, values, and duties you have adopted as relevant. You may recognize them as customs, laws, rules, beliefs, or simply "the way things always were done in my family." Saints and moral heroes have so fully personalized what they learned that they can stand alone in their convictions when opportunities for wrongdoing arise and can make decisions that others admire because they are exemplary. Everyone has a personal morality, however imperfectly internalized.

One task you face as a health professional is to try to understand the personal morality of your patients, clients, colleagues, and others with whom you come into contact. The health professionals treating Drew will not be successful if they fail to take into account the values and rights of the Harvey family, as well as their own values, rights, and duties. Without sensitivity to the differences between your own and their personal moral beliefs and habits you will not be able to communicate or work together effectively.

Reflection

Identify four or five things you consider a part of your own personal morality, because we seldom step back and do this except in times of crisis (e.g., lying is wrong; I should be kind to myself and others; everyone deserves respect).

1. ______________________________

2. ______________________________

3. ______________________________

4. ______________________________

5. ______________________________

If you have time, compare your list with a classmate to see if there are large areas of agreement. Usually there are because you also participate together in a larger societal morality. Discuss your differences and how you think they might affect your life as future colleagues in the health professions.

Societal Morality

Large components of personal morality represent a common denominator of shared beliefs about values and duties called *societal morality*. Some beliefs are generated by culture, ethnic group, or geography. Almost always they spring from deeper religious, philosophic, or anthropologic beliefs about humans: their relationship with God (or the gods in some cultures) or with each other. In the United States, the founding legislators, who had risked crossing oceans and leaving behind almost every security, tried to capture the common denominator of their societal morality in a slogan stating that "all are created equal" and therefore everyone should have an equal chance at "life, liberty and the pursuit of happiness." One characteristic of a democratic society in good working order is that everyone engages in critiquing and refining morality (e.g., laws, customs, and other moral components of the society) to keep it on course, all the while being attentive to the heterogeneity of ethnic and religious traditions.[2]

Almost always some tensions exist between personal and societal morality. These tensions are played out in large societal debates with individuals and groups taking sides. Two current health care–related debates deal with the morality of abortion and physician-assisted suicide. The abuse of the physical environment, sometimes occasioned by health care technology and waste disposal, the status of immigrants, and taxation for purposes of providing health care coverage are examples of other debates that present challenges at the level of social policy.

Group Morality: The Health Professions and Their Institutions

Everyone except perhaps the most isolated recluse joins or is swept into one or more subgroups of society by virtue of being a member of a religious group, a club, an organization, an ethnic group, or other affiliation. This can be termed *group morality.* One such subgroup, the health professions, has some moral values and duties that do not apply to others in society. For instance, citizens in general are not morally required to help another in need. You are. Citizens are not morally required to keep in confidence information they hear about another. You are. Citizens are not morally required to be nonjudgmental about another's character. You are, through your *fiduciary* duty discussed in other parts of this book, notably in Chapter 3.

> **SUMMARY**
>
> You are a member of a group in a special type of relationship because of your professional role, and with it comes special moral expectations arising from your role.

To help inform you about the special virtues, values, and duties of the health professional, you will be introduced to traditional oaths, codes of ethics, and modern customs and standards of professional practice throughout your professional preparation. A careful study of them (together with reading this book and other ethics resource materials and observing your role models) will highlight aspects of this morality. Because the Hippocratic Oath is so well known, it is displayed in Box 1–1 for you to read carefully.

BOX 1–1 HIPPOCRATIC OATH

I swear by Apollo the Physician, by Aesculapius, Hygeia, and Panacea, and all the gods and goddesses, making them my witnesses, that I will fulfill according to my ability and judgment this oath and this covenant:

To hold him who has taught me this art as equal to my parents and to live my life in partnership with him, and if he is in need of money to give him a share of mine, and to regard his offspring as equal to my brothers in male lineage and to teach them this art—if they desire to learn it—without fee and covenant; to give a share of precepts and oral instruction and all the other learning to my sons and to the sons of him who has instructed me and to pupils who have signed the covenant and have taken an oath according to the medical law, but to no one else.

I will apply dietetic measure for the benefit of the sick according to my ability and judgment; I will keep them from harm and injustice.

I will neither give a deadly drug to anybody if asked for it, nor will I make a suggestion to this effect. Similarly I will not give to a woman an abortive remedy. In purity and holiness I will guard my life and my art.

I will not use the knife, not even on sufferers from stone, but will withdraw in favor of such men as are engaged in this work.

Whatever houses I may visit, I will come for the benefit of the sick, remaining free of all intentional injustice, of all mischief and in particular of sexual relations with both female and male persons, be they free or slaves.

What I may see or hear in the course of the treatment or even outside of the treatment in regard to the life of men, which on no account one must spread abroad, I will keep to myself holding such things shameful to be spoken about.

If I fulfill this oath and do not violate it, may it be granted to me to enjoy life and art, being honored with fame among all men for all time to come; if I transgress it and swear falsely, may the opposite of all this be my lot.

From Edelstein, L. (1943). The Hippocratic Oath: Text, translation and interpretation. Bulletin of the History of Medicine, 2(suppl), 3. © Johns Hopkins University Press, Baltimore. Reprinted with permission.

Reflection

Which aspects of the Hippocratic Oath taken by medical doctors still seem relevant to the group morality of the health professions today? What are its shortcomings? Which ones apply to the health professionals treating Drew Harvey?

____

____

____

____

Today, in modern bureaucratized society, much of the morality of the health professions is embedded in the policies, customs, and practices of health care institutions. You probably have an honor code in your educational institution. And when you reach the clinical years you will become familiar with moral guidelines and policies specific to those institutions. Federal and state laws embody and codify moral values and duties that must govern individual and institutional conduct. For instance, laws about informed consent, confidentiality, and the competence required of persons working as professionals are based on moral values, on duties the professional has to society, and on expectations of the type of moral character professionals will have.

Occasionally, the virtues, values, and duties of a person come into conflict with the morality of a subgroup she or he has joined.

Reflection

The Christian Reformation in the 1500s took place when the personal morality of some religious leaders came into conflict with the customs and patterns of moral conduct in the institution of their church. The famous statement, "Here I stand. I can do no other," exemplifies the moral breaking point persons sometimes reach. It is attributed to reformist Martin Luther as he nailed 95 objections to the official church morality regarding a practice called "indulgences" to the door of All Saints Church in Wittenberg, Germany. Can you name other historical instances in which a moral breaking point changed society?

In health care today the accepted professional morality may conflict with the belief and conscience of a professional's personal morality. Abortion is one issue that has caused deep consternation for some health professionals because of their personal morality. Many hospitals and clinics have accepted an interpretation of professional morality that commits the institution to enabling medically safe abortions to women under the conditions detailed in the U.S. Supreme Court decision for *Roe v. Wade* and other subsequent law. Mechanisms to protect personal morality that are built into the professional morality are described at the end of this chapter in the case of abortion and some other important social issues. In another example, such protection is not assured. Some health professionals have objected to treating male homosexual patients with AIDS because of a personal morality that rejects homosexuality. No protection of personal morality of this type currently overrides the professional duty to provide "due care" to everyone whose symptoms and other signs require intervention.[3] The predicament that the health professionals found themselves in regarding Drew Harvey's care presents a big problem because it is safe to assume that most of them would find it personally wrong to lie. At the same time, some of them probably are considering it because the institutional policies seem unfair.

SUMMARY

Moral values, rights, duties, and expectations of character occur at the level of personal life, within one's society (i.e., "group" morality), and, for professionals, within their oaths, codes, and practice guidelines.

From the "Moral" to the "Ethical"

In its barest form, morality keeps individuals and groups directed toward character development, behaviors, and values that assure they can sustain themselves. Beyond that, the positive goal of thriving in a harmonious environment presents itself as a possibility.

I like to think of the path of morality as one that individuals and groups can follow with ease and confidence most of the time because of good customs, laws, traditions, and other markers that have been developed. For an individual the path will be the most trouble-free when her or his personal, societal, and group moralities are identical. However, philosophers, psychologists, and others who have thought about such things remind us that constant vigilance and frequent reflection are needed to keep us clear about the relevance of specific attitudes, values, and duties that are designed to move members of society along certain paths. Whereas the most general standards for the morally good life never change, the ways it is expressed is context-dependent insofar as it is useful only in a specific time and place. The question then is: Are the usual behaviors and attitudes fitting for *this* time and *this* place in history?

Reflection

In recent history, societal self-consciousness about the accepted U.S. morality in regard to some ethnic and other marginalized groups has led to the recognition that not all is well. The U.S. civil rights movement, which required changes in behaviors and values, was one response to this heightened awareness. Can you name some ways this has affected the practice of health professionals?

1. ______________________________

2. ______________________________

3. ______________________________

4. ______________________________

When the fittingness disappears, the experience is akin to stubbing your toe on a rock in your path. You lose your balance. It hurts. It makes you take notice. You probably noted that even in the description of personal, social, and group moralities I raised the possibility of problems and conflicts that could arise at each step of the way.

Ethics is the discipline that provides a language, some methods, and guidelines for studying the components of personal, societal, and group morality to create a better path for yourself and others.

Ethics: Studying and Reflecting on Morality

Ethics is a systematic study of and reflection on morality: "systematic" because it is a discipline that uses special methods and approaches to examine moral situations, and "reflection" because it consciously calls into question assumptions about existing components of our moralities that fall into the category of habits, customs, or traditions. Originally, the systems of analysis were developed as parts of philosophy and theology. Today, the social sciences and other disciplines have added to the number and types of approaches that are useful for such a task. You will have an opportunity to learn more about them in Chapter 3.

Ethics takes as its standard this question: What do human dignity and respect demand? Some second level questions are as follows:

- Do our present values, behaviors, and character traits pass the test of further examination when measured against this standard?
- In situations where conflicts arise, which values, duties, and other guidelines are the most important and why?
- When new situations present uncertainty, what aspects of present moralities will most reliably guide individuals and societies on a sustainable path for survival and thriving?
- What new thinking is needed in such situations and why?

Ethicists have as their primary career activity the work of ethics. At one level they *analyze* issues. They help to clarify the moral character, values, duties, and other aspects of morality in specific situations. (Medical ethicists or health care ethicists specialize in areas of health care.) At another level they work to *resolve* issues. They work as consultants in the design of ethical policies and practices (Fig. 1–1).

The ethicist also consults with persons or groups who are faced with situations of high moral uncertainty or who are experiencing conflict between competing values and duties. In many institutions today *ethics committees* serve much the same purpose and often include ethicists, as well as thoughtful professionals and laypeople. Some people become teachers of ethics in their given area.

But ethics is not the work of ethicists or ethics committees only. Ethics is the work of everybody.

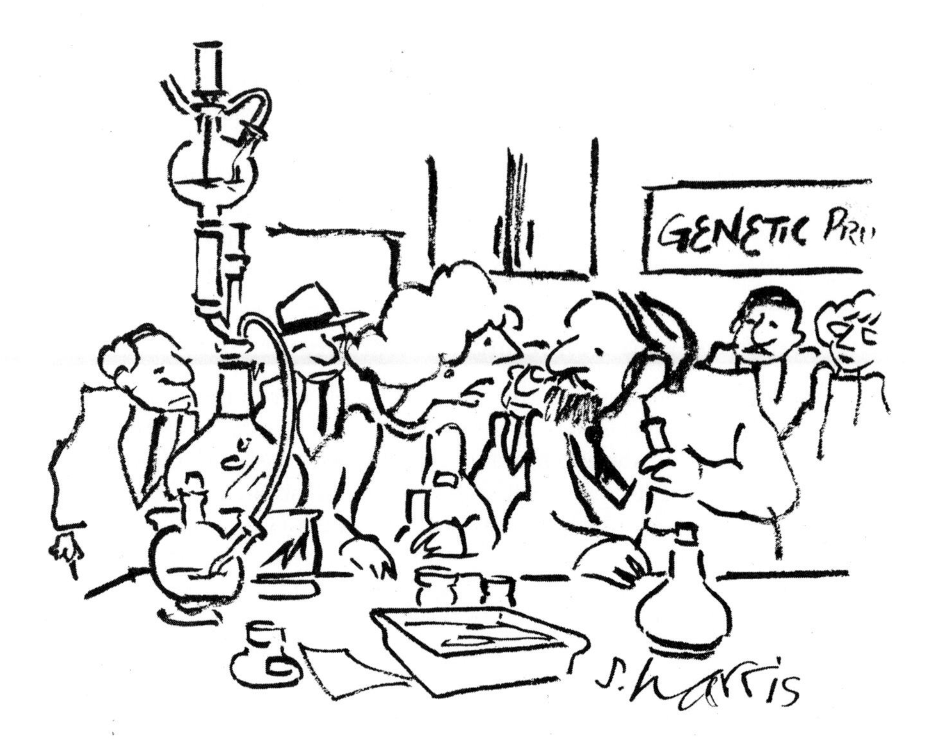

Figure 1–1. *(Courtesy Sidney Harris, with permission.)*

SUMMARY

Ethics is the study of and reflection on everyday morality. It can function as a fundamental part of the life of every thoughtful citizen and takes specific forms when someone assumes a special role such as health professional.

As this book proceeds, each of you will be learning to become a role ethicist—that is, you will become capable of analyzing morality issues within your role as a health professional.

Ethical Issues and Ethical Problems

An *ethical issue* is any situation you believe may have important moral challenges embedded in it that you want to identify. For instance, in the 1950s when the idea of organ transplantation began to be discussed, speculation began immediately that an ethical issue was present because the prospect that one person's (or an animal's) body part would be inserted into another human being raised serious questions about the morality of this type of activity. Still, some types of transplantation could save the life of patients who otherwise would have died. Many asked, Does it support a type of human community that honors cherished moral values and duties that uphold human dignity? Are we playing God?

Had you been introduced to this novel idea and having reflected on it you might have concluded with confidence that the moral value of acting in the presumption of saving human life is expressed through this procedure. If you had answered, but I'm not sure the costs involved for this type of treatment justify the expense to society, or healthy animals should not be sacrificed to extend the life span of a human being, or some types of transplantation may have such poor results that more harm than good will be done to the patient, you would be raising areas of concern about the morality of the procedure that others were raising (and continue to raise).

Reflection

What are some health care technologies that raise serious ethical questions in the minds of many people today just as transplantation did when it was first introduced?

____

____

____

____

An *ethical problem* is a situation that you have reason to believe has serious negative implications regarding cherished moral values and duties and that will pose extremely difficult choices for individuals who want to help support high moral standards. The categories of ethical problems faced by health professionals, patients, and society in the health care environment are discussed in Chapter 2.

The Moral and Ethical Thing to Do

It is common to hear someone say, "That's the moral and ethical thing to do." You will hear the terms "moral" and "ethical" used interchangeably. I suggest you use them more purposefully, however, because after what you have just learned, that phrase should have more meaning for you. The "moral thing to do" means that the traditions, customs, laws, and other markers that an individual and society call on for habitual moral guidance allow you to proceed with confidence in your course of action. Conversely, the "ethical thing to do" means that the course of action that would be taken in the everyday moral walk of life has been reflected on and your moral judgment dictates that it still seems the right thing to do. Fortunately, most situations allow you to act both morally and ethically!

Using Ethics in Practical Situations Involving Morality

The scholarly discipline of ethics has always been interesting from the point of view that its subject matter has immediate relevance for everyday life. Aristotle and others in the classical Greek era called ethics "practical philosophy." This interest has led to the development of ethicists and ethics committees discussed earlier. But we now turn to your formation as an ethicist and potential member of your institution's ethics committee. Earlier in this chapter you read that ethics is about studying and reflecting on moral situations such as the one the health professionals treating Drew Harvey face. In subsequent chapters you will see how the concepts and methods of ethics are tools to help *you analyze* specific moral problems, work toward *resolution* of moral conflicts, and *act* in a manner consistent with high moral standards.

Analysis

Analysis of morality allows you to stand back and identify categories of issues and problems and to delineate which of the aspects of morality are involved in any situation. One type of analysis is the process you engage in when two parts of your own morality collide: "I shouldn't lie to my spouse, but the truth will be bitter, and I shouldn't hurt her either." We already have considered some examples of how your personal set of values and your society's or subgroup's values could collide.

Reflection

The medieval physician Galen fled Rome during the plague. He analyzed his personal morality and decided he had to flee on behalf of his wife and children, whose lives he knew were threatened by the plague, but all of his life he had nightmares about his "failure" because he believed he had also abandoned his patients. In other words, his beliefs regarding his personal and professional duties collided. Do you think his analysis served him well in resolving his dilemma? Did he do the right thing?

The analysis of situations allows one to know *why* there are psychological and other practical consequences of proposed action. Therefore, analysis leads to knowledge that can inform purposive action.

Resolution

Ethical reflection geared to resolving conflict goes beyond solely analyzing a situation and categorizing it. In other words, the knowledge base of analysis is complemented by a process that works toward resolution. One approach to finding resolution is to try to build consensus among the various concerned parties (e.g., yourself, patients, families, the institution). This requires that those involved have analyzed the situation, are willing to hear everyone's point of view, will assist others in clarifying their own view, and are willing to facilitate the building of morally acceptable courses of action. Some ethics approaches focus on how to resolve issues when there is no consensus or when consensus does not seem to fully address the moral challenges embedded in the situation.

Action

Purposive action often can stem from analysis and successful work toward resolution. The health professionals involved with Drew Harvey's potential discharge from their care are looking for an action guide. The party responsible for putting ethics into action is the *moral agent.* You will be introduced more fully to the idea of moral agency in Chapter 2, but you can already begin to see that moral agency is part and parcel of professional decision making. Take, for example, the decisions facing Drew Harvey's caregivers and the one Galen had to make.

SUMMARY

The recognition that ethics can be used for analysis, for resolution of complex situations, and ultimately as a guide for action has led to a resurgence of interest in ethics in various practical contexts. Health care ethics is one such area of applied ethics.

Ethics Research

To understand exactly what is important for ethical analysis, resolution, and action in the health care context, studies are conducted to identify behaviors and beliefs of individuals or groups regarding ethical issues or ethical problems. Social scientists (anthropologists, sociologists, and psychologists) are among the most active in this area of research. For instance, through research we now know that there are differences in cultural and ethnic groups regarding the understanding of and response to the Western European idea of informed consent.

Reflection

What are some topics you think are good areas for research in your chosen field or the health professions as a whole?

Such knowledge can help everyone to gauge the effectiveness of the mechanisms that have been developed to protect important values, character traits, and duties. There also is continuing research on basic concepts of ethical approaches and theory. This pursuit is more in keeping with classical scholarship, which continues to enrich the whole discipline of ethics.

Morality: Ethics and Following Your Own Conscience

In the discussion so far, you have been introduced to some ways that can help you recognize the values, duties, and character traits of your own morality, as well as those with which you will be required to reckon in your activities as a professional. You have also begun your exploration into how ethics will help you when challenges to everyday morality arise. In this section you will have an opportunity to think about institutional and social protections available to you as a professional when and if you encounter a situation (e.g., an instance or policy) that you believe compromises the dictates of your *conscience*.

The Story of the Harvey Family (continued)

Sally Lim is one of the health professionals involved in Drew's care. She is attending the patient evaluation conference called by the home health care coordinator to discuss what to do in relation to discontinuing Drew's therapy. Sally assumes that the only option available to the home health care team is to discontinue him from their care even though she is among those who believe most ardently that he could benefit from more of her interventions and those of other team members. She is prepared to express her difficulty with the reimbursement policy's unresponsiveness to patients like Drew Harvey and her regret and anger that he cannot receive more therapy. She also plans to tell Drew how she feels and to document in his clinical record something like the following: "My judgment is that this patient should not be discontinued at this time since his clinical profile is similar to that of many patients whose progress plateaus for a brief period but after which real progress is realized. Patient discontinued because utilization review recommends this course of action."

The first part of the patient evaluation conference goes as Sally had imagined, the majority agreeing with her assessment of his clinical status. She is comfortable in stating her assumptions and expressing her feelings to the group. However, one of her colleagues, Nick, responds, "What we really *should* do is to bend the truth about his progress just enough so we won't have to discontinue him." Sally begins to protest but finds herself in a minority. She is appalled that her colleagues would consider what she considers outright lying. Finally she blurts out, "I can't believe what you are saying! This is just plain *wrong* – you are talking about lying on his report." Still she feels as if she is being swept along by a flood in which her personal beliefs and convictions will be drowned in the group's decision.

Generally speaking, laws and policies regarding this type of situation maintain that it is wrong to intend to do something that is wrong. Period. Being in a situation in which there is wrongdoing may be inevitable at times, however, when you are not in complete control. Furthermore, sometimes opportunities for achieving a good end and avoiding other greater wrongdoing can depend on cooperating with wrongdoing in some fashion. A common way to think about the justification for cooperation with wrongdoing is embodied in the principle of *material cooperation.*

The Principle of Material Cooperation

The following guidelines are offered in the principle of material cooperation:

- Cooperation with wrongdoing cannot be directly intended. The cooperation can be only *indirectly* not *directly* intended, perhaps occasioned solely by one's position as a member of a group.
- The more remote the cooperation the better.
- Cooperation under these circumstances is easier to justify if the wrongdoing would happen with or without one's personal cooperation.
- The benefit that is attained by the cooperation must greatly outweigh the wrongdoing that will result.

In a specific situation this general set of guidelines for when one might be able to justify cooperating with wrongdoing has to be submitted to further interpretation. From this point of view can Sally's cooperation be justified?

Reflection

A common application of the principle of material cooperation is that sometimes a dying patient will receive pain relief only at the level of painkiller that may also suppress breathing to the point that the person dies. Try to work through the steps using this example.

You can see that in the principle of material cooperation much hinges on the individual's intent to do wrong. In the eyes of the law, actually going ahead and completing the action is a key consideration. In Sally's case, the more she tried to seek other alternatives and to persuade the others not to engage in outright lying, the more justified she would be if the group report was put forward without her being successful in changing their minds. She may decide, however, that her loyalty to her colleagues and coworkers is not sufficient excuse for her to remain silent, and she may decide to write a minority report or go public with the fact of their wrongdoing. In Chapter 6 you will be introduced to the issues of loyalty and reporting others' wrongdoing in more detail.

Protection Through Laws and Policies

As you think about living within the dictates of your conscience in seriously contended issues such as abortion or clinically assisted suicide, keep in mind the following general resources available to professionals through laws and policies.

State Interests

Common law (i.e., unwritten law that comes into practice over time through the lived life of a community) dictates that there is a *state interest,* a responsibility to intervene on behalf of any person under four circumstances: (1) to save their life, (2) to prevent their suicide, (3) to protect him or her from harm as an innocent third party, or (4) to protect him or her as a bearer of the "integrity of the professions." This final cause for state intervention obviously applies to professionals only. It has evolved because of circumstances in which health and other professionals have been faced with requests by patients or clients or have been dictated to by policies to act in ways that are believed by a court to be contrary to the true moral and legal social role of a professional. This protection must be appealed to on a case-by-case basis.

State Licensing Laws

Professionals become certified, registered, or licensed to practice within a particular state or jurisdiction after the completion of all formal professional preparation requirements. Written into the laws governing professional practice are both responsibilities and protections or rights. Among the rights is your right to practice within the dictates of your convictions. This right is weighed against the "reasonable expectations" of patients or clients who come to you for professional help.

Moral Repugnance

Moral repugnance came into the health professions' literature with the Supreme Court decision *Roe v. Wade,* which made abortion a legal right. It is written into a conscience clause that allows individuals who believe it is morally wrong to participate in abortion procedures to be exempt from having to do so. An important aspect of this provision is that the *procedure itself* is key to whether this exemption will be upheld. It is not a protection against, for example, your refusal to treat patients whose lifestyles are morally unacceptable to you. Therefore, it is a limited but important protection. Many have argued that a request to assist in the lethal procedures causing death in capital punishment would fall under the protection of this notion. The same is true should medically administered euthanasia become legal in the United States as it is in the Netherlands. This conscience clause operates as a conscientious objection analogous to conscientious objection in situations of war.

Institutional Policy

Finally, the *policies* of hospitals, health systems, and other health care entities may preclude your ever having to participate in processes, procedures, or other activities that are likely to run counter to the dictates of your conscience. It is always a good idea before accepting a position to be well informed of the job requirements outlined in policies. For instance, Sally may want to talk directly with the Harveys about her decision and place the responsibility for having to discontinue Drew's treatment on his insurance company or the utilization review policies in her institution. The so-called gag clauses preventing her from doing the latter have sometimes created moral challenges for professionals who have signed contracts agreeing not to say anything derogatory about their employer. Because of society's sensitivity to the importance of truthfulness within the health professional and patient relationship, the gag clause condition became the subject of debate and legislation in Congress a few years ago, the outcome being to eliminate it from employment contracts.

Limits of Protection

In summary, society and many institutions that deliver high-quality health care are aware of the need for personal protection in those hopefully rare circumstances in which you will feel compromised. The final burden of proof regarding why you refuse to participate falls on you, but you may be able to find support for your position in one of the above-mentioned legal and policy mechanisms that have been developed. The best recourse is to know your own values and reasons for behavior and have good reasons for supporting them. Fortunately, most health professionals are seldom in a position where they experience the deep, troubling tension of being in a situation they believe compromises their own deep convictions.

It finally all boils down to you, although your social and professional environment can provide significant support.

SUMMARY

Protections allowing you to follow the dictates of your own conscience are provided through federal, state, and institutional mechanisms, although in the end the final burden of proof for your action falls on you.

The development of the ethical dimension of your professional identity requires that you enter into conversation and debate regarding questions of character, value, or duty. Therefore, this first chapter of your journey into professional ethics ends with an introduction to four very basic distinctions that help you place yourself in these larger discussions.

Becoming a Part of the Ethics Conversation

Your familiarity with several basic distinctions that divide ethical theories and approaches will allow you to become a part of the ethics conversation because you will be able to identify where a writer or other person is coming from in an ethics discussion or debate. Once you have identified your own or another's thinking, you will be able to enter into the ethical discussion more confidently.

Deductive and Inductive Theories and Approaches

Deductive theories and approaches propose that the human mind (usually the faculty of reason) is capable of discerning truths about the moral life from a pattern of visible laws in the universe or from some set of general rules or principles that can be discerned by humans through intuition, revelation, or other reliable means. The general truths become a basis to guide action in concrete situations.

Inductive theories and approaches start with concrete experience. Some suggest that these theories and approaches are less a system for guidance and more a rejection of the belief that reliable action guides can be found, the least likely being those found in places where deductive theorists turn.

Between these two extremes are many theories that give credence to some combination of human rationality (or other intellectual resource): one theory is the dialectic approach, which proposes an interplay between abstract action guides and concrete situations; another is a casuistic approach that depends heavily on everyday situations that are related by common ethical themes.

To Do and to Be

Another type of tension has existed through the ages. Ethicists have debated over the question: Does the moral life fundamentally demand of you to do certain right things and avoid other wrong ones? Or, at the basis of morality is there a mandate to be a certain kind of person (i.e., a person of virtue)?

Theories of the former sort are classified as theories of action, whereas those emphasizing character trait formation are virtue theories. Perhaps the correct answer lies in discovering the appropriate relation between action and virtue, although exactly which ultimately takes precedence in the moral life is open to discussion. You will learn more about both sides of this debate in Chapter 3.

Individuals and Communities as Units of Concern

In recent years there has been renewed inquiry regarding the appropriate moral relationship of individuals to the larger community in which they live. Should individual or community well-being be the standard? This is important for many reasons, the most obvious being that the answer to that query will guide ethical practices and policies about right and wrong actions, as well as form the basis for deciding which virtues should be applauded or negatively sanctioned. Individualistic ethical theories and approaches take individual well-being as the standard by which to make correct moral judgments. The individual as the focus of concern is a recent phenomenon in the history of ideas. Protection of individual rights and a focus on individual autonomy and happiness are important goals in this approach. This position is seen in many aspects of modern health care. For example, informed consent is one safeguard for individuals. At the same time, some ethicists are joining others in wondering if modern Western societies have gone awry in placing individual well-being at the highest pinnacle of society's values and duties (i.e., its morality).

In common good theories and approaches the community as a whole is the appropriate denominator of concern. Their strength is their attention to the deep (essential) interdependence among humans. *Communitarians* help to set checks and balances on individual self-interest. These theorists focus on communal arrangements that they believe assure the larger society and its subgroups will survive and flourish. As you might expect, fairness in the distribution of scarce resources and a deep respect for the environment and other resources that sustain human health are an important (although by no means the only) focus of such theories and approaches.

Attempts to strike a reasonable balance between the extremes of these two positions have been made. Aggregate approaches propose that the major criterion for an acceptable moral community is that each and every individual realizes her or his own basic values and upholds her or his own duties. Communitarian approaches depend on reaching agreements (e.g., social contracts, consensus building, utilitarian weighing of benefits and burdens) that are acceptable to all. Both aggregate and communitarian approaches caution that neither unbridled expressions of individual rights or complete neglect of them can be tolerated.

Reason and Emotion for Reliable Moral Judgment

Deductivists maintain that your reason is your internal Web site where you can go and search to find the appropriate ingredients for ethical assessment, movement toward resolution of problems, and action. Of course, different theories and approaches might assert that your reason is informed through direct revelation by God or through intuition or natural laws, but rationalists agree that your use of reason finally does the essential work of ethical reflection.

This approach has led to considerable debate about the significance of emotion in ethical reflection. Strict rationalists view emotion as too subjective and unpredictable to serve as a reliable guide.

At the same time, there are convincing arguments for assigning emotion at least two roles in ethical reflection. First, when you encounter a morally perplexing situation you feel discomfort, anxiety, anger, or some other disturbing emotion. Emotion is an "alert" system. Recall above when Sally Lim became angry and confused because she realized her colleagues were preparing to tell a lie about Drew's progress. Emotion was the painful warning signal that she had "stubbed her toe" on her moral journey through life. Nancy Sherman, a contemporary philosopher working on the place of emotion in morality, proposes that emotions are "modes of sensitivity that record what is morally salient and . . . communicate those concerns to self and others."[4] Your emotions grab your attention. A second role for emotion emerges: it assists you in deciding whom to help and when and where. In this regard, emotions also are motivators. Sometimes it is an emotional response to wrongdoing or tragedy or a heroic act that stirs a person out of lethargy and into action on someone else's behalf. In summary, ethical reflection without the life infused into it by emotional responses to specific situations could be vacuous and misleading.

Despite the caveats traditionally posed by rationalists, many ethicists today acknowledge a positive role for emotion in ethical reflection: it alerts, focuses attention, communicates where the real problems lie, motivates, and increases one's knowledge about complex situations.

SUMMARY

Several ongoing points of difference distinguish ethical theories and approaches from each other. Not all theories or approaches fit neatly into one or the other category. To be "in the know" you would be well advised to watch for signs that a person is appealing his case from a particular approach or theory because it may influence the conclusion the person finds compelling when conflicts arise.

Summary

This chapter is but one step into a lifelong journey in professional ethics. You have chosen a career path that will require complex (and at times perplexing) judgments about morality regarding patient care, health policy, and other aspects of professional life. Many such judgments will have significance in terms of your own moral life, that of your profession, and of society. But the path is not one that you must forge anew every step of the way. This chapter has introduced you to some basic ways of thinking about the sources of morality on which you can draw, the general relevance of ethics to your everyday professional life, and the personal protections you can expect if you are faced with potential compromises of your convictions. You also have begun to make some basic distinctions about major approaches to ethics. As you study the subsequent chapters you will be better able to appreciate the contribution of these considerations.

Questions for Thought and Discussion

1. Imagine a situation that may arise in your professional career that would pose a challenge to your personal morality. What is it about this situation that creates the challenge?

____

____

____

____

2. Using the code of ethics from your own chosen profession, identify three or four basic moral guidelines that you will be expected to follow.

____

____

____

____

3. Search in your newspaper for an article about health care involving ethical issues.
   a. What are the main issues?

____

____

____

____

   b. What types of decisions will have to be made (or have been made) about the right or wrong thing to do in this instance?

____

____

____

____

References

1. Beauchamp, T. L., Walters, L. 1999. *Contemporary Issues in Bioethics.* Belmont, CA: Wadsworth Publishing, p. 1.
2. Turner, L. 1998. An anthropological exploration of contemporary bioethics: Varieties of common sense. *Journal of Medical Ethics* 24:127–133.
3. Sim, J., Purtilo, R. 1991. An ethical analysis of the duty to treat persons who have AIDS: Homosexual patients as a test case. *Physical Therapy* 71(9):650–656.
4. Sherman, N. 2004. Emotions. In Post, S. (Ed.), *Encyclopedia of Bioethics* (3rd ed.). Vol. 2. New York, NY: Thomson Gale, pp. 740–748.

2

The Ethical Goal of Professional Practice and Prototypes of Ethical Problems

Objectives

The student should be able to:

- Identify the goal of professional ethics activity.
- Describe the basic idea of "a caring response" and some ways this response in a professional relationship is distinguished from expressions of care in other types of relationships.
- Identify three component parts of any ethical problem.
- Describe what an "agent" is and, more importantly, what it is to be a "moral agent."
- Name the three prototypical ethical problems.
- Describe the role of emotions in ethical distress.
- Distinguish between two varieties of ethical distress.
- Compare the fundamental difference between ethical distress and an ethical dilemma.
- Define ethical paternalism or parentalism.
- Describe a type of ethical dilemma that challenges a professional's desire (and duty) to treat everyone fairly and equitably.
- Identify the fundamental difference between distress or dilemma problems and locus of authority problems.
- Identify four criteria that will assist you in deciding who should assume authority for a specific ethical decision to achieve a caring response.

New terms and ideas you will encounter in this chapter

a caring response
paternalism/parentalism
locus of authority problem
moral agent
ethical distress
integrity
ethical dilemma

Topics in this chapter introduced in earlier chapters

Topic	*Introduced in chapter*
Ethical problem	1
Role of emotion	1

Introduction

In *The Magic Mountain,* Thomas Mann observes that "order and simplification" are the first steps toward the mastery of a subject.[1] Although most "games" are leisure pastimes and ethics deals with a fundamental component of human well-being, there are certain similarities that are worth considering at this point in your mastery of ethics. First, games have goals. And so does the activity of professional ethics. The goal of professional ethics is to arrive at *a caring response.* Obviously, to "win" *this* game one must thoroughly grasp what a caring response looks like. It will have a certain shape and consistency specific to the situation. If one pursues a lesser goal, or a misguided one, the mastery is incomplete. Second, almost all games present certain "problems" or "challenges" that must be met and overcome successfully. In the activity of professional ethics, the problems present themselves in three major forms or prototypes, each of which may take several varieties. The prototypes are ethical distress, ethical dilemmas, and locus of authority challenges.

In Chapter 3 you will learn some of the approaches and theories that, over the ages, have been developed to help you identify a problem involving morality, analyze it, work toward its resolution, and act to the benefit of the persons involved. Unlike leisure games, however, not all such problems can result in resolution. Mastery is the recognition of, careful attention to, and perseverance to the completion of the problem, with resolution and action the ultimate ideal. The goal of a caring response is met when one has gone as far as possible toward that ideal. The following story sets the stage for our discussion.

The Story of Beulah Watson and Tiffany Bryant

Beulah Watson is a 46-year-old environmental services employee in a large hotel in town. She has been employed for 18 years in this position, and by and large says she has enjoyed her work. In recent years, however, she has increasingly suffered from shoulder and elbow pain that Dr. Taschioglu, the rheumatologist in the hotel's health plan, accredits to her many years of tugging and hauling heavy linens and cleaning equipment required in her work.

Tiffany Bryant is the occupational therapist who has been treating Ms. Watson for the pain and stiffness that has caused her so much discomfort and has increased her absenteeism. Beulah Watson originally was very prompt in keeping her appointments, but recently she has missed almost all of her sessions. Tiffany is concerned about whether Beulah is taking the time off to do other things while telling her workplace that she has a therapy appointment. This idea starts to work on Tiffany, and she gets more and more annoyed with Beulah.

Finally, Tiffany calls the hotel environmental services manager. She tells her about Beulah's missed appointments (five in the last 6 weeks). She also tells the manager that the hotel's health plan is being charged for the missed visits since Beulah has not called to cancel, which is the policy of the institution where Tiffany is employed.

The manager responds that Beulah does not qualify for release time from work for the visits, and because the clinic hours correspond with her work hours, she may not keep all her appointments on that basis. She adds that Beulah probably is worried about the salary loss, even though the treatments are paid for, because she is the sole breadwinner for herself, her disabled husband, and two small grandchildren. The manager says she will talk to Beulah about the unacceptability of her failing to let the Occupational Therapy department know when she decides not to keep her appointment. In fact, if Beulah keeps that up, the manager continues, she will find herself paying for the missed appointments, because the hotel can't be expected to pay for her lack of responsibility. Tiffany responds that maybe Beulah didn't know about the policy. The manager replies, "It doesn't matter. She knows better than that. By the way, she has been here at the times you mentioned, so at least she wasn't off on a shopping trip or anything like that."

A week goes by. At the scheduled time for Beulah's appointment, she does not appear. Tiffany has been uneasy about the conversation with the manager, and when the time comes for her to fill out the billing slip for another missed appointment, she feels positively terrible.

Reflection

In this narrative, what additional information would help you better evaluate the situation? For example, what details of their stories (Beulah Watson's, Tiffany Bryant's, and the hotel manager's) would help you have greater certainty about the ethical problem Tiffany is facing?

____

____

____

____

Do you share Tiffany's feelings that something is not right? If yes, what do you think the problem is?

____

____

____

____

What type of person would you want to be if you were in Tiffany's shoes and knew that professionally speaking you would have to arrive at a caring response?

____

____

____

____

What do you think Tiffany should do to achieve a caring response? Why?

____

____

____

____

In answering these questions you have used basic ideas that you will learn about in Chapter 3: specific ways in which the patient's and others' narratives are relevant to ethics, the importance of character traits, and the duties, rights, consequences, and principles that you can call on when deciding on a course of action. All are necessary as you begin applying your knowledge and skills to actual ethical problems. But in this chapter we examine the goal that puts all of the above analysis and activity into motion.

The Goal: A Caring Response

The central feature of your professional role is "care" activity. Remembering this will always bring you back to the appropriate focus when you are involved in complex or troubling situations. These situations always involve relationships. Sometimes they are relationships with patients or clients, other times with families or professional team members, still other times they are with research subjects, policy makers, or the public. In all of these relationships, the goal of your ethical analysis is to be able to arrive at a caring response and to carry it out.

From time to time you will find yourself torn between more than one claim on your care. Your role as a professional helps to set priorities. Your primary loyalty must always be to the patient or patient groups under consideration. Of course, most ethical problems involve legitimate competing loyalties, so at another time the problem will arise as a conflict between two or more courses of action for a particular patient or two patients. Or it can be a conflict about what is due to an identified patient in relation to other identified, or not yet identified, groups.

SUMMARY

From time to time you will be torn by conflicting claims on you. Your primary loyalty—giving direction to your caregiving activities—always must be to the patient or patients.

Knowing that the goal is care only raises more questions. I placed the term *care* in quotation marks earlier in the chapter because that idea is used to convey a lot of different things. Professional care has several specific characteristics.

A caring response sometimes is identical to the one you would show toward a friend or relative. At the same time, a health professional's relationships are very different, with moral and legal dimensions not fully applicable to other relationships. One point of your caring response is not to cross the physical, psychological, and sexual boundaries that make the person responsible or responsive to you in ways that go outside (or create opposition to) the healing core of the relationship.[2] Therefore, a caring response must mean something more than common, everyday expressions of affections, nurturance, or protection associated with care.

A caring response entails responsibilities that have clinical, ethical, and legal dimensions. Often, this idea is partially captured in common phrases such as "professional responsibility" or "treating the whole patient." In legal language, the term *due care* is used to specify the essentials expected of you in a given situation in your role as a provider of professional service.

A caring response includes professional duty. It shifts the claim on you from a patient's hope that you will offer a kind or even generous response, to making it your duty to respond to the patient's need. At times the most effective response may be to change policies that are unfair to a whole group of similarly situated persons, but usually the immediate response must be for the welfare of the individual. More specifically it places you in a position to aid that person toward maintaining or regaining health (or relief of suffering or a peaceful death) in ways that he or she cannot achieve on his or her own accord.

A caring response is highly individualized. It is the language adopted in the health professions ethical literature to emphasize the imperative that professionals keep a focus on the well-being of the whole person. Although the terms *health care* and *managed care* may simply mean dealing with the patient in the technical sense, ethicists use the term *care* with the broader common connotation of really wanting to *pay attention to what matters to the person* and what the health professions role has to offer in that regard. This focus of attention is frequently challenged in an era of clinical specialization and sophisticated medical technology.

Intervention is so specialized that a particular disease, symptom, body part, or biologic system becomes the focus of attention. Fear of the dehumanizing effect that a fragmented focus will have on both the health professional and the patient is illustrated in Figure 2–1.

In subsequent chapters you will learn to build on these basic ideas of a caring response, which will further enrich your understanding of this goal.

SUMMARY

Fundamentals of a caring response include (1) elements of human nurturance, (2) the patient as the primary focus of loyalty, (3) limits guided by the patient's vulnerability because of the health-related concern, (4) recognition of it as a professional responsibility involving duty, and (5) the condition that it be individualized.

For the time being I leave this idea for your further consideration and turn to the other basic orienting structures for your ethical activity—namely, the components of an ethical problem and three prototypes. An *ethical problem* is a situation that you have reason to think presents serious challenges or threats to important moral values, dispositions, and duties. The situation requires you to reflect on what type of person you should be or on what you should do in a partic-

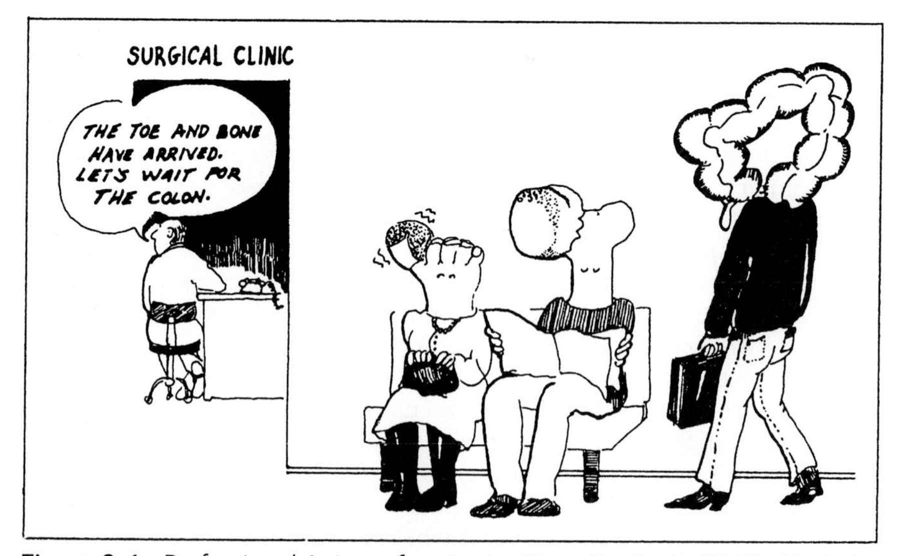

Figure 2–1. Professionals' view of patients. *(From Purtilo, R. [1978]. Kapital II. Att upprätta en relation. In Vård, Vårdare, Vårdad [p. 139]. Stockholm: [translation: Care, Care Giver, Receiver of Care] Esselte Studium.)*

ular situation. Three varieties you will deal with in the ethics dimension of your professional life are the following:

Ethical distress: You face a challenge about how to maintain your integrity or the integrity of the profession.
Ethical dilemma: You face a challenge about the morally right thing to do; two or more courses of action diverge.
Locus of authority problem: You face the challenge of deciding, from an ethical point of view, who should be the primary decision maker.

Components of Ethical Problems

The three prototypes of ethical problems have the following components in common:

A—the moral *a*gent
C—a *c*ourse of action
O—a desired *o*utcome.
Each will be discussed in turn.

The Moral Agent—A

What do you think an agent is? In ethics or law an agent is anyone responsible for the outcome of her or his actions in a specific situation. Obviously, agency requires that a person be able to understand the situation and be free to act voluntarily on her or his best judgment. It also implies that the person intends for something to happen as a result of that action. A *moral agent* is a person who "acts for him or herself, or in the place of another by the authority of that person, and does so by conforming to a standard of right [or wrong] behavior."[3] In the story at the beginning of this chapter there are at least three moral agents: Tiffany, Beulah, and the hotel manager.

Reflection

This book emphasizes your role as a moral agent in the health profession setting because as a professional you must answer for your own actions and attitudes. If you have observed a situation in which someone in your chosen field has had to act courageously, then you have observed moral agency at work. Think about why the responsibility fell to him or her and not to someone else.

The Course of Action—C

The *course of action* includes the agent's analysis, judgment process about the resolution to the moral challenge, and decision. In the story earlier in this chapter, Tiffany Bryant used the information she had to analyze the situation. Her attempt at resolution was to call the hotel manager. This could well have arisen from a sense of moral responsibility she felt not to continue to bill the company for treatments Beulah did not receive. It probably also reflected a concern for this patient's well-being. Afterward, her discomfort may have meant that she was not sure she had exercised the correct moral judgment in making the call to the hotel manager to know if she achieved her hoped for result. However, it seems as if she had some questions about whether it was in fact the right decision.

The Desired Outcome—O

The desired outcome is the intended and hoped for result(s) of having taken a particular course of action. We would need to have more information to know what Tiffany was hoping would happen when she called the hotel manager.

> **SUMMARY**
>
> Three components of ethical problems always involve a moral agent (or agents), a course of action, and an outcome.

Protoypes of Ethical Problems

Having acquainted yourself with the common components of ethical problems, you are ready to explore the three prototypes: ethical distress, ethical dilemmas, and locus of authority challenges.

Ethical Distress: Barriers to Agency

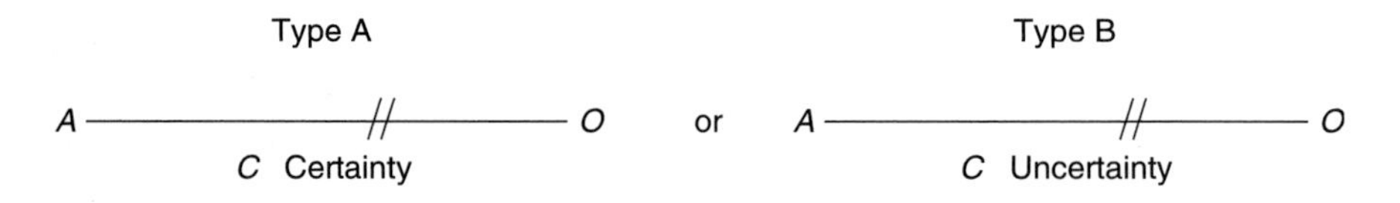

Ethical distress focuses on the agent *(A)* herself or himself. When you are the agent, ethical distress denotes the appropriate emotional or cognitive discomfort, or both, you feel when you are blocked from being the kind of person you want to be or from doing what you believe is right. Agents encounter two types of barriers: types A and B.

Type A: The Barrier Keeping You from Doing What You Know Is Right

A common problem today is barriers to adequate care of individual patients created by the mechanism for the delivery and financing of health care. For example, a hospital policy may be to refuse admission of patients who do not have insurance to fully cover the cost of their treatment, or to discharge patients that physicians, nurses, therapists, or others judge to be unsuited for the rigors of transition to the home environment. Here the morally right course of action *(C)* leading to the desired outcome *(O)* may involve the health professionals talking to the patients to expose the unethical practice or talking with the administration to try to influence the unethical policy. The ethical distress comes precisely because of the repercussions the professionals believe they may have to endure. There are institutional and traditional role barriers keeping them from exercising their moral agency for the good of patients. This does not mean that you will never take into account the larger social context in which you are practicing. For instance, health professionals must always attend to the larger public health considerations in the case of a patient with a serious, highly infectious disease. The patient may experience forced quarantine or be placed in isolation. The health professional's distress at causing this type of discomfort for the good of many other individuals should not be an occasion for ethical distress. Only when you are quite sure you cannot be faithful to the basic well-being of the patient is there legitimate reason for ethical distress.[4]

Type B: The Barrier of Knowing Something Is Wrong, but You Are Not Sure What

The barrier may not be policies or practices, but instead may be that the situation is new or extremely complex. Your only certainty is an acknowledgment that something is wrong; the rest is a big question mark. You may question the morally correct course of action *(C)* or what to work toward as a specific desired outcome *(O)* that should be consistent with your overall goal of making a caring response to this situation. The challenge is to remove the barrier of doubt or uncertainty by further analyzing the problem, using all the tools of analysis available to you as you work toward resolution.

You can see that the psychological response of distress is the first sign to most health professionals that something has gone—or is about to go—wrong, something that will threaten your professional role or your whole profession's integrity.

Integrity comes from the Latin for "fittingness" or "wholeness." A threat to integrity arises when you cannot be the person you know you should be in your professional role or cannot do what you know, for certain, is right. The internal signals are warning you there is something wrong: a knot in the pit of your stomach, a catch in your easy stride, and waking up in the early hours of the morning with the haunting feeling that something is awry. Emotions, feelings, and experience are critical data of the moral life, and now they are trying to work for you to say, "Stop! Wait! Don't! Think twice!"

But you also will need character traits as resources in this situation: compassion, commitment to competence, and courage. The virtues act as motivators, goading you to correct something you know is wrong or to increase your certainty about the right decision to make.

Reflection

Think about Tiffany Bryant. What type of ethical distress is she facing? Tiffany feels uneasy. I asked you to think about why you might feel uneasy too if you were in her situation. I assume that her discomfort partially stems from her wanting to do what is best for Beulah Watson but not being sure she has. She wants to show a caring response that befits a health professional, but she is not sure how to do that. Understandably, she also wants to honor the rules and policies of her workplace, but is not sure she should be charging for Beulah's missed treatments. Her ethical distress is more of type B, as I read her situation. Do you come to the same conclusion?

____

____

____

____

Tiffany's task as a moral agent in this situation is to continue to reflect on and analyze the situation. (In Chapter 4 you will learn a step-by-step method for this analysis.)

SUMMARY

Ethical distress occurs when the moral agent knows what the morally appropriate course of action is but cannot achieve it because of external barriers, or when there is a high level of uncertainty regarding the information needed to arrive at an outcome consistent with a caring response. Integrity is a central notion in ethical distress situations.

As she analyzes the situation, Tiffany thinks about whether her distress also is related to the fact that she is facing an *ethical dilemma*. So that you might join her in that reflection, we turn to the second type of prototypical ethical problem: the ethical dilemma.

Ethical Dilemma: Two Courses Diverging

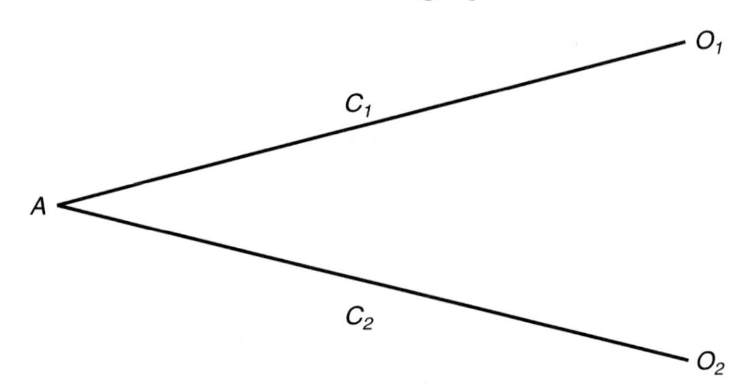

Many people call all ethics problems ethical dilemmas. More correctly, an *ethical dilemma* is a common type of problem that involves two (or more) morally correct courses of action that cannot both be followed—that is, to take course C_1 precludes you from taking course C_2. As a result, you (the agent, the responsible one) necessarily are doing something right and also wrong (by not doing the other thing that is also right). You are between a rock and a hard place, between the devil and the deep blue sea.[5] Again, your integrity feels threatened

Ethical dilemmas involve ethical conduct. Suppose that Tiffany Bryant has just read the above paragraph and realizes that before she called the hotel manager she had an ethical dilemma but did not recognize it at the time. She was aware of her ethical distress and that further analysis was needed. Here is why she now knows she had a dilemma.

On the one hand, Tiffany is an agent *(A)* who has a professional duty to look out for her patient, Beulah Watson, and in Tiffany's role as health professional, the course of action *(C_1)* that will express that respect is in the form of giving Beulah the treatment that is best for her. The desired outcome *(O_1)* is the relief of the patient's pain and stiffness. On the other hand, Tiffany is an agent *(A)* who has a duty to abide by the policies of her place of employment. The course of action *(C_2)* that will express her loyalty is to charge for all treatments that are given or are not officially canceled. The desired outcome *(O_2)* is the financial solvency of the occupational therapy clinic and recognition that patients have a responsibility to show up for their scheduled appointments or to cancel them. Both outcomes are ethically appropriate, taken alone. However, Tiffany Bryant probably caused some negative repercussions for the patient. Therefore, she maintained fidelity to her workplace at the price of doing what would benefit Beulah Watson.

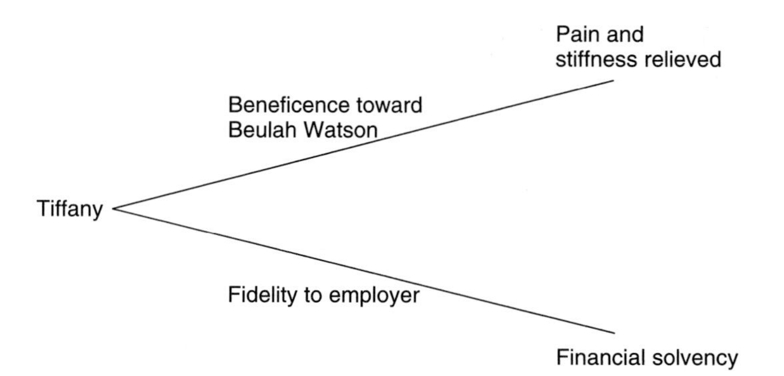

Of course, Tiffany might have thought that charging for missed appointments is wrong under any circumstance, a position being examined in the health profession literature because this practice is increasing in health care institutions.[6]

The Special Case of Paternalism

Sometimes an ethical dilemma presents itself in this manner: The patient's deep preferences conflict with the health professional's judgment of what is best for the patient on the basis of the professional's values, which are not necessarily those of the patient. In other words, the conflict is between the patient's choice and the professional's judgment of what is best for the patient. This type of dilemma is called a situation of *paternalism* or *parentalism.*

This is such an important idea that you will have an opportunity to think about it in several of the stories that follow.

In subsequent chapters you will also have ample opportunity to work with several types of dilemmas because they are the most commonly confronted type of ethical problem.

SUMMARY

Paternalistic or parentalistic decisions are those in which a health professional acts as a parent with all of its negative and positive connotations.

Justice Seeking as an Ethical Dilemma

Another special ethical dilemma arises in regard to searching for ways to allocate societal benefits and burdens fairly and equitably. As in all ethical problems, the agent *(A)* makes a judgment to take a course of action *(C)* that results in an outcome *(O)*. The situation is this: competition exists for a cherished but scarce resource such as a medication, health professionals' time, money to pay for health care, or an organ or other types of life-saving procedures. The agent's *(A)* morally right course of action *(C)* is to give everyone a full measure of the resource to the extent their needs warrant it. In so doing, the outcome *(O)* will be that the patient's legitimate claims are honored. The scarce supply, however, requires that the agent take difficult, even tragic, courses of action, the outcome being that some claimants will get the cherished good and others will not. In summary, it is morally right to give your own patient everything he needs to benefit from your interventions. It is also morally right to spread resources around to the benefit of others. The question of how to treat each person fairly, and to treat groups equitably, becomes a challenge involving a dilemma.[7] You will study about this more extensively in Chapters 14 and 15.

Reflection

Try to think of an example in your chosen field of how you might become involved in a dilemma that requires you to make tough decisions because of scarce resources.

SUMMARY

Ethical distress occurs when a moral agent is faced with two or more conflicting courses of action but only one can be chosen as the agent attempts to bring about an outcome consistent with the professional goal of a caring response. Two special cases of a dilemma involve paternalism and justice issues.

Locus of Authority Problem

A *locus of authority problem* raises the question of who should have the authority to make an important ethical decision. In other words, the question is: Who is the rightful agent *(A)* to carry out the course of action *(C)* and to decide the desired outcomes or results *(O)*?

This kind of problem highlights that it does matter who has decision-making power. For instance, if you work in a situation in which one person or group *always* has the final decision because of a degree after her name or because of a title he holds, then you know the ethical distress that led you to further analysis is coming from that some stake holders (moral agents) have too little or too much authority for what a good outcome warrants. Figure 2–2 graphically illustrates how health professionals who are *not* in appropriate positions to act responsibly sometimes feel.

Locus of authority problems most often arise when roles or other institutional policy or societal arrangements create *ambiguities* about who is in charge. Schematically, the problem looks like this:

Note that two people assume themselves to be appropriate moral agents (A_1 and A_2) and proceed along different courses of action

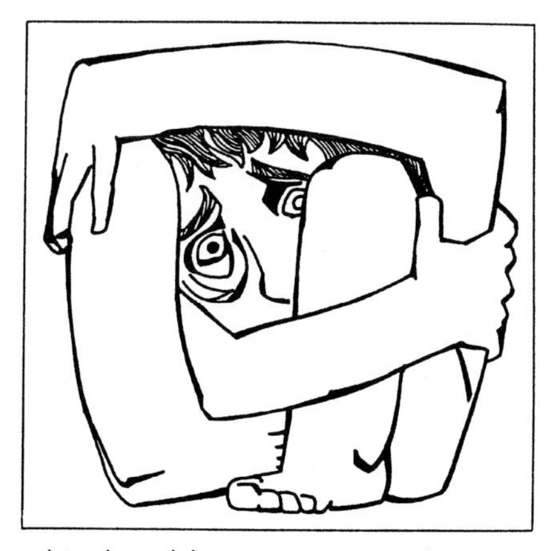

Figure 2–2. Facing ethical problems. *(From Purtilo, R., & Haddad, A. [2002]. Respect. The difference it makes. In Health Professional and Patient Interaction [6th ed.] [p. 13]. Philadelphia: WB Saunders.)*

(C_1 and C_2). As each analyzes the situation they may come to different conclusions about how to achieve the best outcome (O_1 vs. O_2) for a patient.

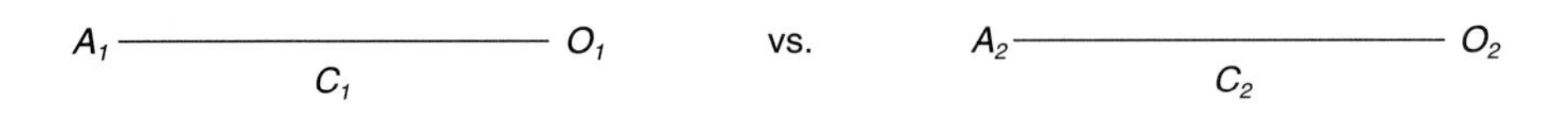

Reflection

In the story of Tiffany Bryant and Beulah Watson, who do you think should make the decisions about whether to charge for missed treatments?

- The health professional providing the service?
- The supervisor of the unit?
- The institutional administrator?
- The government or some other, larger societal regulating body?

Sometimes there is no ambiguity, but reflection on the issue reveals that the wrong person has the authority. The challenge of determining the appropriate locus of authority is the topic of thoughtful reflection by ethicists and other individuals. In the context of health professions, there are at least four ways of thinking about authority in health care decisions:

1. *Professional expertise:* You are in a professional role along with other people in different professional roles. This is the essence of teamwork that characterizes so much of health care today. The role differences mean that you bring different spheres of expertise to the situation. In some areas of the patient's care, each professional is *an authority* on some part of the whole picture. That alone should be a vote for the person who has the most relevant knowledge about the patient's condition and other factors to be the decision maker.
2. *Traditional arrangements:* Traditionally in the health care system the physician has been the authoritative voice in health care decisions by virtue of his or her role as a physician. In other words, the physician is considered *in authority* because of his or her office or position rather than (or in addition to) being *an authority* because of special expertise. From this perspective the medical director of the unit would unquestionably be the one to make a decision about what to do, although he or she may choose to invite advice and counsel from other individuals.
3. *Institutional arrangements and mechanisms:* Sometimes the decision about the authoritative voice will come from special institutional arrangements. For example, some tasks may be delegated to committees. In these instances, the committees or designated individuals assume specific task-related roles.

This is really a variation of the first two, the designated individuals being *in* authority both because of their expertise and the positions they hold. For example, it is possible that the authority for making a decision regarding billing for missed treatments may be referred to a committee designed to deal with humane treatment of patients in unusual situations rather than treating billing solely as a financial issue.

4. *The authority of experience:* A voice of authority may emerge because of the insight that comes from experience. There are always those situations in which we seek the advice of people who have been in similarly perplexing situations and defer to their judgment. Tiffany Bryant may wish to seek advice for the next step from a supervisor, senior member of the professional staff, or other person judged to have the benefit of experience. This is seldom institutionalized as a formal mechanism for dealing with locus of authority problems and is a variation of the professional expertise approach, which assumes that expertise often is refined with experience in a wide range of situations.

None of these approaches should be taken for granted for all situations. The ethical gold standard remains the welfare of the patient, which flows from a truly caring response, and institutional arrangements must follow from it.

SUMMARY

Locus of authority problems focus on questions about the appropriate moral agent in a situation. Conflicts often can be resolved by an analysis of who has the most expertise, the traditional practices regarding who makes what decisions, an appeal to policies, and respect for experience. The goal is to achieve an outcome consistent with a caring response.

Summary

This completes your introduction to a caring response, the basic goal of professional ethics, and three prototypes of ethical problems that will confront you as you attempt to carry out your roles as clinician, administrator, researcher, teacher, and team member. The goal of a caring response includes qualities that distinguish it from other types of responses. The ethical problem prototypes of ethical distress, ethical dilemmas, and locus of authority quandaries will cause you to have to analyze and decide which course of action toward the resolution of the problem is the most likely to work best.

Questions for Thought and Discussion

1. Jane is a medical student who does not want to treat a patient with AIDS in the intensive care unit because she is afraid of contracting AIDS herself. Her supervisor assures her that she is safe as long as she uses the universal precautions designed to make the treatment of patients with infectious diseases safe for everyone. Jane still hesitates saying, "I know it's irrational, but I'm afraid I will not be effective because I'm so scared." Using the prototypes of ethical problems you have learned, what type of ethical problem do you think Jane has?

2. Taking Jane's story above, what do you think are the major considerations she must take into account in arriving at a caring response?

3. Find a newspaper or magazine article this week that portrays an ethical problem and analyze it using the material presented in this chapter.

4. Describe an ethical dilemma that you or someone you know has faced. This does not have to be a problem that arose within the health care context. What did you have to take into consideration as you moved toward a decision about which of the two or more courses of action available to you should be taken? Did it result in a good outcome?

REFERENCES

1. Mann, T. 1927. *The Magic Mountain* (H.T. Lowe Porter, Trans.). New York: Alfred A. Knopf.
2. Purtilo, R., Haddad, A. 2002. Professional boundaries guided by respect. In *Health Professional and Patient Interaction* (6th ed.). Philadelphia: WB Saunders, pp. 207–222.
3. Hurley, A.C., MacDonald, S.A., Fry, S.T., Rempusheski, V.F. 1998. Nursing staff as moral agents. In Volicer, L., Hurley, A. (Eds.), *Hospice Care for Patients with Advanced Progressive Dementia*. New York: Springer Publishing, p. 155.
4. Beauchamp, T.L., Childress, J.F. 2001. Professional-patient relationships. In *Principles of Biomedical Ethics* (6th ed.). New York: Oxford University Press, pp. 283–336.
5. Freeman, J.M., McDonnell, K. 2001. Making moral decisions: A process approach. In *Tough Decisions: Cases in Medical Ethics* (2nd ed.). New York: Oxford University Press, pp. 241–246.
6. Fay, A. 1995. Ethical implications of charging for missed sessions. *Psychological Reports* 77:1251–1259.
7. Daniels, N., Sabin, J. 2002. *Setting Limits Fairly: Can We Learn to Share Medical Resources?* New York: Oxford University Press, pp. 178–191.

3

Ethics Theories and Approaches:

All You Need to Know

Objectives

The student should be able to:

- Describe the usefulness of the basic ethics theories and approaches described in this chapter as tools in analyzing ethical problems and attempting to resolve problems by arriving at the most caring response in the situation.
- Distinguish metaethics from normative ethics.
- List three reasons why your acquaintance with metaethical theories is relevant to your work as a health professional.
- Name five types of normative ethical theories and approaches that help illuminate what a "caring response" entails.
- Describe *how* and *why* the idea of a caring response is central to the health professional and patient relationship.
- Describe a narrative and what it means to take a narrative approach to an ethical issue or problem.
- Assess the contribution of psychologist Carol Gilligan and others who stress relationships.
- Discuss several contributions that feminist and postmodernist approaches have made to our understanding of ethical issues and problems.
- Describe the role of moral character or virtue in the realization of a good life and its significance for health professionals faced with the goal of arriving at a caring response.
- Describe ways the various story or case approaches help one understand what a caring response involves.
- Describe the function of a principle (norm, element) in ethical analysis and conduct.
- Identify six principles often encountered in professional ethics that can help guide one in trying to arrive at a caring response to a professional situation.
- Discuss the meaning of autonomy in Kant's and Mill's theories and the relevance of each to ethical conduct.

- List five reasonable expectations a patient or client has because of the health professional's responsibility to act with fidelity.
- Describe the principle of veracity as it applies in the professional context.
- Describe the basic difference between deontological and utilitarian ethical theories of conduct and the role of each in the health professional's goal of acting in accordance with what a caring response requires.

New terms and ideas you will encounter in this chapter

theories (and approaches)
absolutism
normative theories
foundationalism
feminist approaches
ethics of care approach
character trait
principles or elements
beneficence
fidelity
justice
prima facie duties
teleology
metaethics
relativism
story or case approaches
narrative approaches
postmodernism
virtue theories
moral character
nonmaleficence
autonomy
veracity
deontology
conditional duties

Topics in this chapter introduced in earlier chapters

Topic	*Introduced in chapter*
Three uses of ethics in everyday life	1
Hippocratic Oath	1
Deductive reasoning	1
Inductive reasoning	1
A caring response	2

Introduction

In this chapter you will be introduced to a whole "toolbox" of cognitive tools you will use to accomplish your professional goal of arriving at a caring response in the wide variety of challenges you may encounter. They are presented in the form of *ethical theories* and *ethical approaches*. A complete *theory* is a general overview or statement that begins with an assumption about the very nature of doing right and wrong, of virtuous or vicious character, and includes how humans can go about achieving one and avoiding the other. In contrast, an *approach* does not propose to be a complete system or model, but to be an aid to existing theories or other approaches.

If you are like me you probably take a look at how many pages you have ahead of you for your assignment and you quickly concluded that this is a very long siege of reading! When I titled this chapter "all you need to know" it was with the idea that you will get a "mini book" of ethical theory by reading this chapter. Depending on your course of study your professor may add to these pages with another more theoretical text or may split the chapter into smaller parts. But I encourage you to work your way through it carefully so that the rest of your study of this book will be easier and your preparation in ethics more complete.

More practically speaking, in Chapter 1 I suggested three general ways that ethical tools have usefulness in your everyday life: (1) to analyze moral issues, (2) to help resolve moral conflicts, and (3) to move toward action when faced with a problem. In Chapter 2 you had an opportunity to learn the basic varieties of ethical problems you'll encounter in your professional career. In this chapter you will gain more knowledge and tools enabling you to move skillfully from the identification of a problem, through its analysis, and, hopefully, to its resolution through action that achieves your goal of a caring response. Chapter 4 provides a simple six-step process you can follow as you apply everything discussed in this and the previous chapters. To help set the stage for your thinking, consider the story of Ronald Rachels, Pam Faden, and Metsui Hasagawa.

The Story of Ronald Rachels, Pam Faden, and Metsui Hasagawa

A radiologic technologist, Ronald Rachels, works in a large community hospital. He is responsible for performing many radiologic procedures each day and takes his job seriously. Patients who arrive at his department quickly learn that Ron is a bright spot in their otherwise anxiety-producing ordeal of having x-rays or imaging. He explains everything to the patients in language they can understand and tries to make them comfortable while waiting and during their procedures. If there are necessary delays, he explains why.

Two weeks ago, Ron had an experience that upset him, and he's not sure what to do about it. A young woman, Pamela Faden, had met Ron when her radiographs were taken before her first surgery for abdominal cancer. This day she was brought back from her hospital room. She remembered Ron and greeted him. He learned that this 23-year-old woman had had a difficult time after abdominal surgery and had not been able to leave the hospital. Radiographs were ordered to try to discern the cause of her ongoing problem with the idea that an ultrasound, MRI, or other tests would be conducted if nothing showed up on the x-ray.

The x-rays were developed. Ron happened to walk by the radiology medical resident who was reading the films and was astonished to see a large scalpel in Pamela's abdominal cavity, lodged near her liver. The resident instructed Ron to take several additional radiographs, not explaining why, though Ron, of course, knew. The patient asked, "Did you find something? Why are you taking so many x-rays?"

"We just want to be sure we have all the views," he replied nervously. She said with anxiety, "Is anything wrong?"

"That's what the x-rays may help to tell us," he answered.

After all the x-rays had been developed, Ron heard the resident talking on the telephone to Dr. Metsui Hasagawa, who performed the surgery. A few minutes later Dr. Hasagawa arrived. When he saw the scalpel he muttered, "This is *not* good, *not* good." He gathered up the radiographs and hurried out of the room.

Ron wanted to say, "Are you going to tell her?" but he didn't. He knew Metsui Hasagawa was on his way to see the patient and also was afraid the doctor may have been insulted by such a question.

Today, 10 days after the second set of radiographs were taken, Ron is transferring a portable x-ray unit to another part of the hospital when he sees Pamela Faden in the elevator. She says, "Well, they didn't find anything on those x-rays."

"Did the physician talk with you about them?" Ron asks, feeling tense.

"No—he hasn't said anything at all."

"Well," Ron says, "You have the right to know the results if you want to."

She immediately looks concerned. He wants to say something to reassure her, but the words fail him.

The elevator door opens, and Ron says a hurried good-bye. He feels a gnawing in the pit of his stomach, but he can't immediately figure out what, if anything, he should do next.

It is not surprising that Ron Rachels is distressed, because something definitely is wrong. In fact, we might wonder about a health professional who felt no emotion at all about this situation: a young woman with cancer is suffering; a scalpel has been left in her abdomen; and communication between her and her physician appears to have broken down. Maybe Ron has said too much—or too little—to help this patient and physician, both of whom have had some bad news to confront. He is not sure how far he should go in revealing directly to the patient what he knows.

Reflection

What *is* the caring, morally responsible action in this type of situation?

____

____

____

____

We will return to this story throughout the chapter, so keep your response in mind.

Parts of Ethical Study

The ethical theories and approaches you will use for situations like the one you've just read fall within the dimension of ethics called *normative ethics*. Almost all the ethical reflection you do relevant to everyday life problems is in the area of normative ethics, so several approaches and theories are described in detail in this chapter. However, each theory also is part of a larger approach called *metaethics*, so you will first be introduced briefly to it.

What Is Metaethics?

Metaethics tries to discover the nature and meaning of ethical reasons we propose as valid for making judgments about morality. How do we know if there are ultimate truths about morality? Does the certainty about what Ron Rachels should do come from lived experience? From revelation or Scripture? From reasoning? Is there a "natural law" from which humans can discern truths about right or wrong? These are just some questions with which metaethics deals. You may recognize some of them as belonging to deductive or inductive schools of thought introduced in Chapter 1. An understanding of metaethics requires that you become more aware of your beliefs—religious, philosophic, what you have been taught or told—and how you imagine them to influence what is right or wrong, virtuous or blameworthy, whenever you face a situation with troubling ethical issues like the one you've just read. Anytime you think about the sources that inform your thinking, you are doing important work related to metaethics because the sources of your moral beliefs are the starting point from which your own thinking and action will be justified. Of course, over time, you may modify your understanding of the sources of morality.

An Example of Metaethical Approaches: Absolutism and Relativism

Let's look at the predicament Ron Rachels, Pam Faden, and Metsui Hasagawa are in. Surely you have some idea of what you think ought to be done regarding the situation Pamela and her caregivers are facing. When you first read their story did you feel certain from the beginning that you knew why a particular course of action should be taken? Did you wonder why anyone would ever worry about the alternatives because it was so obvious? Did you think, "There is a good (moral) reason why everyone should *always* do such and such"?

If you answered "yes" to these questions and if your reflection is based on believing that there are clear, unchanging reasons for always taking a certain position on an issue, then you were thinking as an absolutist. *Absolutist metaethical theories* rest on the notion that what is right is based on knowledge that can be known to be a truth. In your consideration of sources of morality, some of you probably stated your religious beliefs as one important source. Religious truths are believed to be absolute truths that can be known to be truths because they are from a divine source, usually recorded in Scripture. Other theories add that truths may become evident through the working of natural forces (natural law theory) or by intuition. Even in these theories, however, there may be differences of opinion about the exact way that these truths provide guidance for everyday decisions. Some (e.g., fundamentalists) argue that there is knowledge from the source to the direct application of any decision. Others (e.g., rationalists) would counter that the faculty of human reason must intervene to discern right or wrong in any given situation, interpreting what the absolute truth requires at any specific moment.

Perhaps you answered "no" to the above questions. You are quite sure that there are no true reasons to guide what is right or wrong, or that if there are such reasons, you could not be sure of ascertaining them. That is, one person's (or group's) morally right judgment is another's wrong judgment. If this is your approach, you are reasoning as a relativist.

Relativistic metaethical theories rest on the assumption that ethical statements are not known to be ultimately true or false. In the end, what any society, group, or individual believes is right can be as legitimately defended as what another society, group, or individual asserts. All is relative, although many different groups *may* agree regarding the course of action that should be taken. *Postmodernism* is one approach holding such a position. You will encounter more about this position later in this chapter. Basically, postmodernism suggests that the richness of our plurality as humans goes to the very root of our makeup and that ultimate truths are conjectures by groups to try to gain power or control over others.

Reflection

Do you think you are basically an absolutist or a relativist? Why?

____

____

____

____

This example of metaethical considerations should illustrate that your acquaintance with the metaethics level of ethical theory is relevant in several ways. First, it is important for you to be aware of the lines of thinking by which you yourself believe that judgments of right and wrong can be made with certainty—or perhaps, never can be made with certainty. Second, in disagreements with professional peers, patients, and others about important moral positions, often it is critical to be able to figure out the basis of their justification for their positions for you to know whether you can hope for a consensus. (It is difficult to persuade someone to change his or her mind if God has spoken directly to that person through revelation or Scripture.) Finally, as an educated person you should have the capability to listen knowledgeably at all levels of ethical reflection in everyday discourse about important ethical issues and problems in society.

SUMMARY

Metaethics deals with the source of the reasons we give for our positions. Acquaintance with metaethics helps you gain insight into your own and others' basis for moral judgments.

For our current purposes this brief discussion of metaethical considerations provides you with an adequate working knowledge of the role such theories play in overall ethical thought. In your lifelong learning you may wish or need to know more about metaethical theories. Most basic ethics textbooks have a section on metaethics or, as it is sometimes called, critical ethics.

What Is Normative Ethics?

Normative ethics asks more concrete questions related to morality. When you assessed the situation described earlier in this chapter you were using the concepts of normative ethics if you wondered, What would be an appropriate expression of care toward Pam Faden? What types of acts are morally right or wrong and therefore should be considered in this case? What are the morally praiseworthy or blameworthy traits (virtues) needed for the individuals or institutions involved in this story to arrive at a caring response? What values are morally good or bad for the harmonious functioning of this group of individuals?

Your encounters with real situations involving patients, colleagues, other people, rules, policies, or practices are what will motivate you to engage in normative ethical reflection and ethical problem solving.

SUMMARY

Normative theories and approaches deal with methods for ascertaining right and wrong actions and morally praiseworthy or blameworthy attitudes and behavior.

The basic normative theories and approaches you encounter in this chapter focus on care as a central concern, the dispositions and attitudes that will help you, principles approaches that provide some moral markers for the general direction your care should take, the role of duties and rights, and considerations that give moral weight to the consequences (i.e., outcomes) of your actions (Fig. 3–1).

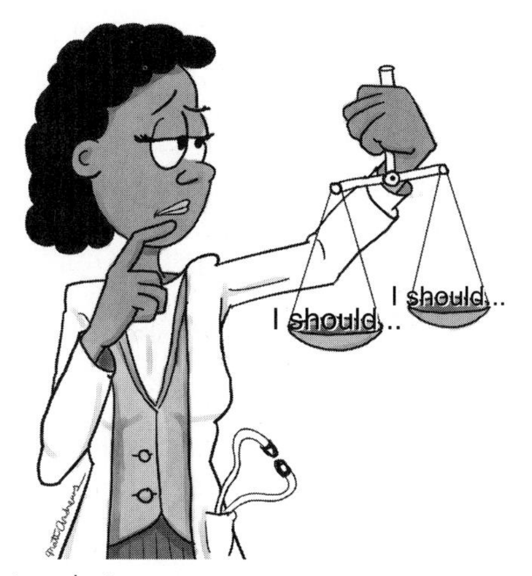

Figure 3–1. Weighing duties.

The Caring Response: Five Theories and Approaches to Help You

You have already learned that the goal of your ethical deliberation is to answer the question: "What does it mean to provide a caring response in this situation?" You have also learned that although you will be faced with legitimate competing loyalties as a health professional, your primary loyalty must always be patient-centered. But all these insights beg for further description about how to actually arrive at the ethically appropriate caring response in a particular situation.

Several normative theories and approaches are relevant to your work of putting together this caring response. Your ethics work differs from an academic philosopher's because you must not only apply clear thinking to the issues, which a philosopher must do, but you must also come to a conclusion that leads to purposive action. Therefore, it is not surprising that both the theories that focus on dispositions or attitudes you should harness and the theories focusing on conduct itself are relevant for parts of your deliberation. The former types emphasize what kind of person you should strive to *be*, the latter what you should *do*. They are presented here in the order in which I find them the most useful for organizing my own thinking for practice within the health professions role. I hope you will also find them useful. As you go through them, remember that by no means will you use all of the theories or approaches covered in this chapter for any given situation. Just as you need to select the correct tool for building anything, the same is true for the tools I am describing.

The first two types, *Story or Case-Driven Approaches* and *Virtue Theories,* emphasize the importance of the kind of person you should strive to be (i.e., your attitudes and dispositions), so that you will be well positioned to find the caring response. Taken together, the several varieties share the common themes of paying attention to the details of stories for their moral content, becoming aware of one's emotions in relation to what is happening in the story, and development of character traits that allows one to be prepared to act in a caring manner. Collectively, they also stress the moral relevance of relationships, both between individuals and with the institutional structures of society.

The last three approaches and theories, *Principles Approaches, Deontological Theories,* and *Teleological Theories,* are geared to forms of ethical conduct itself. Principles approaches have been developed to help people understand general action guides for ethical behavior, some of which are related to duties or rights, whereas others are related to consequences. Regarding deontology and teleology theories, these mouthfuls can be broken down into more digestible pieces by looking at their roots: the root word "deonto" means duty; the root word "telos" means end. Already you can see a distinction developing. Deontologic theories delineate duties (actually duties, rights, or other forms of action), whereas teleologic ones rely on an assessment of the ends or consequences to determine right or wrong. You've heard the expression, "Do the ends justify the means?" Deontologists would say "no"; teleologists would say "yes." As noted earlier, some principles guide you toward duty, others toward the "telos" or consequences. Are you ready to delve into these five theories or approaches in more detail?

Varieties of Story or Case Approaches

In professional ethics the story is the inevitable beginning point of ethical reflection because you encounter the problems in everyday life with everyday patients (or others). As Chapter 1 briefly noted, all inductive approaches to ethics hold that there is morally relevant information imbedded in the story. Therefore professional ethics is inductive by nature.

In professional ethics you also are provided with ethical codes, a tradition, and societal expectations of how you will respond to legitimate requests for your professional services. *Foundationalism,* as it is called, holds that although the appropriate starting place for ethical analysis is the story, there are standards, principles, and other moral guides against which your opinion must be tested when you are deciding on a caring response. It is not simply, "you hold your view and I hold mine and they are on equal footing, morally speaking." Therefore professional ethics also is foundationalist by nature.

Within the inductive, foundationalist context of professional ethics, several varieties of story or case-driven ethical approaches can be found among the writings in health care.

Narrative Approaches

Narrative is the technical term applied to the story's characters, events, and ordering of events (e.g., the plot), although in health care ethics and legal circles you will more often see the term "case." Narrative approaches are based on the observation that humans pass on information, impute and explore meaning in their and others' lives, commemorate and celebrate, denounce, clarify, get affirmation, and, overall, become a part of a community through the hearing and telling of stories. These stories are passed down from generation to generation among families or whole communities.[1] Sometimes the stories have been fictionalized in novels, poems, plays, songs, or other literary forms. Narrative ethicists conclude that good moral judgment must rely on the analysis and understanding of narratives. Kathyrn Hunter, a contemporary leader in narrative approaches to ethics within health care, reiterates this point, noting that through narratives:

> [W]e spin and untangle explanatory accounts of the way the world works and how we and our fellow human beings act in every conceivable circumstance. Memories of the past and ideas of the future are expressed in narrative accounts of how the world was and how it will, or should, become.[2]

Her emphasis on "should" underscores the narrative ethicists' position that future moral choices of individuals and communities are shaped through understanding and taking seriously the information and lessons embedded in stories.

Ron Rachels's situation is revealed to you as a narrative. One thing probably disturbing to him is the fragmented narrative he himself has received. He lacks certain information about the patient, the physician, and their exchanges that he would need to be confident of the moral challenges in the situation. This means that he is not only without facts and details but may feel he lacks pertinent information to make a valid ethical judgment about the real significance and meaning of the events unfolding before him. Looked at from the standpoint of ethical problems, Ron is in a situation of ethical distress.

Narrative approaches also highlight that in complex situations there is not just one but several accounts. Suppose this story simply was titled "The Story of Dr. Hasagawa." What different concerns might Dr. Hasagawa express regarding *his* role, his relationships with the patient Pam Faden and with Ron, or anything else? It may be a different story than the one as told by Ron. Or suppose this story was titled "The Story of Pam Faden." Surely this young patient's account would include details about her personal life and experience, her response to her illness, and her hopes, dreams, and fears. These details would alter inexorably what Ron's story taken alone conveys. Narrative ethics approaches require your diligent effort to consider as many "voices" as possible before interpreting the situation for its moral significance.

SUMMARY

Narrative ethics requires that all voices be considered before the situation is assessed for its moral significance.

Hunter further elucidates the role of narrative approaches by comparing moral reasoning to clinical reasoning. Clinical reasoning requires that you be able to gather relevant information and correctly apply your clinical knowledge and skills in a way that will meet your desired goal of a caring response. To do this well you have to be attentive to the details of each patient's unique history and present situation. Likewise, moral reasoning requires that you be able to gather relevant information and correctly apply your ethical knowledge and skills in the process of ethical reflection. This too requires great attention to the details of each narrative.[3]

Approaches Emphasizing Relationships

Some ethical approaches that rely on story search for the central moral themes of a narrative in an examination of the human relationships revealed in the story. You can immediately see the importance of this insight for health professionals because almost all your work involves relationships. In this approach ethical issues or problems are embedded in the relationships, not just the individual's situation. Not surprisingly, this approach has been promoted and refined by psychologists, particularly those working in the area of moral development.

Carol Gilligan became an important leader in this area in the 1980s, her work having been drawn from a widely accepted model of children's moral development advanced by Harvard psychologist Lawrence Kohlberg. He hypothesized that children go through stages of moral development similar to cognitive development and that children become more independent and autonomous as they mature as moral beings. His work became a, if not the, dominant moral development theory in the early 1980s.[4] At that time, Gilligan, working as Kohlberg's graduate student, noted that his work depended on studies of boys and young men. She repeated some of the work with girls and young women, only to discover that her subjects conceptualized ethical issues and problems differently than their male counterparts. She found that girls had a high sensitivity to how various actions would affect their important relationships (i.e., with parents, friends, teachers, or other authority figures) and concluded that girls' "awareness of the connection between people gives rise to a recognition of responsibility for another."[5] Furthermore, her subjects did not see moral maturity as being characterized by an increasing independence from everyone else, but rather by decisions that would result in deeper and more effective connections and relationships to significant others and the larger community.[6]

Gilligan's work has become one vital basis for ethicists to emphasize anew that relationships figure into morality. Many have worked to refine their understanding of the ways relationships are central within various social settings, including professional relationships. Moreover, further examination showed that although girls and women may be socialized to think in terms of sustaining relationships, the significance of Gilligan's findings are by no means gender-specific.

Reflection

Ron Rachels's reflection on his situation suggests that he believes his relationship with the patient, Pam Faden, has several morally significant aspects. Can you name some of them?

____

____

____

____

Ron Rachels seems to be aware that he has significant power to determine what will happen in Pam Faden's situation because of the nature of his professional expertise, his access to the x-rays and to Dr. Hasagawa himself, and also because of his secret regarding one likely source of her abdominal discomfort. He is aware that the type of "connection" they have might place some responsibility on him to tell her what he knows. In other words, he has some question about who the appropriate moral agent is for addressing that this patient has a scalpel mistakenly left in her abdominal area. In addition to ethical distress he appears to be struggling with a locus of authority problem. He detects that she trusts him and Dr. Hasagawa. Perhaps he wonders if her trust has any relevance in determining what he should do.

Approaches Emphasizing Deep Diversity and Social Structures

Partially because Gilligan's findings initially were assumed to highlight gender-specific differences, her studies led to considerable growth in publications by feminist ethicists. Feminist approaches and theories analyze narratives to make careful critiques of prevailing ethical theories, approaches, and methods, exposing their relevance (or lack of it) for women's experiences.[7,8] They are committed to showing how social practices and institutional structures are important aspects of the spoken (or unspoken) narrative of women's experiences and how many negatively affect women.[9,10]

Postmodernism and Diversity

Some feminists (and others) are postmodernists, the latter being a group who are involved not only in critiquing but also in denying the validity of prevailing theories, approaches, and methods. Postmodernists assert that because there are radical differences among people and cultures, according to their gender, age, ethnicity, or other differences, no one set of moral rules or values is a valid guide "across the board" or even "across a relationship."[11] They are among the thinkers who are not foundationalists. Since I noted earlier in this chapter that professional ethics is foundationalist, it is difficult to reconcile pure postmodernist approaches with the larger social context of professional ethics. At the same time, their contribution is extremely important and points out a possible shortcoming in professional ethics: All too often what passes for a foundation of moral standards is a bias that harms some groups. Our provincialism quickly hems in our ability to make wise judgments about how communities are conceived and operate peacefully and harmoniously. This leads postmodernists to assert that mainstream society fails to respect how deep the diversity of human morality goes, so it simply imposes its own morality, to its own advantage. Therefore, one important contribution of postmodernist thinking to ethical reflection is its urgent call for respectful attention to diversity. In this regard, feminist postmodernist thinkers have made contributions to professional ethics that go well beyond the issues of male versus female gender.

Institutional Arrangements as a Factor

Some feminists join with other thinkers to highlight how institutional and other social arrangements of a society influence individual action and relationships in general. Ethical reflection requires recognition of the powerful influence of each player's and some groups' socially determined "place" in society.

In health care, your recognition of imbalances of power among individuals because of the types of institutions and other social arrangements society condones will be a key factor in your ability to interpret complex situations accurately. If you noted the difference in power between Ron Rachels and Pam Faden or between Ron Rachels and Metsui Hasagawa, because of their relative status and assigned roles within the institution of health care, you were inherently attending to social or institutional influences as relevant considerations in ethical analysis.

In summary, in story-driven, inductive approaches, the first major task is to be attentive to the details of the situation. How is this accomplished? It requires that you not only be humble in the face of rich diversity but also respectful of deep differences and, to the extent possible, show respect for those differences in your relationships with others. It also requires taking seriously the larger social and institutional forces that influence interaction, a topic covered in more detail in Chapter 7.

Ethics of Care Approaches

So far you have been introduced to ethical approaches you can use to:

- Discover the areas of moral relevance by paying attention to the details of a narrative;
- Highlight the moral significance of relationships in the situation;
- Remember to be attentive to deep differences among persons or groups; and
- Appreciate the power of institutional and other social arrangements to influence a situation.

In this subsection you will have an opportunity to examine some ethical approaches that take the idea of care itself as their central feature. There is not *a* "care ethic" at this time but, generally speaking, in an ethics of care approach the major question one asks is: "What is required of a health professional to be best able to express, 'I care'?" As you noted in Chapter 2, care is the language adopted in the health professions ethical literature to emphasize the imperative that professionals must keep a focus on the well-being of the whole person. It is within this context that I have emphasized the goal of professional ethics as being a caring response. Bishop and Scudder describe the core of an ethic of care as residing in the health professional's "caring presence" as follows:

> Caring presence does not mean an emotive, sentimental, or maudlin expression of feeling toward patients. It is a personal presence that assures others of another's concern for their well-being. This way-of-being fosters trust, mutual concern, and positive attitudes that promote good health. When caring presence pervades a health care setting, the whole atmosphere of that setting is transformed so that not only is sound therapy fostered, but patients appreciate, take pride in, and feel part of the health care endeavor.[12]

At least two aspects of a care ethic approach are implied: first, it is dependent on making real contact with the patient as a person, that is, it is deeply relational; and second, it fosters trust.

Baier[13] places trust as one of the central notions for an ethics approach that derives from a perspective of care. That, in turn, suggests that the health professional must bring trustworthiness to the relationship, a notion that will be discussed in greater detail later in this chapter.

As nursing ethics became more sophisticated, the idea of care emerged as a central theme in studies designed to characterize the profession's identity.[14] Since then, additional exciting work by ethicists in many disciplines has helped to refine what caring entails.[15]

For instance, from the beginning maternal activities that foster growth and consciousness have been a key focus, producing advocates and critics.[16] Advocates find deep similarities. Critics voice concern that although caring for others is an activity associated with the maternal, women's traits often are devalued. Therefore, they worry, reliance on the model of motherhood may not fully convey the complexity and importance of caring activities nurses and other health professionals engage in to show respect for the dignity of patients, clients, and others.[17]

Some ethicists worry that an accent on the silver thread of care may deflect attention from injustices woven into the basic warp and woof of the health system, placing all the responsibility to care on individual professionals in the face of policies, practices, and institutions that are unjust. At the same time, Andolsen[18] holds that there is much more overlap in the two themes than many theorists admit.

Story or Case Approaches and a Caring Response

Because an ethics of care is still developing, continue to watch for articles and other opportunities to refine your own interpretation of what a full theory of an ethics of care entails in the health professional and patient relationship. It will be extremely important for you in your quest for a caring response to a wide variety of professional challenges. Story or case approaches combine to include several facets of the overall picture of care. For instance, the vigilance directed to the details of the story and its narrator(s), the emphasis on relationships that shape the story, and a deep respect for the differences that exist among peoples and cultures all are important dimensions of what it means "to care." Approaches that are explicitly termed *an ethics of care* continue to develop and provide you with another opportunity for a rich understanding of what a caring response entails.

We turn now to *virtue theory*. The appropriateness of giving your attention to this theory is expressed by a health professional who in thinking about her profession said, "caring behavior involves the integration of virtue and expert activity of . . . [professional] practice."[19] In other words, an understanding of virtue theory provides an important link between the motivation to find a caring response and the ethical acts or behaviors that will follow from such a disposition.

Virtue Theory

Many varieties of virtue theory have been developed over the ages. The attempt here is to provide you with some basic threads that have created the general tapestry of varieties called *virtue ethics*. Looking back on the early Western development of those theories, Aristotle can be credited with providing us with a basic framework for this thinking.[20] Within the Judeo-Christian theologic tradition that has deeply influenced Western ethics, the virtue dimensions of Thomas Aquinas's theories have had a profound impact on the shaping of virtue theory.[21] Within the health professions and early medical ethics writings, the idea of virtue also was dominant. For example, authors of the Hippocratic School wrote approximately 70 essays on health care in addition to the Oath, several of which discussed character traits. The *Decorum* enjoins that a physician "should be modest, sober, patient, prompt and conduct himself [sic] with propriety in professional and personal life."[22] In short, the professional caregiver will have the moral fiber required to carry out the various duties outlined in the Oath.

Maimonides was a highly respected and renowned Jewish philosopher of the 13th century who wrote extensively about the relationship of medical issues to Jewish law. The prayer of Maimonides is based directly on the belief that the development of certain character traits enables the caregiver to exhibit appropriate moral behavior. In making this promise the physician calls on God for help to have the right motives worthy of this high calling:

> May neither avarice nor miserliness nor thirst for glory nor for great reputation engage my mind, or the enemies of truth and philanthropy could easily deceive me and make me forgetful of my lofty aim of doing good to my patients. May I never see in a patient anything but a fellow creature of pain.[23]

Maimonides believed that important character traits of the health professional are sympathy for the patient's plight, humility, and a devoted commitment to helping others.

From those early influences many normative versions of virtue theory have evolved so that the tapestry of thought today is splendid indeed. The easiest way into the understanding of virtue theory is through the basic idea of character traits and moral character.

Character Traits and Moral Character

A *character trait* is a disposition or a readiness to act in certain ways. Some character traits are supportive of high ethical standards. Some people exhibit character traits that lead an observer to judge that they are of a *high moral character*. In other words, they are a type of person who can be *expected* always to act in a manner that will be praised by others because it upholds high standards. To some extent, our society is measured by the type of people in it. Professionals are judged on this basis more than on any other criterion. Your oaths, codes, and standards of practice declare it. Your state licensing laws will require it of you.

Certain character traits enable you to be the kind of person you want to be as a caregiver.[24] For example, honesty will manifest itself in your trying to refrain from deceiving others for your own comfort or protection. Courage may be required to speak out against injustice or other wrongdoing. Courage combined with honesty will be needed for a therapist to admit that she or he mistakenly took the wrong treatment approach to a patient. Compassion can help motivate you to refrain from thoughtlessly harming vulnerable people.

Recall the health professionals involved in Pam Faden's care. Honesty taken alone would dispose you to encourage Ron Rachels to tell the patient about the medical mistake. Honesty and courage taken together would dispose you to telling her, but also to take every step to assure that she actually receives the correct information. This may involve some risk-taking conduct if Ron believes a cover-up is going on. In other words, the two virtues together will drive him to take measures that assure Dr. Hasagawa will be held accountable for his surgical team's error. These two character traits combined with compassion would motivate you to make sure the information is transmitted in a way that shows respect for everyone involved, even though the outcome was flawed. Taken together, the habitual practice of exercising these traits would create a high moral character that prompts you to do everything possible to diminish harm and foster a morally healthy work environment.

Reflection

Examine the code of ethics in your chosen health field. What character traits are listed or implied? Would your code provide guidance for the attitude you should have toward the situation Ron Rachels is faced with?

____

____

____

____

Probably the most widely esteemed traits are those that convey an attitude of respect for individuals who come to you as patients. The underlying ideal is that individuals should be treated as ends, not as means to some other end.

Both individual and institutional virtues are important within the health professions. In this respect one can speak of the moral character of an individual health professional, as well as the moral character of health care institutions. In addition to the elaboration of specific virtues that should be cultivated, there are several other points about the cultivation of virtue you'll want to know.

First, experience is extremely important. Only through experience can we ultimately learn exactly what contributes to a morally good life (the goal of exercising virtue in the first place).

Second, because the cultivation of virtue depends on experience, we can't simply think ourselves into being virtuous or knowing what virtue consists of. We must add feelings. Emotions must be attended to—they are the motivators toward certain kinds of actions and not others (e.g., Ron Rachels's emotional attachment in the form of sympathy for this patient's suffering figures into his concern about what to do that is right).

Third, in the process of experiencing and feeling what is happening in the situation we ourselves become transformed. When we follow the inclination of virtue we are working at becoming more virtuous. We grow into virtue by acting in accordance with what virtue counsels us to do.

Fourth, a community of persons is vital for discerning virtue in a situation. In this regard, the health professions are one community where such discernment takes place.[25]

Character Traits and a Caring Response

This discussion of virtue illustrates that "caring," in the context of professional ethics, incorporates more than common ordinary dimensions of the notion of care, although those are important. Several positive character traits may be called into play at one time or another to prepare you attitudinally for the action you will have to take. Understandably, the development of habits that allow you to move easily into a caring response will serve you well. Being able to live a life of moral excellence requires exercise, but I believe Aristotle was correct in saying that high moral character is the key component to a good life overall.

SUMMARY

The early crafters of the idea that professionals must exert high moral character through the cultivation of virtues made good common sense when viewed through the lens of the professional's moral task of achieving an outcome consistent with a caring response.

We have come considerable distance already in this chapter. Although the professional ethic takes the story and your disposition to what you learned from it as the fundamental starting point, the ethical challenge does not end there. The caring *response* requires that you become a certain type of person (i.e., of high moral character) *to do what is right*. Therefore, because professional ethics requires action, as well as dispositions and character traits, we turn now to ethical theories and approaches collectively termed *action theories*. They include principles approaches, deontology, and teleology.

Principles as Guides

When you move to purposive action, it is helpful to be able to say, toward what end? Ron Rachels will ask, "What guidelines can I use to help know if my action is in the (morally) right direction?" This concern, and the recognition that guidelines are needed, led to the development of approaches that emphasize *principles*. In most professional ethics literature (as well as modern social ethics writings) they are called *principles,* but I also think of them as *elements* because they do for ethical theory what the basic chemical elements do for chemistry theory: they provide a way to see something concretely that is quite abstract. As you know, a chemical element can be combined with other elements. Sometimes they combine to form a new compound that looks and acts differently than each of the units taken individually. Sometimes they clash. Often, two or more elements have different relative weights so that one is heavier than the other(s). The principles are shown in Table 3–1 for your future reference.

There is more to the story than Table 3–1 indicates because "I" may be a person, a group, or even an institution. Principles can help you know how an individual, group, or institution stands in relationship

Table 3–1 Ethical Principles

Principle	*When Applicable*
Nonmaleficence (refraining from potentially harming myself or another)	I am in a position to harm someone else.
Beneficence (bringing about good)	I am in a position to benefit someone else.
Fidelity	I have made a promise, explicit or implicit, to someone else.
Autonomy	I have an opportunity to exercise my freedom in a situation.
Veracity	I am in a position to tell the truth or deceive someone.
Justice	I am in a position to distribute benefits and burdens among individuals or groups in society who have legitimate claims on the benefits.

to other people, morally speaking. The British philosopher David Hume[26] justified this position in his belief that we incur obligations to act in certain ways because we have received positive responses to our own needs to be treated humanely: "I have benefitted from society, and therefore ought to promote its interests." Some philosophers argue, correctly I think, that principles help to identify what we should do in special relationships regardless of whether we have received benefits from the other person (or from society). Some such relationships, Hume says, are between parent and child, spouses, faculty and student, or citizen and society. The health professions have emerged as another source of special relationship, with patients.

Several principles are extremely important in the health care context. For example, the principle of nonmaleficence, or "do no harm," was an explicit theme in the ancient Hippocratic Oath and ever since has been viewed as an overriding moral principle guiding health professionals' conduct toward patients. Because of their importance you have this opportunity to examine several in more detail.

Nonmaleficence and Beneficence

Primum non nocere ("First, do no harm") is thought to be at the nexus of traditional health care ethics and often is attributed to the author of the Hippocratic Oath. It is at the very heart of what is meant by a caring response! The principle of *nonmaleficence* is the noun used today to talk about this type of action. You can figure out the general meaning of the term by breaking it into its prefix, *non*, and the root, *maleficence* ("mal, bad, or evil"). The difference in power between professional and patient alone helps to support the instinctive wisdom of this strong call to refrain from abuse. Furthermore, Western societies in general usually attribute greater significance to a harmful act done out of deliberate intent than out of neglect or ignorance. It is difficult to believe that a society could survive if people went around trying to harm each other, and the laws of our land take seriously the necessity of stemming the potential for harm to go unchecked. The early purveyors of professional ethics left nothing to chance, warning health professionals that there was no room whatsoever for acting in ways designed to bring about harm.

In professional ethics, not harming and acting to benefit another are treated as separate duties. Sometimes philosophers treat them as different levels of the same principle or element. When duties are thought of in this latter fashion, at least four types fall along the continuum of the same principle:

Do no harm.

Prevent harm.

Remove harm when it is being inflicted.

Bring about positive good.

Professional ethics limits *beneficence* to the last three on the list.

Reflection

Before you leave the principles of nonmaleficence and beneficence, think again about the story in this chapter. Ron is worried about what has happened to the patient, Pamela Faden. He believes she has been harmed by having a scalpel left in her abdominal cavity and then by the surgeon's failure to tell her about the surgical error.

Is Ron following the principle of nonmaleficence by his actions so far? The principle of beneficence? What evidence do you have that he is or is not? In your opinion what would he have to do to be beneficent in this case, given the level of his authority and his knowledge, skills, and compassion?

____

____

____

____

Because these two principles are so pervasive in the everyday decision making by a professional, you are well advised to think about their relevance in every new situation you encounter.

Autonomy

The principle of *autonomy* is the capacity to have the say-so about your own well-being, "the capacity to act on your decisions freely and independently."[27] Some call this the principle of self-determination. Obviously the principle applies to you whether you are acting in your professional role (professional autonomy) or as a citizen (social autonomy) or have become a patient (patient autonomy). Much of the discussion that follows focuses on the important arena of patient autonomy.

We know that patients' basic health care needs have not changed significantly over the decades, but our idea of what fully constitutes a caring response has changed. Today so many clinical interventions are possible that the type and number of interventions alone may lead to suffering. A few years ago the health professional who did everything clinically possible for a patient was seen as being beneficent. Today that same professional could find that the process leads to moral regret: the patient or patient's family may charge that harm has resulted because the interventions have gone beyond what the patient wanted or could tolerate.

In light of this situation, the last several decades have seen the emergence of the patient as a more active negotiator regarding health care decisions. The patient's *autonomy,* say-so or self-governance, has come to be accepted as a legitimate moral claim to be placed in the balance with the health professional's independent judgment about what is beneficent. Some suggest that autonomy has too much emphasis, creating a monopoly on our moral attention.

The principle of autonomy (or self-determination) and its role in morality have been developed from the views of diverse and colorful figures in philosophy. Two who have been especially influential are the deontologist, Immanuel Kant, and one of the crafters of a consequence-oriented theory, John Stuart Mill (both of whom will be discussed further later in this chapter). Both of their interpretations of the principle of autonomy have been adopted in health professions usage. Kant[28] emphasized the role of being in control of making one's own choices in accord with a moral standard that could be willed valid for everyone. Therefore, his main contribution was his discussion of self-legislation: the reasons for actions. Conversely, Mill[29] focused his thought more on the context of the freedom of action, arguing that an individual's actions legitimately can be restricted only when they promise to harm someone else. Up to that point, he contends, each person should be permitted to act according to his or her own convictions. Therefore, his main contribution was to highlight the social and political context in which the exercise of autonomy can thrive.[29]

The two interpretations together point to our assumption today that a patient's input can be rational and that the context of decision making must be conducive to the patient's exercising his or her real and informed wishes. Anything less fails to meet the criterion of a caring response (Fig. 3–2).

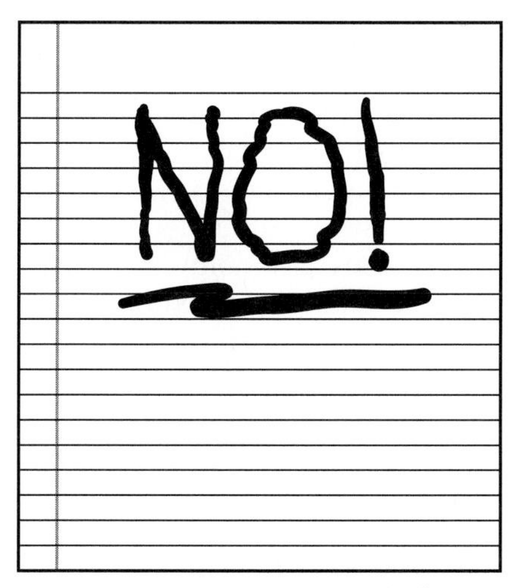

Figure 3–2. This statement was written on a pad of paper by a 27-year-old hospitalized woman with ovarian-breast cancer syndrome. She could not communicate verbally because she had a tracheostomy and therefore could not speak. The physician had explained that he wanted to reimplement chemotherapy for a tumor that had appeared in her remaining ovary. She had already undergone an oophorectomy and hysterectomy and had received radiotherapy and chemotherapy for the previous tumors before their removal.

Gilligan, whose theories were introduced earlier in this chapter, is among those who criticize a focus on autonomy because it requires that a person be treated as an isolated unit standing alone, over and against all other people, whereas, as you recall, she emphasizes the importance of relationships for the moral life.[30] This is a serious criticism. She is correct in her observation that we understand ourselves as moral beings largely within the context of our relationships. Be that as it may, we also live in a society that is highly individualistic in its behavior and laws. The principle of autonomy provides direction in those situations in which an individual is in a position to make a claim on others to respect his or her selfhood. In fact, sometimes the claim for autonomy is given the power of a right.

Currently, there is a lot of discussion about autonomy in regard to decisions about the timing and type of death one will have, a topic you'll encounter again in Chapter 13. Underlying the idea of a right to die is the more fundamental belief in the right to autonomy or self-determination. But the principle of autonomy has much broader applications than end-of-life situations. For instance, it undergirds the idea of informed consent. And in the predicament in which Ron Rachels finds himself at the beginning of this chapter, he is hemmed in by the physician's decision not to share the news about the medical mistake with the patient. You might say that Dr. Hasagawa's autonomy has led to the diminution of self-determination for both Ron Rachels and the patient Pam Faden.

The principle of autonomy (or self-determination) is a helpful principle, but, like all of the principles, it is not absolute in the delicate complexity of real life situations. For example, Mill would put his foot down at the point when Metsui Hasagawa's exercise of autonomy results in direct harm to Pam Faden or to Ronald Rachels. If I want to hit you, my autonomy ends where your nose begins. Should the physician's autonomy end where Pam Faden's troubled question begins? You will revisit the principle of autonomy several times later in this book. Watch for it.

Fidelity

The principle of *fidelity* comes from the Latin root *fides,* which means faithfulness. Being faithful to the patient entails meeting the patient's reasonable expectations. The patients come with all kinds of expectations. What can be counted as a *reasonable* expectation?

First, there is a reasonable expectation that basic respect will be shown to anyone, anywhere. Sometimes health professionals have been criticized for failing to show basic respect, such as respecting the modesty of a patient.

Second, the patient has reason to expect that you will be competent in what you do.

Third, the patient has a reasonable expectation that you will adhere to statements you have subscribed to as a member of a profession. The most public of these statements is your code of ethics.

Fourth, the patient has a good basis for believing you will follow the policies and statements adopted by your place of employment, as well as laws that are designed to protect patients' well-being.

Finally, the patient has good reason to expect that you will honor what the two of you have agreed to, such as the promises involved in any informed consent form the patient has signed, verbal agreements, or serious conversations.

Can you think of others? A caring response cannot be affected if you fail to meet the reasonable expectation of your patients and others.

Veracity

The ethical element of *veracity* binds you to honesty. Veracity means that you will tell the truth. This principle is more specific than, say, beneficence or fidelity. For this reason some would call it a second level principle directing you to engage in a specific type of behavior, which in turn can support your intent to be beneficent or to maintain your fidelity in relationships with patients and others. Kant gave veracity a central role, taking the position that veracity is an absolute to which no exception can be made "however great may be the disadvantage accruing to yourself or another." The lie, he argues in one place, always is wrong because the practice of lying is something that weakens the entire human fabric.[31] Most others would weigh veracity heavily regarding its potential for benefiting others but would not make it the absolute or governing duty above all others.

In our story, Ron Rachels understandably seemed depressed about the possibility that Pamela Faden was not being told the truth about the surgeon's mistake. The situation was made more complex by the different professional roles of the radiologic technologist and the physician.

Reflection

Given his role, do you think that as a radiologic technologist Ron personally should have acted according to the principle of veracity and told her about the scalpel? Do you think that the surgeon had a moral obligation to tell her the truth? If not, what other principles would you weigh against veracity in this situation that leads you to your conclusion?

____

____

____

____

Later in this book (see Chapter 10) we return to the important matter of truth telling as it relates to your professional task of disclosing different types of information in general.

Justice

Patients do not always get all the treatment and attention they deserve or need because of a lack of resources, and anyone who worries about that is worrying about the principle of *justice* in the situation. Discrimination against some individuals or groups may appear to be shortchanging them, and anyone who worries about that is worrying about the justice of the situation. A lack of due process regarding who receives priority in situations of conflict may cause concern, and anyone who worries about that also is worrying about the justice of the situation. In general, their concern is that all similarly situated individuals receive their fair share of benefits and assume their fair share of burdens. The caring response is achieved when individuals or groups are treated fairly and equitably.

Justice can be thought of as an arbiter. It is called on when there are problems regarding what is rightfully due a person, institution, or society. Three types of justice have particular importance in professional ethics situations: distributive, compensatory, and procedural. We take up the complex issues of justice more fully in Chapters 14 and 15.

Principles and a Caring Response

This concludes our list of the ethical principles you will most often encounter in your professional roles. As you can see, they still are very general, but, importantly, they move you in the direction of action according to some guidelines. In their particularity they are instrumental in helping you further delineate the conditions that must be met if you are to show a caring response toward the patient. For instance, you know that you must honor the patient's reasonable expectations, you must do it truthfully, and so on. The principles themselves force you to consider who the patient is as an individual different from all others.

SUMMARY

Principles provide general action guides in the search for a course of action that will result in an outcome consistent with a caring response.

You may have noticed that some of these principles are more oriented toward a duty-driven ethic. They include fidelity, autonomy, truthfulness (veracity), and justice. Others, namely beneficence and nonmaleficence, require you to weigh the most favorable (or least damaging) consequences in a situation. Does this sound vaguely familiar? It should. The "duty" theory of deontology naturally would appeal to principles that help delineate what a particular duty (e.g., veracity) entails. The consequence-oriented theory of utilitarianism uses the principle of beneficence or nonmaleficence as a guideline.

Both deontologists and teleologists express the need for individual or group actions to be guided according to principles. However, you have not yet had the opportunity to look more closely at these two major theories that have been the most influential in traditional professional ethics approaches. We turn to them now.

Deontologic and Teleologic Theories

Taking Duties Seriously

Ron Rachels faces a perplexing dilemma regarding loyalty and honesty. One approach would be to identify whether there is a duty that can help him decide what to do. In his search for a duty (or duties) he is appealing to deontologic theories.

One place where duties are codified is in statements that comprise codes of professional ethics. For example, currently you will find statements such as, "respect a patient's dignity" or "honor the patient's [or client's] right to consent to a potential treatment." When you look more closely, the statements or axioms imply fundamental ideas about humans—namely, that we stand in relation to each other in a number of morally significant ways. In this regard, deontologists agree with Gilligan and others whose theories have been discussed in this chapter regarding the centrality of *relationship* and the importance of paying attention to the details of a patient's (or another's) story. Deontologists hold that there are basic concepts that individuals and societies recognize and agree on that give rise to a shared sense of duty or right. These could be arrived at through *reasoning* about such things or, others might argue, we *intuit* them (i.e., have intuition; note the deductive assumptions discussed in Chapter 1). Although a narrative approach correctly helps to focus attention on particular details of a story, the deontologist goes further to say there is a concept of duty informing (or at least available to) all individuals. In other words, this is consistent with a foundationalist approach described earlier in this chapter—that is, the foundation being in the various duties.

Deontologic theories hold that you are acting rightly when you act according to duties and rights. In other words, duties and rights are the correct measuring rods for evaluating action. There are many versions of deontology. The person most often identified with deontologic approaches is Immanuel Kant, whose philosophies were introduced in the discussion of the principle of autonomy. His basic premises still figure strongly in arguments within health care ethics today. He held that every person has an inherent dignity and on that basis alone is entitled to respect. Respect is shown by never *using* people to achieve goals or consequences. He thought that duties help to determine how respect toward others can be expressed. It follows that the morally correct thing is always to be guided by moral duties, rights, and responsibilities. He concluded that some actions are intrinsically immoral, no matter how positive and beneficial one might judge the consequences to be, and that other actions are intrinsically moral, no matter how negative the consequences might be. In short, he said that one cannot judge the moral rightness or wrongness of an act on the basis of its consequences alone.[32] Whatever his conclusion about what Ron Rachels or Metsui Hasagawa should do, Kant would arrive at his decision by a process of determining what their duty should be, not simply whether there would be overall better consequences achieved by one type of act or another.

Reflection

Do you think that this appeal to duties is the correct moral tool to use in the situation in which Ron Rachels and Metsui Hasagawa find themselves? What important moral considerations are taken into account in this approach? What could be overlooked if they appealed to their sense of duty alone?

____
____
____
____

As you can begin to see, there are some challenges to applying this approach in its "pure" form. For instance, the idea that we ought to do the right thing, informed by duty, is general. **How** to show respect for individuals still needs further interpretation in any situation. What do we do when duties or rights themselves come into conflict? Deontologic theories require that a method of weighing be available to determine what to do when conflicts arise, and critics charge that there is no obvious way to weigh them. Such a process is not self-evident. Thus, the appeal to **principles** discussed in the previous section is one attempt to provide further detail and interpretation to the general idea of duty and to order, or give varying weight to conflicting duties, rights, and responsibilities.

Absolute, Prima Facie, and Conditional Duties

We have seen that from a deontologic viewpoint principles can assist in interpreting one's duty. Principles that carry the weight of duties may be absolute, prima facie, or conditional. *Absolute* duties are binding under all circumstances. They can never give way to another compelling duty or right. *Prima facie* duties or rights allow you to make choices among conflicting principles. For instance, the prima facie duty of veracity is actually binding if it conflicts with no other duties, or rights, that are weightier in a given situation. But it is not an element that is absolute either, because other elements may be more compelling. In the discussion of the primacy of "do no harm" over "beneficence" in the clinical ethics context, it was suggested that each is being treated as a prima facie principle, and the mandate not to harm is more compelling than the mandate to bring about some positive good. A *conditional duty* is a commitment that comes into being only after certain conditions are met. For example, the Americans with Disabilities Act outlines certain rights and responsibilities that apply solely to individuals who have disabilities.[33]

However binding a principle or element is deemed to be, it has the role of providing a marker to guide the conduct of individuals and groups wanting to live a good moral life.

Paying Attention to Outcomes

Partially because of some of the criticisms of deontology, *teleologic theories* emerged, placing the focus on the ends brought about and the consequences of actions. The most important teleologic theory for our consideration of health care ethics is *utilitarianism*. This word takes its root from the idea of *utility* or usefulness.

In utilitarianism an act is right if it helps to bring about the best balance of benefits over burdens, in other words, the best consequences overall.* This approach was developed first by two English philosophers, Jeremy Bentham (1748–1832)[34] and John Stuart Mill (1806–1873).[35] Note that they are roughly contemporaries of Kant. In fact, they were vigorous opponents of Kant's position.

Consider Pam Faden's question about why she is having so much difficulty. How should one decide what Ron Rachels or Metsui Hasagawa should do? From a utilitarian point of view, first you must consider what several different courses of action could accomplish. You might say, "The goal is to treat Pam Faden in such a way that everyone else will be able to have the same type of care she gets," or "The goal is to be able to live with my own conscience." If both these goals can be attained by taking one, single course of action, it should be taken. If this is not possible, the course of action you believe will bring about the best consequences overall should take priority.

One important task of this approach is to distinguish alternate paths of action and then predict as accurately as possible the consequences of each path. As you can begin to see, this approach also has

---

**Rule utilitarians* are sometimes thought of as a hybrid of duty-oriented approaches, which rely on certain forms of actions, and pure utilitarians, who think about consequences solely in the specific details of each situation. A rule utilitarian would hold that you will always bring about more good consequences by following certain "rules" or duties. What the rules should be then becomes the task for these theorists.

some inherent challenges. How can anyone predict all the potential consequences of an act? Moreover, doesn't this approach ignore that at least sometimes humans do think in terms of their duties, rights, and responsibilities to one another?

Duties, Consequences, and a Caring Response

The deontologic and utilitarian normative theories have been helpful to health professionals because they set a general framework for thinking about specific moral issues and problems in health care settings with a focus on the action that needs to take place. Probably as you were reading you were thinking, "Well, both the idea of duties and rights *and* the idea of consequences are important in my attempt to arrive at a caring response." In fact, most of us do draw on both to make practical, everyday moral decisions. Only occasionally does it make a big difference in what you judge to be right if you follow a deontologic line of reasoning or appeal to consequences only. Fortunately, most of the time you can take action that is in line with your sense of duty, honor others' rights, *and* consider the outcomes you are bringing about without any conflict among the three. But it is in the occasional moment during which the means and the ends seem to be competing that it may become necessary to plant your feet firmly in one theory or the other and be able to justify why. See Table 3–2 for a summary of deontology and teleology.

Summary

This chapter introduces you to ethical theories and approaches that will help you the most when faced with ethical problems in your role as a health professional. The ability to absorb a narrative for its moral content and the development of moral character will help you to be ready for the hard times when no answers seem to be forthcoming or when you are confronted with something that is not easy to face. You also have learned the most important principles or norms of ethics that you need to understand the ethical aspects of your life as a professional person. Duties and rights are tools for recognizing and working to resolve problems that arise in your everyday practice. Although traditionally much of the language of health care ethics has been that of what is owed the patient (i.e., the language of duties), the importance of character traits and attitudes

Table 3–2 Theories of Deontology versus Teleology

Deontology	*Teleology*
Duty-driven	Goal-driven
Means count	Ends count
Kant	Bentham, Mill (utilitarians)

and, more recently, the ideas of patients' (as well as professionals' and society's) rights have enriched the understanding of professional ethics with its goal of ascertaining a caring response. With this basic framework at your disposal you are well positioned to engage in the six-step process of ethical analysis and decision making introduced in the next chapter.

Questions for Thought and Discussion

1. This is an opportunity for the class to create a narrative of a patient, Esther Korn. It is a group exercise about a health care situation that came to the attention of the hospital ethics committee. The whole class can participate in the discussion as members of the ethics committee, and five people will assume various important roles.

   The ethics committee has been asked to give advice on whether Esther Korn should be sent back home or to a nursing home.

   Esther Korn, a 72-year-old woman, has been admitted to the hospital with a diagnosis of dehydration and serious bruises from a fall sustained in her home. She was found by a neighbor, Anna Knight, who says she stops by Esther's home daily because Ms. Korn has lived alone with her eight cats since being discharged from a state mental institution with a diagnosis of involutional paranoia, which is believed to be under control with medications. From the degree of dehydration, the health professionals believe that Ms. Korn was very dehydrated before she fell and that she had been lying on the floor for at least a day. The emergency medical team who brought her to the hospital described her home as "filthy, full of dirty dishes and clothes strung all over, with cat droppings everywhere."

   Now, 5 days later, Ms. Korn seems confused about where she is, but she does know her own name. She says over and over, "Let me out of here! I want to go home!" Her sister, whom she has not seen "for years" (according to Anna Knight), has a telephone message service and does not return the nurses' calls. The nurses are not in complete agreement, but most of the staff believes that Esther would be better off placed in an institution for her own safety. Anna Knight and the local priest, who visits her regularly, also have strong opinions about where Esther should live.

   Five people will be "storytellers" to provide some missing parts to her story: one will be Esther, the other four will be significant others in her life. Together the class can create a fictional story that fills in information about who she is and what may, in fact, be in her best interest in this difficult question facing the ethics committee:

Person A — Write a few paragraphs about Esther from her neighbor Anna's perspective and what Anna thinks should be done.
Person B — Write about her from the Episcopal priest's perspective and what she would recommend.
Person C — Write about her from the perspective of her long-lost sister and what she would recommend.
Person D — Write a report from the point of view of the primary nurse and what he thinks.
Person E — Speaking as Esther, give some background as to what kind of person she believes herself to be, what is important to her, and so on.

When each of the five storytellers has completed this part of the exercise, read the notes aloud to the ethics committee (i.e., rest of the group). After everyone has heard the "bigger picture," answer the following questions:

- What should be done?
- What influences your thinking the most?
- Which values do you think are the most prominent in this discussion?
- Did anything that was said in these stories change your mind about your initial thoughts regarding what should be done? If so, explain.
- Discuss what the health professionals must do to show caring in their relationship with Esther Korn.

2. Cite an example from health care in which a conflict could arise between your sense of duty to the patient and the negative consequences your act might have on someone else.
3. Elva, a 370-pound, 62-year-old woman, is in a nursing home after complications of diabetes and several small strokes. Although she has been obese all her life, she now is at a weight where it is impossible to move her without a lift. Elva, however, refuses to be moved by it, claiming, "I'm not a piece of meat."

   It is possible to transfer her to a chair using four or five of the staff. The administration, however, is worried that the staff could be injured while moving her physically. Her daughter insists that it is a violation of Elva's dignity and an unnecessary compromise of her autonomy to submit her to "the indignity of the mechanical lift."

   You are the supervisor of the unit. What ethical principles presented in this chapter can help you to assess what to do in this situation? What should you do?

___

___

___

___

4. Walter is a resident in the same nursing home with Elva. He is a 78-year-old widower who has been on antidepressants since the sudden death of his wife 5 years ago. He, too, is visited often by his daughter. The staff of the nursing home inadvertently threw out his dentures with the sheets while making his bed. He had a habit of leaving them on the bed, and although the staff usually noticed them, a new employee failed to do so.

   Since then Walter has adamantly refused to have his teeth replaced. The nursing home administration is more than willing to fit him with a new set of dentures and to pay all costs. His daughter is very much in agreement with the administration that he should have his teeth replaced. They are all aware that his nutrition is suffering, as well as his ability to be understood when he tries to talk.

   Should Walter be allowed to continue without his dentures? What principles and other considerations of ethics should you, as a nursing home administrator, bring to bear on your decision on how to proceed in this situation? What should you do?

References

1. Hunter, K. 2004. Narrative. In Post, S.G. (Ed.), *Encyclopedia of Bioethics* (3rd ed., vol. 4). New York: Macmillan, p. 1875.
2. *Ibid*. p. 1876.
3. *Ibid*. p. 1877.
4. Kohlberg, L. 1981. *The Philosophy of Moral Development: Moral Stages and the Idea of Justice*. San Francisco: Harper and Row.
5. Gilligan, C. 1982. *In a Different Voice—Psychological Theory and Women's Development*. Cambridge, MA: Harvard University Press.
6. *Ibid*. p. 30.
7. Warren, V.L. 1989. Feminist directions in medical ethics. *Hypatia* 4(2):73–87.
8. Moody-Adams, M. 1991. Gender and the complexity of moral voices. In Cord, C. (Ed.), *Feminist Ethics*. Lawrence, KS: University Press of Kansas, pp. 195–212.
9. Wolf, S.M. (Ed.). 1996. *Feminism and Bioethics. Beyond Reproduction*. New York: Oxford University Press.
10. Lindemann Nelson, H. 2004. Feminism. In Post, S.G. (Ed.), *Encyclopedia of Bioethics* (3rd ed., vol. 2). New York: Macmillan, p. 884–889.
11. Gillett, G. 1997. Is there anything wrong with Hitler these days? Ethics in a post-modern world. *Medical Humanities Review* 11(2):9–20.
12. Bishop, A., Scudder, J. 2001. Caring presence. In *Nursing Ethics: Holistic Caring Practice* (2nd ed.). Sudbury, MA: Jones and Bartlett Publishers, pp. 41–65.
13. Baier, A., 1995. The need for more than justice. In Held, V. (Ed.), *Justice and Care*. Boulder, CO: Westview Press, pp. 47–58.
14. Fry, S., Killen, A.R., Robinson, E.M. 1996. Care-based reasoning, caring and the ethic of care: A need for clarity. *Journal of Clinical Ethics* 7(1):41–47.

15. Gastmans, C., Dierckx de Casterle, B., Robinson, E.M. 1998. Nursing considered as moral practice: A philosophical-ethical interpretation of nursing. *Kennedy Institute of Ethics Journal* 8:1,43–69.
16. Ruddick, S. 1989. *Maternal Thinking: Toward a Politics of Peace*. Boston: Beacon Press.
17. Condon, E.H. 1991. Nursing and the caring metaphor: Gender and political influences on an ethics of care. *Nursing Outlook* 40(1):14–19.
18. Andolsen, B.H., 2001. Care and justice as moral values for nurses in an era of managed care. In Cates, D.F., Lauritzen, P. (Eds.), *Medicine and the Ethics of Life*. Washington, DC: Georgetown University Press, pp. 41–56.
19. Bradshaw, A., 1999. The virtue of nursing: the covenant of care. *Journal of Medical Ethics* 25:477–481.
20. Aristotle. Nichomachean ethics. 1984. In Barnes, J. (Ed.), *The Complete Works of Aristotle* (Vol. 2). Princeton, NJ: Princeton University Press, p. 1729.
21. Aquinas. Summa Theologica. 1945. In Pegis, A.G. (Ed.), *Basic Writings of St. Thomas Aquinas*. New York: Random House.
22. Hippocrates. Decorum. In *Hippocrates II* (W.H.S. Jones, Trans.). Cambridge, MA: Harvard University Press, Loeb Classical Library, pp. 267–302.
23. Maimonides. 1927. Prayers of Moses Maimonides (H. Friedenwald, Trans.). *Bulletin of the Johns Hopkins Hospital* 28:260–261.
24. Loewy, E.H. 1997. Developing habits and knowing what habits to develop: A look at the role of virtue in ethics. *Cambridge Quarterly Healthcare Ethics* 6(3):347–355.
25. Marton, M. 2002. Personal communication. National Endowment for the Humanities Seminar on "Justice, Equality and the Challenge of Disability." Bronxville, New York, June 24, 2002.
26. Hume, D. 1976. On suicide. In Gorowitz, S., Macklin, R., Jameton, A. (Eds.), *Moral Problems in Medicine*. Englewood Cliffs, NJ: Prentice Hall, p. 356.
27. Beauchamp, T., Childress, J.F. 2001. *Principles of Biomedical Ethics* (5th ed.). New York: Oxford University Press, pp. 259–260.
28. Kant, I. 1963. *Lectures on Ethics* (L. Infield, Trans.). New York: Harper and Row, pp. 147–154.
29. Mill, J.S. 1939. On Liberty. In Burtt, E.A. (Ed.), *The English Philosophers from Bacon to Mill*. New York: Random House, pp. 1042–1060.
30. Gilligan, C. 1982. *Psychological Theory and Women's Development*. Cambridge, MA: Harvard University Press.
31. Kant, I. 1963. *op. cit.*
32. Kant, I. 1949. In Beck, L.W. (Ed.), *Critique of Practical Reason and other Writings in Moral Philosophy*. Chicago: University of Chicago Press, pp. 346–350.
33. Americans with Disabilities Act. 1990. H.R. Rep. No. 485 (II), 101st Congress, 2nd Sess. at 22 12.
34. Bentham, J. 1939. An enquiry concerning human understanding. In Burtt, E.A. (Ed.), *The English Philosophers from Bacon to Mill*. New York: Random House, pp. 792–856.
35. Mill, J.S. 1939. Utilitarianism. In Burtt, E.A. (Ed.), *The English Philosophers from Bacon to Mill*. New York: Random House, pp. 895–1041.

4

A Six-Step Process of Ethical Decision Making in Arriving at a Caring Response

Objectives

The student should be able to:

- Identify six steps in the analysis of ethical problems encountered in everyday professional life and how each plays a part in arriving at a caring response.
- Describe the central role of narrative and virtue theories in gathering relevant information for a caring response.
- List four areas of inquiry that will be useful when gathering relevant information to make sure you have the story straight.
- Describe the role of conduct-related ethical theories and approaches in arriving at a caring response.
- Describe why imagination is an essential aspect of seeking out the practical alternatives in an ethically challenging situation.
- Discuss how courage assists you in a caring response.
- Identify two benefits of taking time to reflect on and evaluate the action afterward.

New terms and ideas you will encounter in this chapter

chemical restraints
rounds

Topics in this chapter introduced in earlier chapters

Topic	*Introduced in chapter*
A caring response	2, 3
The importance of story or narrative	3
Ethical distress	2

Ethical dilemma	2
Locus of authority problem	2
Paternalism	2
Ethics	1
Deontology	3
Teleology	3
Utilitarianism	3

Introduction

You have come a long way in laying the foundation for identifying prototypes of ethical issues and problems and in identifying the ethical tools available to you for analysis in your search for resolution of conflicts as you work toward a caring response. In this chapter you will have an opportunity to apply what you have learned and to use a problem-solving method to analyze and resolve problems. The story of Anthony Carnavello and Alexia Eliopoulos is a good starting point for this discussion.

The Story of Anthony Carnavello and Alexia Eliopoulos

Alexia Eliopoulos, a physical therapist, has just begun working in a municipal nursing home. The facility has a reputation for maintaining high standards of care. When Alexia was interviewed for the position, she made a thorough tour of the home and talked with several employees and residents. Everything seemed "in order," and she took the job.

It is now near the end of her second week of work. Alexia goes to the nursing home office to read the personal record of a resident who may be transferred to another facility because of his apparently worsening mental status. She learns that Mr. Anthony Carnavello is 76 years old and has diabetes. Recently, his left leg was amputated because of complications from a fracture of his left femur sustained in an accident. According to the record, he fell in the corridor of the nursing home after tripping over a chair. Reportedly he is "confused" most of the time and is kept quite heavily sedated "to keep him from becoming violent." He is almost blind. There is no neurologist's report in the record.

Alexia decides to introduce herself to Mr. Carnavello before going to lunch. When she finds Mr. Carnavello's room she is surprised to see a shriveled-up little old man lying in bed staring at the ceiling. Alexia introduces herself and tells Mr. Carnavello that she will be coming back to treat him in the afternoon.

Mr. Carnavello squints in an effort to see Alexia. Abruptly he raises up on one elbow and says, "I'm so scared! They keep giving me shots and pills that make me crazy! Can you get them to stop?"

Just at that moment a nurse comes into the room with a syringe on a tray. "Anthony!" she says in a firm, loud voice. "Turn over on your side, please. It's time for your shot!"

Mr. Carnavello protests that the pills and shots are making him "crazy as a hoot owl." But the nurse has exposed one loose-skinned buttock and is deftly injecting the solution before Mr. Carnavello succeeds in resisting. He tries to take a swipe at her, but she backs off quickly. She pats his bony hip, saying, "There now, you're okay, Tony," and leaves immediately. Mr. Carnavello lies back on the pillow and sighs. He grabs the rail, pulls himself up toward Alexia, and says, "See what I mean!" Alexia thinks that Mr. Carnavello seems to be in genuine anguish. She reaches out to pat his hand, but he pulls it away and falls back against the sheet.

Alexia is angry and confused. There is a gnawing feeling in her stomach that something is wrong in the way Mr. Carnavello is being treated. At lunch she shares her concern with Annette Carroll, the nursing supervisor for the entire home. Annette is highly respected by residents and staff alike. Alexia tells Annette it seems that Mr. Carnavello is not being treated with the dignity that the residents deserve. She doubts that Mr. Carnavello is "violent" but can't put her finger on why she felt so much anger at the nurse who efficiently and without undue harshness gave him the injection. Maybe it is because she believes the medication is being used to "dope" Mr. Carnavello unnecessarily. As she recounts what happened, she can feel a seething rage rising up in her. She decides, on the spot, that she will talk to the nursing home administrator and announces that intention to Annette.

Annette listens attentively. When Alexia pauses for a few disinterested bites of her sandwich, she says, "Alexia, you have been here only two weeks. I can understand your uneasiness at what you thought you saw happening. And maybe you are right—maybe Mr. Carnavello is not being treated with the respect he deserves. But remember, being new here, there is much that you don't know. We are doing for him what we think is best, as well as trying to protect our staff from his dangerously aggressive behavior. He was worse before we started him on Haldol."

Alexia doesn't feel any better after lunch. She'd like to talk to someone and decides to call a social worker who works in another nursing home.

As in most actual situations, Alexia's first encounter with what appears to be an ethical problem has left many questions unanswered. The path from Alexia's first perception to possible action consistent with a caring response traverses a six-step process.

The Six-Step Process

Ethical decision making requires your thoughtful reflection and logical judgment even though the situation usually presents itself in a mumbo jumbo of partial facts and strong reactions. The following steps allow you to take the situation apart and look at it in a more organized, coolheaded way while still acknowledging the intense emotions everyone may be experiencing about the situation.

In Chapter 1 you learned that ethics is reflection on and analysis of morality. Therefore, this step-by-step process is, overall, a formalized approach to reflection. In the context of health care your professional ethics dictates that the reflection is directed toward arriving at a caring response in a particular situation. However, it goes beyond reflection, too. As a professional you must assume the role of moral agent; therefore, the reflection and ensuing judgment is geared toward action.

Step 1: Get the Story Straight—Gather Relevant Information

The first step in informed decision making is to gather as much information as possible. Anyone viewing this situation might ask the following types of questions:

- Does Mr. Carnavello have organic brain disease that might explain his behavior?
- What tests have been conducted to confirm the type and degree of brain involvement?
- What does his "violent" behavior consist of?
- What might have happened in Mr. Carnavello's history to make him afraid of the nursing staff or the whole setting and, therefore, to react in a hostile manner?
- Has the Medical Director been made aware of Mr. Carnavello's complaints about the effects of the medication?
- What is the recent history of the exchanges between Mr. Carnavello and the staff?
- What other approaches (besides medication) to Mr. Carnavello's ostensibly violent behavior have been—or could be—attempted?
- What evidence is there that approaching the nursing home administration will create problems for Alexia, Ms. Carroll, or others?
- What other information about physical and chemical restraints (i.e., medicines that tranquilize the patient) in nursing homes should Alexia seek out?

Reflection

Are there other questions you thought of as you read the story?

____

____

____

____

The necessity for close attention to details takes you back to Chapter 3, which introduced you to the importance of the story or narrative.

Without knowing as much as possible about the story line it is impossible to ascertain the attitudes, values, and duties embedded in it. As you probably recall, the theories and approaches to ethics have important clues about how each of these is an important consideration if you are going to be able to arrive at a caring response. The fact-finding mission is absolutely essential as a safeguard against setting off on a false course from the beginning.

Some of the benefits of seeking out the facts in the situation described earlier are that you may be able to determine whether Alexia's perception of Mr. Carnavello's treatment is accurate and to understand why the various players in this drama are acting as they are. Although Annette Carroll's comments are difficult to interpret, she may be implying that Alexia's response would be tempered by more knowledge of the situation. Often, what initially appears to be a "wrong" act is, after all, a right or acceptable one once more of the story is known.

Fact finding also could help Alexia identify the focus of her anger more specifically. What triggered the response? Was it Mr. Carnavello's apparent helplessness in the situation? The nurse's actions? What Alexia has read about misuse of chemical restraints?[1–3] Why has Mr. Carnavello been labeled as "confused" and "violent" when Alexia believes he showed no signs of being either?

The following general checklist for data gathering and adding specific questions will help you organize your thoughts around your specific situation. They are adapted from a handbook designed for clinicians.[4]

1. *Clinical Indications*
   a. What is the diagnosis or prognosis?
   b. Is the illness or condition reversible?
   c. Is life-saving treatment medically futile?
   d. What is the present treatment regimen?
   e. What is the usual and customary treatment for this type of condition?
   f. What is needed to relieve suffering or to provide comfort?
   g. Who are the primary caregivers?
   h. What can you learn about this patient's medical and social history?
2. *Preference of the Patient*
   a. What does he or she want in this situation?
   b. Who has communicated the realistic options to the patient?
   c. What was the patient actually told?
   d. What evidence do you have that what the patient said has been heard by key decision makers?
   e. Is he or she competent to make decisions about this situation?

   f. If not competent, does the patient have a living will, advance directive, or other document indicating his or her considered preferences?
   g. If not competent, is another person speaking as a legitimate legal substitute for this patient?
3. *Quality of Life*
   a. What are the patient's beliefs and values that make up his or her personal value system?
   b. What quality of life considerations are the decision makers bringing to this situation, and how are their biases influencing the decision processes?
   c. Is there any hope for improvement in the patient's quality of life?
4. *Contextual Factors*
   a. What institutional policies may influence what can be done?
   b. What are the legal implications (court cases, statutes, and so on) regarding this issue?
   c. Are scarce resources an issue?
   d. How will these services be paid for?

Reflection

This general checklist is extensive but not exhaustive. Jot down some other types of information you think will help Alexia to accurately analyze this situation.

____

____

____

____

SUMMARY

Gathering as much relevant information as possible sets the essential groundwork for analysis and action.

When you have searched out the information you and others deem relevant or are convinced no additional helpful information will be forthcoming, you are ready to proceed to the next step.

Step 2: Identify the Type of Ethical Problem

Even while the initial fact finding is taking place, Alexia can begin to *determine the type of ethical problem (or problems)* she is facing and in that regard make significant progress toward arriving at a caring response. You know that in the beginning her worry was something like this:

> Mr. Carnavello is a human being. Human beings always should be treated with dignity. Part of being treated with dignity includes

allowing a person to take part in his or her own treatment decisions whenever possible, and in Mr. Carnavello's case includes at the very least being treated with sensitivity to the anguish that he appears to be experiencing. To ignore his distress shows a lack of compassion, if not outright cruelty, and reduces him to the status of an object. I think that Mr. Carnavello is not being treated as a person ought to be treated.

This is where the prototypes of ethical problems you encountered in Chapter 2 begin to work for you.

Ethical Distress

You know that Alexia is experiencing *distress*. She has witnessed a scene that baffled her, and she finds herself not able to forget about it. My guess about the fundamental basis of Alexia's distress is her perception that Mr. Carnavello is not being treated with the dignity he deserves as a human being. The distress, then, arises from Alexia's role as a professional with a moral responsibility to help uphold human dignity. In other words, she is an agent in a situation that she surmises involves morality and that, because it is worrying her, merits further attention. If she tries—but fails—to put more information in place, she may confirm that her distress is, in fact, *ethical distress type B*. You also can presume that she has the virtues of a compassionate person. Otherwise she would not be worried about what she witnessed.

Ethical Dilemma

Goaded by her character traits and the awareness that she is experiencing ethical distress, Alexia is well positioned to assess whether she also has an ethical dilemma (or dilemmas). Do you think there is an ethical dilemma here?

Alexia learns that quite a few of the staff (but not all) believe the medications are being used disproportionately to the amount of "violence" Mr. Carnavello has been demonstrating. In fact, some of the staff confide that they believe he is being sedated to keep him more in line with the conduct of the other more docile and cooperative residents. Of course, the nursing home is shorthanded, and the administrator makes this point when Alexia finally goes to talk with her. Her argument is that if everyone took as much time and extra attention as Mr. Carnavello does (when without medication), no one would receive a fair amount of treatment. Mr. Carnavello also seemed very agitated and suspicious at times, and the medication has helped to improve his feeling of security. Finally, the administrator mentions that some of the staff are afraid of Mr. Carnavello, and she has a responsibility for their safety, too.

There are several issues here that Alexia, as an employee and team member, may be implicated in as partial agent. Foremost of these is whether the employees, as a team, are acting ethically in the use of restraints under any circumstances. The one ethical dilemma that falls squarely on Alexia's shoulders at the moment, however, is this:

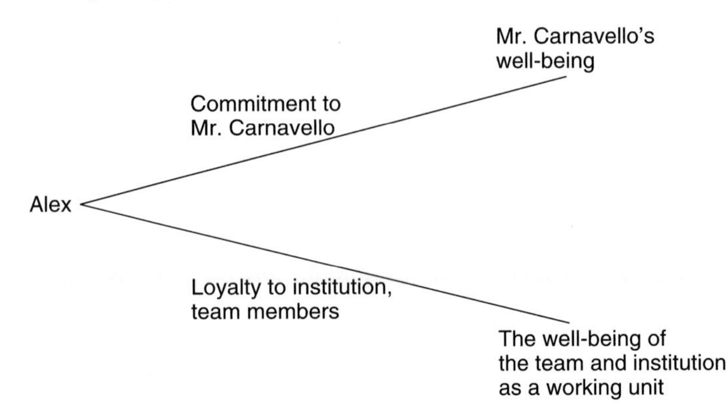

Alexia's dilemma arises from the fact that she has become more persuaded that she was right about what she saw happening to Mr. Carnavello. She believes the principle of beneficence is being compromised. But also she can agree with the points made by the administration and some of the staff regarding fairness to other residents. She is experiencing difficulty in deciding what to do that will honor the several principles guiding professional action in this situation. In summary, she has an ethical dilemma.

Locus of Authority Problem

If Alexia decides someone other than herself, the administration, or the team should be making decisions regarding any aspects of Mr. Carnavello's treatment (or the nursing home policies regarding treatment), she also faces a locus of authority ethical problem. For instance, although the story does not give you the benefit of knowing whether Mr. Carnavello's input is being included in the decision, Alexia could decide that the authority for this decision should rest with Mr. Carnavello. From what we have been told we can assume that the staff and medical director have determined that the patient is not competent to make such a decision, and therefore they are acting paternalistically.

> **SUMMARY**
>
> An essential step in analysis is to identify the type or types of ethical problems that you face.

Step 3: Use Ethics Theories or Approaches to Analyze the Problem(s)

In Chapter 3 you were introduced to normative ethical theory and approaches. You have seen in the preceding pages that the narrative approach, which keeps relevant details of the story at the center of Alexia's deliberation, is the most crucial for her eventual decision to be consistent with professional ethics. She also needs certain basic attitudes to help guide her on the path of a caring response as she deals with her own anger about what she observes. Therefore, virtues such as compassion are among her most fundamental resources. You learned that situations requiring the health professional to be an agent (i.e., take action for which she or he is morally accountable) draws on ethical theories that focus on principles, duties and rights, or consequences. In other words, they are the action theories.

To jog your memory take a minute to review these action theories:

1. Utilitarianism
   focuses on the overall consequences
   is a particular type of teleology
2. Deontology
   focuses on duty

Alexia's story may make it easier to compare the two theories than when they were presented in Chapter 3.

If agent *(A)*, Alexia, is like most health professionals guided by the principles of duty and rights in her professional role, she probably will decide that her weightier (i.e., more compelling) responsibility is to Mr. Carnavello.

If agent *(A)*, Alexia, approaches it from a utilitarian standpoint, she will spend less time thinking about duties and will be guided by the desire to bring about the overall best consequences in this situation. The overall best consequences may be to "leave well enough alone" and not to make waves with the nursing home administrator or others.

Reflection

Which approach do you find yourself leaning toward in Alexia's and Anthony Carnavello's situation? Why?

____

____

____

____

SUMMARY

In Step 3 the tools of ethical analysis further help move you toward resolution and action that is consistent with a caring response.

Step 4: Explore the Practical Alternatives

Alexia has decided what she *should* do. The next step is to determine what she *can* do in this situation. She must exercise her imagination and confer with her colleagues regarding the actual strategies and options available to her. Suppose she decides that her initial perceptions were correct and that she must act on behalf of Mr. Carnavello, even though the staff sees no problem.

At this juncture many people oversimplify the range of options available to them. They tend to fall back on old alternatives when under stress, a behavioral pattern you can probably recognize from your own stressful situations. Therefore, imaginative pursuit of options is a big challenge—but an invaluable resource—in resolving ethical problems. In recounting Alexia's story we learned that she believed her range of options was to confront the nursing home administrator or do nothing. A diligent search for other options can now make the difference between her doing the right thing and allowing a moral wrong to go unchecked.

Reflection

Applying your own imagination to her situation, list all the alternatives you believe Alexia has. Try to identify at least four.

1. ______________________________

2. ______________________________

3. ______________________________

4. ______________________________

Having listed them, which one do you think is the best? Why?

____

____

____

____

Often, it is a good idea to try out some of the more far-fetched alternatives with a colleague whom you trust and with whom you can share the situation without breaching the patient's confidentiality. Alexia did this with the nursing supervisor. We do not know how the supervisor's counsel helped in the end, but we are sure that her words led Alexia to further examination of what her next step should be.

SUMMARY

Imagination enhances ethical decision making by allowing you to think more expansively about the alternatives.

Step 5: Complete the Action

Think of all the work Alexia has already done: She responded to her initial feeling that something was wrong, followed her compassionate disposition that motivated her not to let the matter go unnoticed, reasoned about and decided on the type of ethical problem(s) she was encountering, carried out an analysis using one or more of the ethical theories and approaches, and exercised her imagination to identify practical options needed to effect a caring response. She also shared her worry with at least one other person she knew commands her respect and that of others. Now she has one more task, but it is the crucial one, and that is *to act*.

If Alexia fails to go ahead and act, the entire process so far will be reduced to the level of an interesting but inconsequential philosophic exercise or, worse, may result in harm to Mr. Carnavello. Of course, Alexia may consciously decide not to pursue the situation any further, but insofar as it involved her deliberate intent, it is different than simply failing to follow what seems a correct course of action. If harm comes to Mr. Carnavello or others because of Alexia's inaction or unnecessarily narrow focus, she will be an agent of harm by her own omission or neglect. The solid ethical foundation she laid in Steps 1 to 4 will have been of no use.

Why would anyone fail to act in this type of circumstance? Mainly because it is sobering to be an agent in such important matters of meaning and value in others' lives.

SUMMARY

The goal of your analysis is finally to act!

Some decisions are literally life and death decisions; all are of deep significance to the people facing the particular situation. Although the previous step required imagination, this final step requires courage and the strength of will to go ahead, knowing there may be risks or backlashes. As Alexia becomes more experienced she will be increasingly aware that her integrity of purpose must be supported by her compassion and courage.

Step 6: Evaluate the Process and Outcome

Once she has acted, it behooves Alexia to pause and engage in a reflective examination of the situation. The practical goal of ethics is to resolve ethical problems, thereby upholding important moral values and duties. The extent to which Alexia's decision led to action that upheld morality, however, is knowable only by reexamining what happened in the actual situation. This evaluation is germane to her growth and development as an ethical professional and is essential if the outcome she hoped for was not realized.

In the clinical setting, a widespread mechanism for addressing interventions that go awry is morbidity and mortality (m and m) rounds. If you have not yet been in the clinical setting the term *rounds* may be new to you. Rounds is the general term used for meetings of clinicians. Some are held sitting in a room (sit-down rounds), and others are held walking from patient to patient (walking rounds). The morbidity and mortality rounds allow health professionals whose interventions did not yield the hoped for results to present the case to their peers for further evaluation. Sometimes ethical committees or your own unit staff meetings conduct *ethics* morbidity and mortality rounds to have a group review of a particularly difficult situation that seemed not to meet the ethical goal of a caring response.

Suppose you, like Alexia, have just been through the process of arriving at a difficult ethical decision and have acted on it. Some questions you might ask yourself are the following:

- What did you do well?
- Why do you think so?
- What were the most challenging aspects of this situation?
- How did this situation compare with others you have encountered or read about?
- To what other kinds of situations will your experience with this one apply?
- Who was the most help?
- What do the patient, family, or others have to say about your course of action?
- Overall, what did you learn?

All of these will serve you well in your preparation for the next opportunity to decide what a caring response entails in *that* new situation.

SUMMARY

Reflection on your action prepares you for how you can continue to learn from your experience.

Summary

If you studied this chapter carefully, you will have identified the six-step process that anyone faced with an ethical problem can apply in searching for a caring response:

1. Gather as much relevant information as possible to get your facts straight.
2. Determine the precise nature of the ethical problem (if Step 1 confirms that there is one).
3. Decide on the ethics approach that will best get at the heart of the problem.
4. Decide what should be done and how it best can be done (explore the widest range of options possible).
5. Act!
6. Reflect on and evaluate the action.

Questions for Thought and Discussion

1. The first step in ethical decision making is to gather as much relevant information as possible. The information-gathering process, however, can become so extensive that it becomes an end in itself and could actually deter one from proceeding to action at all. What types of guidelines would you use to decide that you have as much information as you need or can obtain?

___

___

___

___

2. A necessary step in ethical decision making is to act on one's own conclusions about what ought to be done. Under what conditions, if any, would you decide *not* to act according to your own best moral insights and judgment? That is, what, if any, are the limits to your willingness to act ethically?

___

___

___

___

3. In your professional practice you would much prefer always to act ethically. What type of supports or assurances within your work setting would enable you to so act?

___

___

___

___

References

1. Fletcher, K. 1996. Use of restraints in the elderly. *AACN Clinical Issues* 7(4): 611–635.
2. Farrell-Miller, M. 1997. Physically aggressive resident behavior during hygienic care. *Journal of Gerontological Nursing* 23(5):24–35.
3. Omnibus Budget Reconciliation Act PL100-203 (1987) Subtitle C. Nursing Home Reform. 1987. Washington, DC: United States Government Printing Office.
4. Jonsen, A., Siegler, M., Winslade, W. 2002. *Clinical Ethics: A Practical Approach to Ethical Decisions in Clinical Medicine* (5th ed.). New York: McGraw Hill, pp. 1–12.

Section II

Ethical Dimensions of Professional Roles

5

Surviving Student Life Ethically

Objectives

The student should be able to:

- Describe some barriers to achieving a caring response through ethical decision making peculiar to the student role.
- Identify six areas where students have full moral agency in the professional practice setting.
- Discuss two types of wrongdoing students may encounter and what should be done in each case.
- Assess the availability and usefulness of policies, procedures, and practices designed to enhance students' ethical development and decision making.

New terms and ideas you will encounter in this chapter

legal fraud

Topics in this chapter introduced in earlier chapters

Topic	*Introduced in chapter*
Postmodernism	3
Ethical distress (types A and B)	2
Role of emotion	1, 2
Ethical dilemma	2
Utilitarianism	3
Ethical elements, principles	3
Veracity (truth telling)	3
Beneficence	3
Six-step process of ethical decision making	4
Moral agency	2
The story of Anthony Carnavello and Alexia Eliopoulos	4

Introduction

The ethics foundation presented in Section I of this book will serve you well during your student days and throughout your life. This chapter and Chapter 6 focus on your personal moral development and the need to exercise ethical decision making throughout your career, beginning with the time you are a student. It is especially important to include your role as student and some of the particular opportunities and stresses of this period because no matter your age, the student years are the time your approach to ethical decision making in your professional role takes shape.

Special Challenges of Student Life

As a student you have the advantage of coming into a situation with a fresh perspective and can raise issues that more seasoned professionals would miss or might gloss over. At the same time, a situation sometimes is misjudged solely because students do not have the advantage of having served in a professional role or in a particular setting for a long time.[1]

The story in this chapter highlights some ethical challenges inherent in your role as a student.

The Story of Matt and the Botched Home Visit

Matt Weddle is a nursing student in his next to last year of professional education. He has enjoyed his professional training and especially enjoys being in the actual patient care environment. Today, however, he went to bed discouraged and wondering if he has made the correct career choice.

Matt is on a home health care rotation. He has an excellent supervisor, Ms. Needleman, who has tried to provide him with a wide range of learning experiences and proper supervision during his time with her. This has not been an easy task: the census for the home care association is high, and with major cutbacks in professional staff she has been busier than usual. He is sorry to learn that she is going on vacation tomorrow and that his supervision will be turned over to another nurse, Eugenia Cripke.

Today Ms. Needleman asks Matt if he would stop by Mrs. Bedachek's apartment to check on her son and be sure his wound is healing well. "If necessary, the wound may need debridement and a bandage change. You can make the judgment about whether to change the bandage, since I changed it myself yesterday on my way home from work." He is somewhat uncomfortable about going alone to see a patient he has not seen before. He also remembers being told by his academic clinical coordinator at school that under no circumstances should he go into a patient's home unsupervised. But he agrees to do so, not feeling free to question Ms. Needleman about whether this is correct procedure. Instead, he assures her that he has done this procedure enough times under her supervision that he feels he should be able to do it. She agrees.

When he knocks at the Bedacheks' door a large woman in a filthy house dress peers through a crack in the door. At first she doesn't want to let him in, but when he shows her his name tag as identification that he is "the nurse," she admits him. He introduces himself with his name and says he is a student nurse. Mrs. Bedachek is already walking laboriously across the room toward the other occupant, an equally large man with mental retardation. The man strains to peer at Matt from a large armchair set up in the midst of the clutter in the small living room. Matt knows the man's name is Tom, but he is unprepared for the greasy-skinned person drooling onto the front of a mucus-stained shirt.

When Matt tells the patient what he has come to do, the man grunts. The woman says, "I don't want you to touch that bandage. It's fine." She draws up the man's shirt for Matt to see. Matt is surprised at the size of it and concerned about the dark seepage around the bottom edge. Mrs. Bedachek says, suspiciously, "Who are you again?" Matt repeats his name. "At least you're not a student," she says. "They're the worst." Matt says nothing. He feels uncomfortable about this whole situation. He reaches toward the bandage to touch it, and she suddenly pulls the shirt back down over her son's trunk. The stench is making Matt feel woozy.

"Really, it's fine," she says.

Matt replies, "Okay," and leaves.

When he gets back to the office, Ms. Needleman is there, clearing off her desk. "How did it go?" she asks. "Fine," he says. "Well, you did wonders. I didn't want to tell you, but most people can't get through the front door. I went myself yesterday. I thought the wound looked really good except for that distal edge."

Matt had meant to tell her immediately about the whole scene, but for some reason her comments unnerve him and he feels like a failure. He says, "Yeah, I agree."

She comes over to him. "Thanks so much for getting me through that squeeze. I knew you could handle that bandage change, and I was worried about letting it go." She continues, "Sometimes I think it's not worth trying to go on vacation!" She pauses and extends her hand, saying "I have enjoyed working with you as a student. You will make a fine nurse. And you will enjoy working with Eugenia Cripke."

She leaves hurriedly, saying she has to pick up her son at daycare and get packed. Matt takes Tom Bedachek's record from the drawer and writes, "Wound debridement, bandage change. Purulent exudate around the distal rim of wound."

Almost everyone would agree that both Ms. Needleman and Matt Weddle exercised poor ethical judgment. As you look at the story through Matt's eyes, what do you think are the reasons he is feeling discomfort after the day's events?

As soon as you begin your onsite education in the setting where you will pursue (or are pursuing) your professional career, the opportunities to use ethics knowledge and skills present themselves. With that in mind, you have an opportunity in the next few pages to walk in Matt's shoes and explore the ethical implications of his situation.

The Goal: A Caring Response

You have already learned (see Chapter 2) that for a person to be held morally responsible for her or his actions the person must be the moral *agent* in the situation. The health professional's agency revolves around creating a caring response in a variety of health-related situations. In your student role you may have had to sign a student honor code. Many universities have such honor codes and other ethical guidelines detailing the range and scope of your moral agency and accountability generally (e.g., plagiarism, other types of cheating and deceit, use of illegal substances, disrespect of others). Agency becomes a bit more complex in professional educational programs in which moral responsibilities related to your role as a student professional are added. For example, an analysis of Matt Weddle's story reveals there were times he felt he was in a position to take full responsibility for his choices and other times when he knew he was not the agent or was not sure if he was. Some factors in his variable degrees of agency are the nature of his role as a student, the character of the student–professor relationship, and his inexperience regarding some life situations in general.[2]

Fortunately, the degree of agency you have as a student professional is not totally ambiguous or random.

Reflection

Before reading on, think about Matt's experience, or an experience of your own, and write down some areas where his/your moral agency was clear. This will give you a good basis for comparing your judgments about a student's agency with the suggestions in the paragraphs that follow.

Overall, you have a moral responsibility to *take full advantage of your student role to refine your ethical decision making under supervision.* Only then can you assure yourself that you are preparing adequately for making independent decisions consistent with a caring response.

Most of Matt's experience was characterized by this type of situation. Until their last day together Ms. Needleman gave him ample opportunity to practice his skills under her supervision in a variety of settings. He had the benefit of continual discourse and feedback from her. By actually taking the opportunities seriously he was acting responsibly by learning as much as he possibly could before having to make such decisions on his own. Once you graduate you will no longer have the formal ethical and legal supervision to help protect you from making poor judgments that you have as a student.

The Six-Step Process as a Student

As Matt's experience also illustrates, things do not always go smoothly. In the next few paragraphs we will walk through the six steps of ethical decision making so that you can see an example of how each step is involved in highlighting where moral agency resides in your role as a student. Taken together, these examples can be summarized as follows. You have a moral responsibility to:

1. Express serious doubts about your qualifications to your supervisor if you have been given the authority by that person to act independently and you feel ill equipped to do so.
2. Share what you know about the patient and other aspects of the situation with the health care team in an attempt to identify any ethical problems.
3. Refrain from acts that would be wrong for anyone to commit.
4. Be ready to help identify the best alternatives possible for patients, or clients, and others who are faced with difficult situations.
5. Remain faithful to your own convictions and exercise the will and courage to act on them.
6. Give yourself the opportunity to reflect on your action.

Having listed these six guidelines, let's go back to the story to give you an opportunity to move step by step through the six-step process.

Step 1: Gather Relevant Information

As you recall, the first step in ethical decision making is to gather all of the relevant facts. As a student you are practicing under supervision because it is assumed that you will have little knowledge gained from experience and likely also have partial classroom knowledge and skills. You probably have had some training in what to look for, how to interview, and also had an opportunity to observe others' conduct. But if you have doubts about either your knowledge or skills, it is your responsibility to express it at the outset.

In retrospect, you can see that Ms. Needleman used poor judgment in sending Matt to the Bedachek's home alone. Even though she thought he was capable of completing the technical procedures competently and independently, she had not thought through all the ramifications of the situation he might encounter. For instance, she was not being responsive to the literature that warns how differently patients might react to an unexpected visitor in the home care treatment environment, the environment in which most patients' autonomy is at its greatest.[3] It was her moral responsibility to do so, especially in her role as supervisor, and in that respect she failed to exercise it well. In fact, if Matt's actions (or in this case, failure to act) led to litigation against the caregivers, she would have been held legally responsible for what "her" student did or did not do.

Nonetheless, that does not leave Matt Weddle in a position of having no moral responsibility. *Students' moral agency extends to the point of telling a supervisor if he or she feels a serious lack of knowledge or capabilities.* Likely this awareness is also one of the reasons Matt feels so disquieted at the end of the day.

Step 2: Identify the Type of Ethical Problem

A second step in ethical decision making is to be on alert for ethical problems in the situation. *You have a moral responsibility to share what you do know with others who must be accountable for the patient's care in an attempt for all, working together, to identify any ethical problems.* By the time he has completed his first visit, Matt Weddle knows how Mrs. Bedachek feels about students. He knows how hard it will be for other students to go into the Bedachek home and be able to do what they are supposed to do for Tom. That fact alone could be critical information for the home health care team as they plan their schedules. During this one visit, what other information did Tom gain for the future that you would consider relevant to good patient care?

Sometimes students are great reservoirs of information. Although I mentioned previously that patients or clients may be hesitant to let students treat them, the converse often is true as well. Some patients feel safe in telling a student things they do not want to say to professionals. In such moments you are a key member of the team in regard to planning optimal treatment approaches.

Reflection

This is your opportunity to identify some of the ways in which Matt's situation fits the ethical distress prototype. Think about why it is an ethical distress situation before proceeding.

One of the barriers to Matt's doing the right thing is that he does not feel at liberty to question his supervisor's request to go to the Bedachek's home alone and, apparently, also does not feel able to tell her the truth after his botched visit. But why? Ms. Needleman has not presented the situation in such a way that he has reason to fear her disfavor: She does not appear to be motivated to wield her power unfairly or to be punitive. Also, nothing else we know about Matt leads us to believe he is devious, lazy, or dishonest. In fact, his anxiety and subsequent behavior may be at least partially explained by the nature of the student–teacher relationship in which the imbalance of power between the two is built into the structure. Matt's situation is an example of why some of the approaches you encountered in Chapter 3 (e.g., some postmodernist approaches) place so much stress on imbalances of power within institutional structures themselves. This explanation would fit the prototype of *ethical distress type A* in which there is a "structural" barrier to Matt's doing what his better moral judgment would dictate.

He also may be experiencing *ethical distress type B.* He knows a lot but is still in training. Understandably there are unknowns related to the limited professional experience Matt brings to the setting. He knows how to change a bandage and to débride a wound. But the larger *narrative* of the story leaves many gaps for him to fill in as he goes along. For instance, perhaps he has had limited experience talking with people like the Bedacheks. He may never have seen a person with the degree of mental impairment Tom Bedachek manifests and may not know what type of impairment it is. He is not sure how to instill enough confidence in either of them to figure out how to get on with the wound debridement. He also is being forced to reckon with his new realization that in home care a professional is going into the very private "sanctuary" of a person's home and that adaptation to their home environment is essential if a caring response is going to be possible.[4]

SUMMARY

As a student you may not do the right thing because there may be psychological, structural, and knowledge barriers to your acting on what is right. This type of ethical problem is called ethical distress.

In Chapter 1 you studied about the role of emotion in ethical decision making. Matt is frustrated, afraid, and angry, but those responses do not indicate that he is uncaring. His being overwhelmed by the enormity of the unknown and being insecure in his judgment about what to do are not unusual student responses. As a student yourself you may recognize a tendency to discredit your own feelings, intuitions, and judgments. The worst outcome of this student-related stress is that you may assume you are completely unable to evaluate a situation correctly or even to get enough information to make a sound judgment about it. One expression of intense emotion seldom discussed is crying. One article notes of medical students:

> Students often cry in isolation. They run to the bathroom or the stairwell. Some cry in their car or when they get home. Some cry to their spouse, friends or parents. . . .
>
> Crying may be a response of a student who is emotionally raw and fighting for equilibrium and control. It may also be the response of an emotionally mature student experiencing the poignancy of the extraordinary human drama that characterizes the practice of medicine. By ignoring or suppressing crying that springs from feelings of care, physicians risk suppressing those feeling of care.[5]

The best outcome is to use emotion as an opportunity for support and discussion. The student years are the time to become as well prepared as possible, and good teachers will know that "it is not appropriate to ignore situations that call for guidance and recognition of compassionate responses. It is not appropriate to ignore sadness, grief, loss, and hurt. . ."[6]

Let us continue to analyze Matt's problem, considering whether he also has an *ethical dilemma.*

Reflection

This is your opportunity to describe an ethical dilemma that also faces Matt. Take a minute to think about it before moving on.

One dilemma that seems directly related to his student nurse status arises around Mrs. Bedachek's comment about how students are "the worst." When Matt first introduced himself, he identified himself as a student nurse. We do not know his motivation for remaining silent when she later made the derogatory comment about students. He had an opportunity then to reaffirm his student status, which definitely would have been the right thing to do. Let us give him the benefit of the doubt, however, and assume that his reason for remaining silent was that he truly believed this was the only way he could hold on to the little bit of confidence Mrs. Bedachek had in him and that allowing this deceit would benefit Tom Bedachek.

Sometimes patients are less comfortable with students than with others; therefore Matt's judgment to remain silent as a way to allow the patient the benefit of feeling comfortable is consistent with his duty of beneficence. Of course, the motivation might also be to bolster his own confidence, which is not in itself a bad thing.

Step 3: Use Ethics Theories or Approaches to Analyze the Problem

A third step in ethical decision making is to apply the principles and other ethical guidelines available to you in your role. Again, as a student your first response might be that you're not sure how to apply them in your new role. At the same time, if you look closely at Matt's quandary you can conclude that his situation includes morally wrong or illegal acts that are not specific to his role responsibilities as a student professional. These are actions for which he would be held equally accountable as a citizen. It also includes refraining from the exercise of hurtful character traits that would be harmful in any relationship in which someone trusted Matt to treat him or her fairly and with respect. *You have a responsibility to refrain from acts that would be wrong for anyone to commit.*

Reflection

What is an example of Matt's failure to exercise his moral agency and take responsibility for his actions that would have been the same in any relationship?

You may have found several places where you think this happened. I assume you agree that one occasion was his deceit by silence and lying. The more glaring example of this was his decision to report on Tom Bedachek's record that he had performed the therapeutic procedure when he had not. His deceitfulness and dishonesty are not applicable only in the health professional and patient relationship, intentional lying is harmful in any relationship and veracity is supportive of them. There seemed to be no circumstance that would excuse him from this important principle of morality. Making himself look more responsible than he was could not justify his lying.

Entering false statements on a medical record also is illegal. He is committing *legal fraud* because the home health care agency will be paid for treatment it did not perform. This act could cost him his professional career and lead to criminal sanctions as well. What are some of the reasons this breach of professional responsibility is viewed as so serious by society as a whole?

If you are reasoning about this as a *utilitarian,* you are on the path to legitimating his course of action on the basis of the overall good consequences you believe will result. Within professional ethics, however, the commitment to truth telling *(veracity)* is vital as a means to maintaining the patient's confidence or trust. Therefore, to the extent that Matt understands his role as a health professional, he cannot easily justify withholding key information without understanding that he is engaged in wrongdoing. He may decide to forego veracity to honor his duty of beneficence, but believing he has compromised an important ethical principle, he cannot comfortably carry out his course of action. As you should recall, an ethical dilemma creates the type of difficult decision in which you have to allow something wrong to happen (i.e., in his case, withhold the truth from Mrs. Bedachek) while you are also making something right happen (i.e., provide needed treatment to her son, Tom).

SUMMARY

As a student you are not protected from ethical dilemmas in which you have to weigh conflicting moral principles and decide how to act in the specific situation.

During your formative years as a student you have an opportunity to refine your ethics skills even though at times they make you feel uncomfortable.

Step 4: Explore the Practical Alternatives

Yet another step in ethical decision making is to seek the viable alternatives toward finding the one that most fully approximates or achieves a caring response.

One of the reasons health professionals enjoy working with students is that students often provide creative approaches to old problems. Professionals who have been facing similar issues for years get bogged down in habit or become discouraged because attempted solutions have not been successful in the past. (How many times have you heard, "We've tried that before, and it didn't work"?)

Your unwillingness to offer suggestions is not a morally neutral act. Sheer robustness, arrogance, or ill-placed criticisms are not welcome. At the same time, *your moral agency as a student extends to your readiness to voice your thoughtful opinion when you are invited to do so* and taking a posture of readiness to contribute such ideas rather than standing by passively and keeping your insights to yourself.

Although Matt has seriously breached the responsibilities consistent with his moral agency as a student, he can still offer suggestions from the perspective of what he observed in the Bedachek family. Of course, he also has a moral responsibility to contribute his thoughtful ideas regarding all the other situations he has had the opportunity to witness and participate in during his tenure in this clinical setting.

Step 5: Complete the Action

The fifth step in ethical decision making is to act. Students' responsibilities include the four forms described in the following paragraphs.

Act within the Limits of Competence and Self-Confidence

Always seek to balance your knowledge, skills, and abilities with the need for supervision. This will help assure that the patient will be the beneficiary at all times. With this overriding guideline in mind, the next three forms are simply logical complements.

Act According to Your Convictions

Some general protections for health professionals to avoid moral compromise were introduced in Chapter 1. Similar protections should apply to students. For instance, during your student experience you have a moral responsibility to make your convictions known so that you are never placed under pressure to participate in a procedure that undermines your religious or other deeply held convictions. Religious observances may pose another reason for you or your fellow students to want special consideration—for example, to participate in holiday traditions and rituals. Every professional educational program should have a formal or informal mechanism in place to assure that you and your student colleagues are able to offer rationales for wishing to abstain and to have an appeals process in place for disagreements. Of course, you have the responsibility to inform your educational program administrators and supervisors in advance of any such situation so that patient care is never compromised. Whenever possible there should be plenty of lead-in time for your request to be heard and considered in a timely manner.

Right Any Wrongdoing You Have Committed

Another dimension of living according to your convictions is to right any wrongs you yourself have done in regard to a patient's or other's situations within your student professional role. No one enjoys having to do damage control after wrongdoing, but there is no better investment than taking care of yourself by keeping your conscience clear.

Reflection

Matt should admit his wrongdoing of lying about the wound dressing as soon as possible. If you were Matt, how would you go about correcting this serious error in moral judgment?

You must begin to practice during your student years if you are going to be able to admit shortcomings and mistakes throughout your career. Nothing is more harmful to you professionally and personally than to get into the habit of "covering up" your mistakes or deceits. Some ways this practice will backfire on you are discussed in Chapter 6 under the topic of self-deceptions. When approached thoughtfully, professors and supervisors almost always are forgiving of student missteps and stand ready to discuss and help prevent such breaches from happening again.

Address Others' Wrongdoing Constructively

This arduous moral task of addressing others' wrongdoing constructively is also a part of everyone's responsibility in the health care environment, including yourself and your fellow students.

Quiet, diligent observation is a reliable guidepost in your assessment of wrongdoing by your fellow students or by professionals. As we have noted, a legitimate worry about expressing your concern arises because as a student you may be aware that you do not have full knowledge of the situation. Branch's[7] study noted that medical students tend to question their own moral judgment when faced with differing values expressed by authority figures. During my many years of working with students in other health professions, I have found the same response to be true, generally speaking. In Chapter 4, Alexia Eliopoulos, who had completed her physical therapy preparation and was an employee, hesitated after talking to Ms. Carroll because she was warned that she "did not have all the facts." To make certainty more elusive, as a student you are not an actual employee of the institution in which you are placed, and therefore are unfamiliar with its policies. You probably do not know the in-house mechanisms that employees use for resolving concerns and conflict, and even if you do, they may not apply to you.

In the end, these challenges should not keep you from addressing ethical wrongdoing. For instance, Matt knows with certainty that Ms. Needleman acted wrongly in sending him to the Bedachek's home alone, no matter her rationale. Rather than the two of them maintaining a conspiracy of silence, he can help report his own wrongdoing in the context of acknowledging that she, too, was a partner in the way this situation unfolded.

Step 6: Evaluate the Process and Outcome

In the sixth and final step of ethical decision making, the moral agent steps back from the heat of action and goes over the process to think about what can be learned about a truly caring response, how it might be done better next time, or how it applies to other situations. Only through this conscious process will your own moral development be enhanced.[8] By now you are aware that a caring response in regard to present or future patients should ultimately drive your motivation at all times. If any action or inaction flew in the face of this basic core of your professional identity, that path should not be taken again.

Your reflection also should include an acknowledgment that you are "in it together" with your clinical faculty—their job is to guide you in ways that will encourage you, not discourage you. A study of 272 nursing students in a baccalaureate educational program showed that when clinical faculty as individuals were themselves "caring [toward students], gave encouragement and positive feedback, demonstrated . . . new procedures, encouraged critical thinking, clearly stated faculty expectation of students, and conducted pre- and postconferences," students learned the important dimensions of their clinical role more effectively.[9] If on reflection you are experiencing that type of treatment, you will want to model your own behavior toward others in your work situation in the future on how you yourself were treated.

Given the situation that Matt finds himself in he certainly owes it to himself to reflect on what happened and why. He also has a moral responsibility to future patients not to let this negligence and the deceit that followed happen again. He has a moral responsibility to himself to regain his self-respect by gaining more insight into the incident.

SUMMARY

If you go back over Steps 1 through 6, you will see that a student's moral agency applies at every step of ethical decision making.

Strategies for Success as a Moral Agent

The student role has more vitality and enjoyment built into it than risks and challenges. The opportunity to apply your ethical knowledge and skills in real life situations will help your confidence grow and experience deepen. The most difficult situations are those involving the report of wrongdoing, one's own and that of others. Therefore, a few notes on strategies for such disquieting student moments are offered here.

It is advisable to use the channels set up for students in your professional program. You should be made familiar with them before going into your clinical education experiences. If you do not receive this orientation and you run into trouble, your clinical supervisor and academic supervisor are two obvious sources for information. Most educational programs have institutional policies and procedures to protect students who follow the processes designed for reporting concerns.

A good rule of thumb is to honor the confidentiality of everyone involved, reporting only information that is relevant to the situation, containing the report to documented evidence. Understandably, if you report on an error in judgment you made, you may be asked to justify how it happened and work with your supervisor or others to rectify it.

Summary

In summary, there are special ethical challenges during your student years that involve both the peculiarities of the student–supervisor or student–professor relationship and the limits of your own knowledge and experience. At the same time, the story of Matt Weddle's experience in the Bedachek's home illustrates several ways you may exercise your moral agency and be accountable for what you have done or what you observed. It is the mutual task of students, classroom faculty, and clinical supervisors working together to ensure that students trust their abilities, understand their role as moral agents, and act appropriately to help assure that a caring response consistent with the demands of professional responsibility are exercised. In fact, the purpose of this book is to help you think clearly about a wide variety of ethical situations before you are faced with the more weighty responsibilities associated with professional practice after completion of your studies.

Questions for Thought and Discussion

1. Sandra is in her final year as a student in the clinic. For some reason this particular internship setting has been full of rough edges. Sandra and her supervisor have just never really hit it off, but when she talked to her academic coordinator about her feelings, the coordinator urged Sandra to "keep trying." Moreover, the coordinator claimed that the supervisor thought Sandra was "doing great." When her final evaluation came, it was barely passing. For Sandra the most disturbing comment on the report was that she has an "attitude problem." She believes it must be because she reported her dissatisfactions to her academic coordinator, whom she has always trusted. Now she feels betrayed and alone.

   Does Sandra have an ethical problem? If so, what is it? What should she do in this situation? What are the moral responsibilities of each of the people involved?

   ____

   ____

   ____

   ____

2. This morning Andrea, a student working in the outpatient clinic, notices two men sitting in the waiting area. She recognizes one as her dad's business partner, Mr. Brown, and greets him. She recalls that in a recent visit she made to her parents' home for dinner her father had expressed concern about Mr. Brown's failing health, which has begun to interfere with his earnings. Mr. Brown and the other man are chatting amiably despite that they make a striking contrast—the silver-haired Mr. Brown and the seamy young man with a torn leather jacket. She remembers her dad's admiration for Mr. Brown's ability to "cross classes" and have friends in all walks of life. She goes to hang up her coat and when she returns to the waiting area the other man has disappeared and Mr. Brown is sitting alone.

   Andrea is somewhat shy about her assignment to take Mr. Brown's clinical history. Mr. Brown seems relaxed about it, however, and even a little bemused as she earnestly questions him and checks off the answers on her sheet. She leads him to the dressing room where he will undress for his tests. While heading back to her desk she notices that something had fallen from his pocket just before he entered the dressing room. She rushes back and picks up the packet. Inside the brown bag are a syringe and a small plastic bag of white powder. On the outside of the bag, written in a smudged scrawl on a piece of white tape, it says, "Brown, $450." She feels panic rising up in her chest and hopes beyond hope that her suspicion is unfounded.

   If you were in Andrea's situation, what do you believe you should do or not do? Does her role as a student professional dictate what she should do in regard to sharing this information with her father? Her supervisor? The police? That is, would it make any difference if she had met Mr. Brown on the street when her terrible discovery had been made?

   Discuss the steps you would take in arriving at your decision, emphasizing the professional moral duties, rights, and character traits that will help to inform and guide your decision, as well as the special challenges you face as a student professional in this setting.

____

____

____

____

3. You overhear a fellow student say to another colleague, "I just pretended to treat her. She was sleeping and will never know the difference anyway. It's such a drag to have to treat someone who's out of it."

This student has cheated a patient out of her treatment. Is this different from cheating on a classroom test? If so, why? If you observed classroom cheating, should your response to it be different than it would be to your knowledge that the patient was not treated? In each case, what should you do?

---

4. You have learned in your preclinical professional education that use of a certain procedure has been discontinued almost everywhere because of a dangerously high incidence of harmful side effects. You observe it being performed regularly in the setting where you are currently assigned, a place with a good reputation (apparently well deserved, generally speaking). In fact, as you observe patients' responses to the procedure, you become convinced yourself of good reasons *not* to use it. Now you have only 1 week left in this rotation and raise your concern with your supervisor. She responds, "Actually, we know that, and we don't like it either. Our health plan, however, does not allow us to use the newer procedure because it is four times as expensive as this one."

   Do you have a moral responsibility to recommend this site be discontinued for students? Why or why not? Do you have a moral responsibility to do anything in this situation? If yes, what?

---

5. Your friend who is serving in the same clinical setting with you stops you in the hallway to ask you what he should do. His wife has called, crying, saying she feels really sick and would like him to come home right away. He has already missed several days because his uncle died, and he also had a bout of the flu. The supervisor spoke with your friend this morning about how they would have to try to make up for some of the absences by providing special opportunities for him to cover areas he has missed. In fact, she told him that she has arranged for him to assist in an evaluation that starts at noon and will take about 4 hours, but from which he will benefit tremendously. He cannot get home and back in time for the beginning of the procedure.

How should you respond? Why?
What do you think he should do? Why?

____

____

____

____

6. This chapter focuses on your *clinical* education experiences. What are some ethical problems that students may face in the *classroom* during their professional preparation? Discuss one using the tools you have acquired from your study of ethics so far.

____

____

____

____

References

1. Purtilo, R., Haddad, A. 2002. Respect for yourself as a student. In *Health Professional and Patient Interaction* (6th ed.). Philadelphia: WB Saunders, pp. 69–83.
2. Branch, W.T., Jr. 2000. Supporting the moral development of medical students. *Journal of General Internal Medicine* 15(7):503–508.
3. Arnold, R.M., Fello, M. 2000. Hospice and home care. In Sugarman, J. (Ed.), *20 Common Problems—Ethics in Primary Care.* New York: McGraw Hill, pp. 118–128.
4. Collins, J., Bessner, K.I., Krout, K. 1998. Home health physical therapy: Practice patterns in Western New York. *P.T. Magazine* 78(2):170–179.
5. Angoff, N.R. 2001. Crying in the curriculum. *JAMA* 286(9):1017–1018.
6. *Ibid.* p. 1018.
7. Branch, W.T., Jr. 2000. *op. cit.*
8. Bankert, E.G. 2002. Care and traditional ethics: Enhancing the development of moral reasoning among nurses. *International Journal for Human Caring* 6:1,25–33.
9. Brewer, M.K. 2002. Being encouraged and discouraged: Baccalaureate nursing students' experiences of effective and ineffective clinical faculty teaching behaviors. *International Journal for Human Caring* 6:1,46–49.

6

Surviving Professional Life Ethically

Objectives

The student should be able to:

- Describe what "a caring response" entails when the object of care is you.
- Discuss the place of self-esteem and self-respect in your ability to survive professional life ethically.
- Evaluate the phrase "you owe it to yourself" from the standpoints of a duty to be good to yourself, aspirations for yourself, and responsibility to yourself as a caregiver.
- Describe three components of a personal values system and its relationship to personal integrity.
- Evaluate your own personal values system.
- Identify two types of threats to personal integrity encountered in the health professions and some strategies for meeting them ethically.
- Define self-deception and identify five types of self-deception that can threaten your personal integrity.
- Describe two societal mechanisms designed to legally protect health professionals faced with professional situations that would undermine their personal integrity.
- Discuss two key responsibilities to yourself that help health professionals lead a good life.
- Identify three types of responsibility to improve yourself that are relevant to your professional career.

New terms and ideas you will encounter in this chapter

self-respect
responsibilities to yourself
duty of general obligation
self-deception
impairment
a duty to be good to yourself
personal values system
duty of special obligation
aspirations regarding self-fulfillment

Topics in this chapter introduced in earlier chapters

Topic	*Introduced in chapter*
A caring response	2
Duties	3
Personal integrity	2
Cooperation with wrongdoing	1, 5
The principle of material cooperation	1

Introduction

You have come a long way in thinking about the ethical dimensions of professional practice in a general way, and in Chapter 5 you focused on them in relation to your role as a student. This chapter gives you an opportunity to think about loyalty to yourself as you assume your professional role and throughout your professional life. Unlike in most of the subsequent chapters of this book, you will not walk step by step through the six-step process, rather this is a chance to think about yourself as the moral agent who is always having to think about others. How can you take care of yourself in ways that prepare you to not only be strong when ethical problems arise but to flourish in your professional role? Janice K.'s story helps to focus this discussion.

The Story of Janice K. and the Policies of Her Workplace

Janice K. is a dietitian employed by a community health clinic affiliated with a large multihospital health plan. Part of the mission of the clinic is to provide nutritional counseling and services for people in an underserved area of her community. She believes that part of her professional responsibility is to help assure that people in such areas have the same access to health care benefits as everyone else, and she is delighted to have found this position. Janice is distressed, however, when she learns one day that the health plan has designated her clinic as a site where abortion counseling and services will be added to its family planning programs. Janice has strong religious convictions that abortion is murder and that this practice should be stopped by whatever means possible.

Janice is trying to decide what to do. She has been talking with her religious advisors, friends, and colleagues about her feelings, all of whom were well aware of her position before the announcement. They have different ideas about what her response should be. Among the suggestions she has received are the following:

1. Distribute antiabortion pamphlets around the clinic.
2. Talk with clients in the clinic to get their opinion and be guided by their needs.
3. Quit working in a place like this and find another job.
4. Pray about this turn of events.

5. Call some groups who will come and picket the clinic in protest.
6. Talk to the administrator of the clinic and try to persuade those in authority not to include this service.
7. Tolerate the situation—it is a pluralistic, diverse society, and some people who could not receive it elsewhere will want to take advantage of the abortion service.
8. Go about her work diligently and not get involved in taking care of any of the abortion patients.

This story could lead to many interesting and important ethical discussions, but in this chapter we will focus on the prime importance of your personal morality as the ethical wellspring of survival in your professional career. You have had some opportunities to think about your personal values and personal morality already in the course of reading this book. In Chapter 1 you were introduced to the idea of cooperation with wrongdoing, the principle of material cooperation being used as a guide, and some ways in which society tries to protect professionals. In Chapter 5 personal morality was raised again in regard to areas where you must exercise your moral agency as a student. So far every story in this text has posed an ethical problem to you as you try to put yourself into the shoes of the person who is the moral agent. Now you have an opportunity to step back and focus on yourself directly.

Reflection

Janice is confronted with an ethical challenge, and you can try to help her think through her strategies. You read what other people advised her to do. What do you believe she should do?

The question was phrased as what you *believe* she should do, not solely what you *think* she should do, because any answer you provide will require you to draw on your beliefs to arrive at a satisfactory answer.

Her beliefs are powerful resources to guide her thinking about her duties and what kind of character traits she should strive to develop. You can call this the process of finding a caring response when the object of care is yourself.

The Goal: A Caring Response

At the center of a caring response to yourself is self-respect. Respect for the dignity of individuals is an overriding virtue in professional ethics. But respect is almost always understood as referring to the deference one pays to another person, particularly the patient. Where in professional ethics is there a way to incorporate respect for oneself?

Traditionally, there has been very little about *self*-respect in the professional ethics literature. It has taken an understanding of modern moral psychology to bring together the roles of self-esteem, self-respect, and respect for others. An American moral philosopher, John Rawls, has relied heavily on modern psychology to help clarify the relationship of self to others.[1] Unlike other analyses that make respect solely another-regarding virtue, Rawls interprets self-respect as the engine that drives the whole social system toward human flourishing. This is not the kind of self-respect that might be confused today with simple self-satisfaction in an egotistic sense. Although he ties self-respect to the psychological idea of personal self-esteem, he is not just concerned with individual satisfaction: Self-esteem is a resource that boosts self-respect in very particular ways in modern societies; it helps an individual makes choices that are not good only for himself but for everyone. Self-respect helps an individual become a force in helping to assure human flourishing, not the least of which is his or her own flourishing. Self-respect is not gained in a social vacuum. This understanding of one's worth within the larger societal context allows one to have high regard for the societal tasks one has to assume.

I believe an understanding that you deserve self-respect because of your willingness to respect others (required by your special professional role) will have the very practical effect—that is, that you will come to recognize that a lack of self-respect will psychologically undermine your ability to work successfully in your job. This issue is taken up in some detail in Chapter 7, which discusses the challenges of working in institutions. Moreover, as a member of a whole group of self-respecting professionals, you will be more likely to demand that practices and policies are consistent with your personal values and what you judge as your appropriate moral role in society. In short, the often overlooked idea of self-respect and self-esteem is an extremely important dimension of a caring response toward oneself.

You Owe It to Yourself

How is one to interpret this odd phrase, "You owe it to yourself"? Does this mean that you have *a duty to be good to yourself* and to live by your values? In Chapter 3, duties were placed under the umbrella of society's expectations of moral conduct between individuals or social institutions. They describe commitments that individuals should make to *other people or groups* to act in certain ways that are believed to uphold the moral life of the community. In the context of health care you have learned that the goal is to create an environment of caring responses. Ethical theorists often delineate duties more fully in the language of the specific principles or elements. Therefore, it is unusual to talk about a duty to *yourself,* although I will give you an example of one philosopher who has done so.

W. D. Ross,[2] a British philosopher writing in the early 1900s, was influential in developing the idea of moral obligation, and he included the "duty of self-improvement" among his list of duties. He believed that the duties of beneficence (toward others) and *self-improvement* arise because we should produce as much good as possible. He called both beneficence and self-improvement *general obligations* in contrast to special obligations. *Special obligations,* he said, arise from the special relationship in which we stand to each other (e.g., parent–child, professional–patient or professional–client, teacher–student) and include nonmaleficence, fidelity, gratitude, and reparation, among others. General obligations rely less on specific relationships. In other words, Ross treated self-improvement as a duty in that it brings about good generally, but, of course, you are the major beneficiary![2] In short the idea of a duty to oneself seems awkward to most ethical theorists, but Ross contributed to our understanding of the moral life by reminding us that we should have a strong commitment to ourselves and others if our search for moral excellence is to succeed.

Reflection

Can you think of some examples in your everyday life when you felt you were not being "good" to yourself? What are reasons you chose to cheat yourself this way?

The idea of a duty to oneself seldom is reflected in ethics codes of the professions, probably because of the "other-directedness" of the professions' orientation. An important exception is the American Nurses Association Code of Ethics for Nurses that states, "the nurse owes the same duties to self as others, including the responsibility to preserve integrity and safety, to maintain competence and to continue personal and professional growth."[3]

Another way to think about the idea of owing it to yourself is less related to duty and more to giving yourself permission to rejoice in having achieved an aspiration. An *aspiration* is an ideal standard of excellence toward which you strive, and when you have attained that standard you have gained a point toward your self-fulfillment. Anytime you realize such an aspiration, you deserve (i.e., owe it to yourself) to reward yourself. For example, when you have aspired to lose weight or make a high grade in a course and you achieve it, you may owe it to yourself to acknowledge your success by going out to buy a new pair of jeans or taking time from studying to read a novel. Similarly, in the realm of the moral life you may aspire to be courageous, to go the second mile, or to set an example of high moral character for others. Has there been a time recently when you experienced this kind of self-satisfaction? The primary reward in this case is in seeing the good you are capable of bringing about and knowing you have made a stride in developing a high moral character. You owe it to yourself to enjoy the good it has done for others. You owe it to yourself to be aware that next time it will be easier.

SUMMARY

Reinforcing in yourself the good you have been able to do will help you be prepared to do it again.

Yet, a third way of conceptualizing what it means to owe something to yourself is to think of *responsibilities to yourself*. Note that in the item from the nurses' code described earlier the idea of "duty" and of "responsibility" are used interchangeably. That is correct, strictly speaking, but I prefer to separate them because duty focuses on accountability above. Responsibility includes accountability but also has the root idea of responsiveness embedded in it.[4] In other words, it has the force of commitment that the language of duty captures, but it also entails the idea of responding to your aspirations to live according to your personal ideals. I find this notion of responsibility the richest way to understand that we owe something to ourselves insofar as it places a claim on us to act in certain ways that will benefit us and gives us permission to celebrate that we have developed the moral character disposing us to do so. The following discussions introduce you to two responsibilities to yourself that will serve you well throughout your professional career: the responsibility to *maintain personal integrity* and the responsibility to *engage in self-improvement* as an individual.

The Responsibility to Maintain Personal Integrity

You have been concentrating on your responsibility to think clearly about complex ethical situations before acting. Part of the way to achieve this skill is to learn about and honor the duties, rights, and character traits required in your professional role. But here is the rub: as the cases so far have clearly illustrated, these helpful approaches to analyzing professional conduct sometimes come into conflict, and an ethical problem arises in the form of ethical distress, a dilemma, or a locus of authority concern. As introduced in Chapter 2, when faced with any of these types of problems, your personal integrity feels (and often is) threatened. Because in this chapter we are discussing ways to take good care of yourself, this is an appropriate place to consider the tools by which you can succeed in maintaining your integrity. The most fundamental resource is your own *personal values system*. This moral compass will help you decide what to do.

Integrity and Personal Values Systems

What *is* a personal values system? A personal values system is the set of values you have when you have reflected on and chosen values that will help you lead a good life. Usually people adopt personal values that partially overlap with societal values and that are in harmony with them. Elsewhere I have represented and explained them in more detail according to the following scheme[5]:

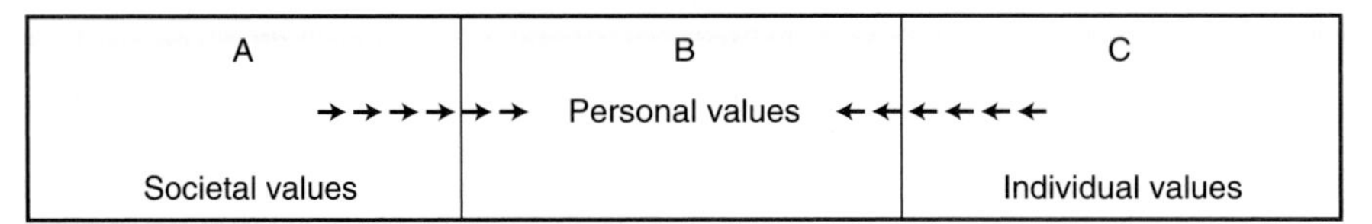

Figure 6–1. Personal values system.

In Figure 6–1 area *A* represents values developed by society. Many times we accept these values because we want to live peacefully and harmoniously in society. Examples include obedience to traffic laws or other laws, adherence to etiquette, and willingness to pay taxes. Area *C* represents individual values that are important to you simply because you value them individually. You receive personal benefits from them. The area of overlap, area *B*, represents values that you have internalized so that they not only are shared by other people in society but also are perceived as your own values. The motivations for accepting them are that leading a good life includes not only living harmoniously in society but also experiencing personal satisfactions and self-fulfillment. For many, some of these values include friendship, economic independence, and the realization of certain character traits such as fairness or courage. Most people integrate these three into a lifestyle and personal values system, drawing at times on all three areas: *A*, *B*, and *C*. As you study to become a professional you will incorporate some professional values into your personal values system. That process has already begun, and for many, there were values brought into professional preparation that help to make one's career choice fitting within the context of one's life.

SUMMARY

Personal values systems are our most fundamental resource for maintaining a sense of personal integrity.

Your personal values system enables you to act on your own convictions in a meaningful way for your own life. At the same time, conflicting ideas may arise that cause you to think deeply about which values are the *most* important. The conflicting ideas for Janice K. are: (1) continuing to work in a setting that provides abortion services when she believes that abortion is wrong, (2) refusing to work there, or (3) disrupting the center's functioning in an act of protest.

Opportunities to Strengthen Your Personal Integrity

It is important to identify any parts of one's professional life that threaten to undermine one's integrity because integrity is so central to psychological and physical well-being over time. The stresses of work life sometimes arise out of the culture of the professions themselves. This is illustrated in a study of physical therapists who incurred work-related musculoskeletal disorders. The investigators found that the therapists' need to continue behaviors they believed best expressed care for the patients, together with their desire to appear knowledgeable and skilled in their ability to remain injury free, sometimes worked against their recovery from injury. These therapists had to leave the profession because of disturbing symptoms associated with their injury, a loss for them, their patients, and the clinical environment of health care.[6] A part of the terrible irony of this situation is that the American Physical Therapy Association is a sponsor of Decade, an international, multidisciplinary initiative to improve health-related quality of life for people with musculoskeletal disorders. Members of this and other professions often have been unable to "practice what they preach," with high prices to pay for it.

At least two major forces may challenge your personal values system and, consequently, threaten your personal integrity. At the same time, they present opportunities for professionals to examine and further strengthen their personal value system by taking advantage of how new information sometimes can lead to refinements of personal insights. Each is addressed in turn, with strategies for strengthening your resolve to lead a good life guided by your highest values.

The Challenge of "Bad" Laws, Policies, and Regulations

Personal integrity can be threatened by *bad laws, policies,* or *regulations.* These might be poorly stated, therefore providing poor guidance, or, worse, they might be morally wrong in their emphasis. In Janice's situation, the center's general policy of providing access to persons in underserved areas is consistent with her personal values system and convictions. Only when the abortion services are added does this new policy become a threat to Janice's personal integrity. She has done the wise thing in seeking the counsel of her friends, colleagues, and others in thinking about this threat, although she undoubtedly has encountered differences of opinion. She wants to know what her role should be in trying to maintain her personal convictions in the face of this new policy.

One factor that will influence her decision is her sense of personal integrity that requires her to try to work within the system to bring about alternative policies she believes best serve the population they are designed to serve. Another factor is her judgment about what of value will be lost if she actually leaves. A third factor is her assessment of whether there is any way she can indeed influence the administration to change the policy. To come to a decision she will have to consider the priorities in her own values system. She may need to write down her priorities and let her actions be guided by those that have top priority.

Moving beyond Janice's story you can think more broadly about this idea of how policies and regulations can threaten your own integrity.

Every health professional should read the play, *The Dark at the Top of the Stairs*, by the great American playwright William Inge, because it is a fine illustration of how individuals sometimes are unwilling or unable to interact with the "powers that be" who make and revise policies. The setting for the play is the home of the Rubin Flood family in a small Oklahoma town, where he, his wife Cora, and their two children are living. It takes place in the 1920s, during a prosperous time for this area because of an oil boom. What we see of the Flood's house is the living room, but there is a flight of stairs at one side, and at the top of it is a second floor landing. Some of the most vital activities in the play, the moments that set direction for the rest of it, are played out on that landing, but the Flood family never integrates those activities into the process of resolving the small sorrows, tragedies, and missed opportunities that finally threaten their integrity as individuals and as a family.[7]

Many policies that cause consternation because they appear to challenge one's personal integrity can be challenged and changed. One source of data that will strengthen your resolve to be an agent of change is a marked increase in the health professions literature of how threats to personal well-being affect patient care. For example, new concerns about the effects of fatigue[8] and of staff shortages[9] are being expressed. Still relatively lacking in the professional literature, however, are studies of the price professionals pay for not being able always to remain comfortably within the boundaries of their own religious or other beliefs. Be that as it may, awareness of the important value of maintaining personal integrity should provide an opportunity for cooperative effort aimed at changing such policies even though maintaining your integrity may mean getting involved with the higher-ups of your institution.

Reflection

Can you think of a health care policy that would present an opportunity to engage in policy revisions that would strengthen your personal integrity? If so, jot it down before going on so that you can think about it as you read further.

An opportunity to examine the specific components that make up your personal integrity may come from your self-perception of your professional role and what is required in it. For example, if Janice perceives her role as a dietitian as being one that has no place in changing policies not directly related to dietetics, she will feel more vulnerable and may believe that her only option is to leave. At the same time, if she discerns that a part of her role generally is to question policies in her workplace that threaten her personal integrity, she will feel more empowered to act within the system. In the latter case, she must be prepared to present her ideas to the people who are involved in making and revising the family planning policies, understanding that her beliefs and convictions may not prevail in the final outcome. At the very least she will know she has made an effort to stop a practice that she thinks is morally wrong. By being willing to speak her mind within the system, she may also have an opportunity to hear the arguments on the other side and learn the reasons why other people are supporting them even if she is not persuaded to support them herself.

The Challenge of Self-Deception

Self-deception also can pose a challenge to your personal integrity, although it has nothing to do with policies or the perception of your role in an institution.

Self-deception is engaged in by all of us at one time or another. The Christian scriptural text instructs one not try to remove the mote in another's eye until you have removed the beam from your own.[10] The Russian novelist Gogol (*Dead Souls,* 1842) observed, "Do not blame the looking glass if your face is awry." Unfortunately, sometimes a challenge to personal integrity comes from within, the result of engaging in self-deception about what is best for yourself or others. When a person's self-esteem is threatened, he or she may resort to the extreme measure of self-deception to try to protect himself or herself. This, of course, backfires. In one of the only books on this important topic, *Morality and Self Deception,* Martin provides the following paradigm of self-deception:

1. Willful ignorance—absence of true belief.
2. Systematically ignoring—distraction of unpleasant thoughts to more pleasant ones.
3. Emotional detachment—protection of self-esteem by detaching oneself emotionally.

4. Self-pretense—a struggle to believe that something is not true.
5. Rationalization—belief that one's own view is necessary regardless of whether it is substantiated.[11]

In short, self-deception is blindness to self-acknowledgment. "To thine own self be true" or "Know thyself" are old adages attributed to Shakespeare and Socrates. Recall that knowing oneself is the result of, and in turn promotes, self-esteem. When self-esteem falters, self-respect plummets. The need to protect a faltering self-esteem by engaging in what we know is a counterproductive coping response that does not work in the end.

Reflection

Can you remember a time you engaged in self-deception? Given what you have just read, how would you categorize it? Can you think of ways to substitute a more caring response to yourself the next time it occurs?

Self-deception should be treated as a form of *impairment*. Institutions have methods for dealing with impairment that include team conferences, support groups, and in-house counseling and education for dealing with uncertainty. Because self-deception hides the need for this type of help from the person who requires it, input from a caring colleague or supervisor usually is required for the problem to be addressed. Offering insight and support to your colleagues and employees in these situations can help the development of their and your own moral character.

SUMMARY

The challenges to your personal integrity occasioned by bad laws or policies and your own self-deception are not impossible to overcome.

Societal Safeguards Revisited

Near the end of Chapter 1 you were introduced to several ways that moral compromise of your values can be minimized by safeguards that society provides for persons in their professional role. Now that you have examined how personal integrity is at the root of your ability to survive ethically in your professional role, it is fitting to review some of those societal safeguards briefly.

First, in situations in which the courts become involved, one of the state's interests is to protect the *integrity of the professions*. This means that as a group you may refuse to engage in a practice that is legally permissible or that society wants you to do because it is your professional judgment that this practice runs counter to the ethics of your profession or goes beyond your area of professional competence.

In addition, as an individual, abstaining on the basis that you find a procedure *morally repugnant* may be allowed if you can show why you believe it will threaten your personal integrity to participate. This idea was developed when abortion first became legalized in the United States because it was known that some professionals would judge the procedure to be morally wrong. It also has been applied to other situations by individual professionals, notably their refusal to engage in medical euthanasia or clinically assisted suicide and to take part in the administration of a lethal injection for purposes of capital punishment.

Both of these lines of reasoning could be used by Janice K. She would not be personally involved in performing the abortion procedure, but she could argue on behalf of her physician and nurse colleagues who are afraid they will be directly involved in having to participate in abortions. The rich interplay of society and an individual in the professional role continues to work itself out through such laws. Fortunately, the cherished value of personal integrity is not overlooked in society's understanding of what you should or should not be required to do.

Personal Integrity and Personal Vigilance

In this chapter the difficult and often heated subject of abortion is used as an illustration of how some individuals' integrity may be challenged. The question of how to maintain personal integrity arises in many more subtle situations as well. The autonomy and elevated status of being a professional, together with society's willingness to protect you from participating in activities you believe are wrong, provide safeguards for you so that you can maintain personal integrity in the practice of your profession.

> **SUMMARY**
>
> At the heart of being able to maintain your personal integrity is to know your own values, to pay attention to when they are at risk for being compromised, to learn to modify them as new insights and experience counsel, and to be prepared to defend and weigh them.

At the same time, societal safeguards cannot identify the content of your beliefs and values. You are the only one who can maintain the vigilance necessary to treat your personal integrity with the care it deserves as your most precious resource. Sometimes conflicting values come into play when you are trying to protect your sense of personal integrity in your professional role, just as you surely face them in your other roles. For instance, the religious values that led to Janice's position about abortion may come into conflict with values that have led her to become a professional or to take this job in the first place. Her values and beliefs may also prohibit her use of violence and confrontation as forms of resistance.

The Responsibility to Improve Yourself

Another responsibility is to continue to become a better professional and to learn more about how your professional role provides an opportunity for self-fulfillment and service to others. Each can be viewed as a charge.

The Charge to Remain Competent Professionally

A professional is required to continue to maintain a high level of professional competence by taking continuing education courses and by demonstrating proficiency in other ways. Sometimes relicensure or recertification examinations are required after a number of years to assure that you have kept up your knowledge and skills. Almost all states require you to demonstrate that you have taken steps to engage in lifelong learning professionally. The goal of these requirements is to safeguard your patients, but for most people the idea of being competent on the job is closely related to their feelings of accomplishment and satisfaction. In that case, your self-improvement in professional areas involves consideration of both your patients' and your own well-being. Recall Ross's observation that if there were a duty of self-improvement, it would flow from that we should bring about as much good overall as we can, including more good for ourselves!

The Charge to Improve Yourself Personally

Beyond improvement in professional areas, there is a charge to improve your personal healthfulness, skills, and interests. Do you have hobbies or other interests? A well-rounded person always makes a better professional insofar as he or she has relief from the demanding routine of professional work. One of the best safeguards against becoming bored or burned out is to have outside compelling interests that require concentrated attention and provide delight. It is not an accident that many application forms for programs of study or jobs include a question about your interests, hobbies, and personal skills unrelated to work.

Reflection

What are your most cherished ways of spending your time outside of your work and study? List them in order of priority.

SUMMARY

Self-improvement involves creative projects within *and* outside of the work environment.

I have heard it said that as part of the professional responsibility of self-improvement you and I have a responsibility to be exemplars in maintaining a healthy lifestyle. An exemplar is someone who demonstrates a quality to an unusually high degree, therefore becoming an example to others. In contrast, a dietitian who is obese because of poor dietary habits, a physically unfit physical therapist, a respiratory therapist who smokes cigarettes, a social worker or psychologist who does not attend to personal emotional problems, or a nurse who consistently gets too little sleep would be soundly criticized on the basis of being a health professional who should "know better." The health professional does know better, strictly from a knowledge perspective, about the deleterious effects of obesity, unfitness, mental stress, driving oneself, and other abuses or neglects of the body and mind. But what do you think?

Reflection

Do you think health professionals should be more responsible than the general public for maintaining a healthy lifestyle? Why?

I am still thinking through my own position, but I do have several thoughts on this issue. It is difficult to defend the idea that personal excellence in their field is a special responsibility of health professionals. That position begins to sound too much like a duty to oneself. In contrast, it is an aspiration toward which everyone profitably *could* strive for their own sense of healthiness and well-being. Sometimes people who choose a health profession have it as a component of their own personal values system to be fit, maintain healthful eating and sleeping patterns, and take steps to remain in good physical and mental health. In this regard, a health professional may experience a sense of personal responsibility to continue to improve his or her own healthfulness. In summary, health-related improvements can be considered important components of self-improvement but are not a responsibility as such.

Challenges Regarding Personal Integrity: Vigilance Revisited

We return to the story of Janice K. to complete this chapter and to consider one more facet of a professional's responsibility for self-improvement. Does Janice's predicament have anything to do with her responsibility for self-improvement? The answer is yes because every challenge to her personal values system provides an opportunity not only to act in accord with her beliefs but also to respond optimally. In the preceding discussion you were introduced to the idea that vigilance is required for maintaining personal integrity. It should now be easier to understand how such vigilance will help determine Janice's overall degree of self-improvement as a moral being. Vigilance is alertness and watchfulness. If she is alert to the details of past challenges to her personal integrity and uses them wisely as a teacher to help guide her in what she should do in each new situation, she will have taken advantage of a grand opportunity for improving her odds in the direction of her hoped for results. Over time Janice's practiced attention to what works best will better prepare her not only for moral leadership in her profession but also for all of life's difficult choices.

SUMMARY

If vigilant, each of us can become better equipped to respond more effectively, efficiently, and caringly with each new situation.

Summary

A focus on the well-being of others often is the sole emphasis in health care ethics. Chapter 5 and this chapter propose that to survive ethically requires self-awareness, experiences (and reflection on them), a commitment to living according to your personal values system, vigilance in maintaining personal integrity, and strategies for fulfilling responsibilities to yourself. In Chapter 7 you will have an opportunity to examine how colleagues and the institutional mechanisms for support and accountability in health care are relevant to your survival ethically.

Questions for Thought and Discussion

1. Melissa Y. is a nurse who works in the neonatal intensive care unit. She has become distressed in the last month because she is increasingly convinced that one of her longtime colleagues is "siphoning off" some of the narcotic medications intended for the patients. Her personal integrity dictates that she pursue the issue. If you were Melissa, how would you proceed? With whom? Why?

2. Some of the physicians who participated in the Nazi medical experiments testified that their activities did not run counter to their feelings of personal integrity. When asked how this could be, they stated that they were simply "doing their job." Discuss the limits of using an individual's personal conscience,

convictions, or understanding of his or her professional role as the ultimate standard of moral judgment. What, if any, higher standard is there? What types of checks and balances do you want to have in place to minimize wrongdoing in an institution or society?

3. Some days it would be better to just stay in bed. Bob started out the day by oversleeping, thereby missing his first patient appointment. When he went out for lunch with Bill, his colleague at work, his car was rear-ended at a stoplight. Now he is treating a patient who has just been diagnosed as having lung cancer. Bob expresses his sympathy regarding this bad news. The patient retorts, "You shouldn't sympathize. It's people like you who are part of the problem! You preach about health, but you smoke like a chimney. If you can't be a better example than this to poor common folks like us, you should get out of the health care field and leave it to someone who knows how to take care of his own health." Bob, who has been fighting the cigarette habit, suddenly feels guilty. He wonders if his smoking really is that bad of an example for his patients. He wants to respond to the patient but can't think of what to say regarding this indictment. Can you help him make an appropriate response? Why do you think your idea is an appropriate remark? Is the patient right?

References

1. Rawls, J. 1971. *A Theory of Justice*. Cambridge, MA: Harvard University Press.
2. Ross, W.D. 1930. *The Right and the Good*. Oxford: Clarendon Press, pp. 26–27.
3. American Nurses Association. 2001. *Code of Ethics for Nurses with Interpretive Statements*. Washington, D.C.
4. Niebuhr, H.R. 1963. *The Responsible Self*. New York: Harper & Row.
5. Purtilo, R., Haddad, A. 2002. Respect. The difference it makes. In *Health Professional and Patient Interaction* (6th ed.). Philadelphia: WB Saunders Company, pp. 14–17.
6. Cromie, J.E., Robertson, V.J., Best, M.O. 2002.Work-related musculoskeletal disorders and the profession of physical therapy. *Physical Therapy* 82(5):459–472.

7. Inge, W. 1968. *The Dark at the Top of the Stairs*. In *Four Plays*. New York: Grove Press, pp. 223–304.
8. Gaba, D.M., Stevens, S.K. 2002. Fatigue among clinicians and the safety of patients. *New England Journal of Medicine* 347(16):1249–1255.
9. Needleman, J., Buerhaus, P., Mattke, S., Stewart, M., Zelevinsky, K. 2002. Nursing staff levels and the quality of care in hospitals. *New England Journal of Medicine* 346(2):1715–1720.
10. Matthew 7:3.
11. Martin, M.W. 1986. *Self Deception and Morality*. Lawrence, KS: University Press of Kansas, pp. 6–30.

7

Living Ethically within Health Care Organizations

Objectives

The student should be able to:

- List three areas addressed by *organization ethics.*
- Define the term *mission statement* and the role of mission statements in the organizational life of contemporary societies.
- Describe what policies are and what they are designed to accomplish within health care and other organizations.
- Discuss several ethical elements that can be applied to an assessment of whether a policy is based on sound moral footing.
- Describe what it means for individuals to have a prima facie obligation to honor policies.
- Identify some ways in which the utilitarian approach to health care organization policy serves everyone well and conditions under which serious shortcomings may arise from relying on this approach.
- Identify three obligations that organizations have to individuals.
- Name some virtues of organizations and why they are important in today's evolving health care system.
- Critique key policies and administrative practices in the health care institution where you are training.
- Describe four areas in the business and management of an organization that require ethical reflection.

New terms and ideas you will encounter in this chapter

organization ethics	business ethics	policies
mission statement	cost-effectiveness	

Topics in this chapter introduced in earlier chapters

Topic	*Introduced in chapter*
Values and duties as constituents of the moral life	1
Ideals or aspirations	1
Prima facie and absolute duties or obligations	3
Utilitarian theory	3
Beneficence	3
Justice	3
Autonomy	3
Ethos	1
The six-step process of ethical decision making	4

Introduction

So far we have been focusing on the individuals most involved in the issues giving rise to ethical challenges in your professional environment. In this chapter, we turn to the organizational dimensions of your professional encounters focusing on your ethical roles, responsibilities, and rights in relation to health care institutions. An emerging area of ethical reflection in health care is organization ethics. *Organization ethics* pays attention to the character traits, rights, values, and duties expressed in the following formats:

Mission statements
Policies and administrative practices
Business priorities

Organization ethics for institutions that deliver health care and those that regulate health professionals and health care practices, professional associations, and profit or not-for-profit enterprises are of relevance here. These entities concerned with the larger social and bureaucratic organization of modern health care have goals that are not limited solely to the ethical goals of individual health professionals. For instance, a business goal of increasing the profit margin each year is legitimate for the type of entity a business is. *Business ethics* addresses the *conditions* under which a profit can be ethically realized and the *amount* of profit that is acceptable for the type of services. The overall goal of business, however, is to make money, which in itself is not wrong. Robert Hall[1] notes that health care institutions have ethical problems that in many ways are similar to good business management anywhere, but because of the special place the professions have in society, these businesses must be styled to fit the type of role its employees and "clients" play. As a member of a health care organization your challenge is to assess whether organization rights, values, and duties affect your professional practice positively or negatively when measured against the standard of your professional values and duties. To illustrate one version of how the ethical challenges of working within an organization affects the individual health professional, consider the following story.

The Story of Angelica Gomez and the Management Discussion Group

Angelica Gomez is the chief physical therapist at Redfield Hospital in a small Midwestern city of 26,000 people. She has enjoyed working in a bilingual environment and is proud of the good services the physical therapy department is able to provide the largely indigent population who has relocated to this area to work in agriculture and as employees of meat packing plants. She credits the department's success in part to the fact that she is bilingual and has hired an administrative assistant and physical therapy assistant, each of whom is fluent in Spanish.

The transition to treating a more diverse population has not always been smooth. Most Redfield Hospital employees are of German and Eastern European descent, second- or third-generation immigrant farmers who resent the influx into "their county" of the new wave of immigrants and undocumented workers. There have been several ugly altercations between the employees and Spanish-speaking patients or family members. To help provide guidance to the top administration on matters pertaining to this challenge, the hospital CEO, Audrey Frankenthaler, has adopted an operational strategy that includes establishment of a management discussion group of hospital administrators. The purpose of the group is to analyze ethics problems that arise because of current policies or organizational arrangements and to make recommendations to her and the hospital trustees for changes that will help guarantee all Redfield Hospital patients are treated with respect and receive the same high quality of care as more traditional clients.

Angelica is pleased to be invited to serve on this committee that meets every week. Although it is a lot of work, she feels confident that this dimension of her work is as important as the direct therapy services she and her physical therapy colleagues provide. At the same time, she is concerned that the model adopted by the CEO is merely advisory, lacking authority to assure implementation of the recommendations. Her experience in the past has been that other recommendations have gone unheeded.

At the end of 2 months the group makes its recommendations, the centerpiece of which is that the hospital administration should make the following changes: (1) hire several Spanish interpreters or bilingual personnel to work in key areas of the hospital, such as the admissions department, the surgical waiting room, and human resources; (2) offer a basic Spanish "language and culture" course to employees at all levels; and (3) provide signs in both English and Spanish around and within the hospital.

Several weeks have now gone by and Angelica realizes that none of the recommendations has been implemented. Last night, a Spanish-speaking patient who presented to the emergency room with a gunshot wound was turned away and almost bled to death, although the admissions clerk insists that the seriousness of his wound was not explained adequately. A newspaper in the large city 75 miles west of the town ran a damaging account of this incident in the morning paper. Angela figures this is the time to follow up with Ms. Frankenthaler, with whom she has had a very cordial relationship both in and outside of the work environment, about the progress on the recommended changes. When she expresses her concern, the CEO replies, "We were appreciative of your hard work, but frankly the management group's recommendations were too costly for the hospital. We have to continue to do the best we can with our usual ways of doing things. I think in time the problems will iron themselves out. Right now we aren't used to having so many foreigners around, but they will eventually blend in."

This is the first time that Angelica has been informed that no steps will be taken to implement their recommendations. As she walks to the physical therapy department she begins to feel that the ethically right thing is not being done. She thinks that the failure to implement any of the changes will only leave too much room for increased misunderstandings and tensions between the old and new populations, and these problems will begin to flow over into the good practices she believes the physical therapy department has adopted. Even with the changes the management group recommended, they believed those changes represented only the first steps of what should be done.

Reflection

What do you think are the major ethical challenges the management group is facing in this situation? What challenges do the CEO and trustees face? What are the serious differences in priorities and perspectives? What are the areas of mutual concern and overlap in their priorities?

The Goal: A Caring Response

Just as health professionals' ethical judgment should be guided by the goal of a caring response in the health professional and patient encounter, so must this goal govern in situations involving the organizations of health care. However, the character traits, needs, and rights of the institution itself must be taken deeply into the equation as a part of the analysis. The "voice" of the institution is expressed through the administrators and other business "stakeholders" (i.e., the CEO and CFO, trustees, and, in privately owned institutions, the stockholders).

The Six-Step Process in Organizational Matters

Given this more complex set of moral agents, you will gain some important insights by walking with Angelica through her story, using the six-step process of ethical decision making as a framework.

Step 1: Gather Relevant Information

Angelica's ethical problem will require her to gather data in places she may not have to appeal to so fully in the search for a caring response between herself and an identified patient or family. As noted at the outset of this chapter, the "situation" of institutions can be found in their mission statements, policies and administrative practices, and business priorities.

Mission Statements as Relevant Information

A *mission statement* is an institution's or professional organization's brief description of its ideals and aspirations. Because the mission statement is stated in general terms, the employee often ignores it completely when joining the group. It is from these ideals and aspirations, however, that goals, behavioral objectives, and expectations of all users (e.g., patients and all employees of a hospital or other health care institution) are derived. Sometimes the values of the entity are reflective of religious assumptions. In the United States, there are many hospitals and schools owned and operated by religious groups, a situation visitors to other parts of the world may not see. Such an organization will make reference in its mission statement to its understanding of the relationship of humans to God and each other and to the way in which the organization views itself as participating in the larger cosmic and social scheme of things. Figure 7–1 contains an example of a mission statement.

Reflection

What does the mission statement in Figure 7–1 tell you about the nature of this institution? What does this document not tell you? To what audiences do you think it is directed?

From reading the mission statement, what types of guidance from it might Angelica and the management group reasonably expect when dealing with their charge from the top hospital administration?

What would you ask if you were new to the Redfield Hospital area and were trying to choose a hospital for your family?

If you have not already guessed, the hospital is a Catholic hospital. You may have missed that it is also owned by a for-profit organization. Because mission statements become the basis for more specific policies and expectations, it is prudent and responsible to check the mission statement with as much care as you have read the Saint Joseph Hospital statement before becoming part of an institution or

Mission Statement

Saint Joseph Hospital is committed to the prevention of illness,
the restoration and improvement of health,
and the compassionate care of the suffering.
We are dedicated to the preservation and enhancement of life
by providing leadership in patient care,
education, and research
responsive to the health needs of our community.
We will pursue our vision
with the Judeo-Catholic heritage
as our foundation
and the hospital values
as our guide.

SAINT JOSEPH HOSPITAL
AT CREIGHTON UNIVERSITY MEDICAL CENTER
SJ

Figure 7–1. 1999 Mission Statement from Saint Joseph Hospital. *Courtesy of Saint Joseph Hospital at Creighton University Medical Center, Tenet Healthcare Corporation, Omaha, Nebraska.*

organization. This checkpoint should enable you to avoid ethical distress or dilemmas further into your affiliation with this body and its policies and practices if you do not subscribe to the overall nature of the organization's mission.

SUMMARY

Like codes and oaths, mission statements are organizations' public statements designed to declare to all the type of organization it is.

Policies and Administrative Practices as Information

Policies are statements designed to establish formal and informal guidelines for practice within an organization context. Policies should be consistent with the values of the entity. They also should be specific expressions of how the ideals in the mission statement can be carried out by the people in the organization and those the organization hopes to attract or serve. If policies are to be followed, they must also be clear, practical, flexible, and consistent with the values of the people or groups to whom they apply.

Currently, policies in health care reflect both traditional health care ethics and business ethics. As I heard one group whose mission was to deliver high-quality patient care comment, "No money, no mission." This is the perspective from which Audrey Frankenthaler, the CEO, was responding to Angelica's query about the management group's recommendations. The goals of the organization often are not fully met simply by focusing on the model of a single patient and health professional. As you can imagine, the picture is not always rosy because an organization's policy may come directly into conflict with professional ethics standards. In fact, it is often at the level of policy that goals for individual patients' well-being or justice among groups come into direct conflict with business interests. Recently, I was conducting a workshop in a private health care facility that had adopted a "no AIDS patients" policy because of the high costs of services for many such patients. The health professionals were distressed because the facility was in the process of building a new multimillion dollar reception area and surrounding gardens with the hope of its beauty being the draw to "beat out the competition." This decision by the trustees of the facility was interpreted by my professional colleagues as being a triumph of profits over patients.

SUMMARY

Few health professionals today will be in situations where they can ignore organization policies. Still, professional values must guide decisions.

Glaser[2] maintains that partially because of the changes in the health care system, all ethical issues involving patient care now also have business/administrative and larger societal dimensions. These three realms of ethics (individual, institutional, and societal) always are present.

Step 2: Identify the Type of Ethical Problem

A *prima facie obligation* to honor policies is an expression of your willingness to become a part of the larger environment in which your professional commitments can be met. Without a posture toward policy that demonstrates your willingness to follow it, chaos could ensue, and even patient care could suffer dramatically.

When faced with a prima facie obligation to honor a policy, you should assess whether it is ethically supportable. If it isn't, but it seems nothing can be done to change it, you will experience ethical distress. More often you, like Angelica and members of her management group, will face an ethical dilemma. They were placed in a consultative role, asked to make recommendations to help ensure a caring response to all patient groups using the facility. They did their job well and had a reasonable expectation that some changes would be forthcoming. Now that changes will not be made, the members of the group still have an obligation to honor the existing policies and practices. At the same time, Angelica is among those who judge that *not* to make changes is resulting in harm to some groups of patients. She is on the horns of a dilemma with two right courses of action facing her, but to subvert the decision of the top administration by encouraging (or implementing) some important changes will require her to *dis*honor the duty of loyalty to her employing institution. Her and her colleagues' sense of compassion and fidelity toward the new population of patients may help to determine her course of action, although they are well advised to be sure they understand all the issues and have applied the appropriate ethical approaches for resolution of this problem.

Step 3: Use Ethics Theories or Approaches to Analyze the Problem

Several ethical norms are important to consider when a policy decision is being assessed. Some are familiar in clinical ethics decisions. To highlight the ones important for policy you should ask the following questions:

Do the guidelines in the policy appear to encourage practices that will do more good than harm overall? If so, the policy could be supported from a utilitarian approach to ethics.

Is the policy aimed at preventing harmful discriminatory practices in the distribution of benefits and burdens? If so, it honors the principle of justice.

Does the policy encourage respect toward everyone involved? If yes, then it is consistent with the overarching duty to treat people with respect or dignity.

Does it allow some members to be rewarded for conduct that is exemplary in terms of improving patient satisfaction or employee morale or demonstrating good stewardship of environmental or other resources? If so, this policy encourages beneficence.

The obligation to follow policies is better understood in light of the fact that from the *institutional* standpoint an ethically supportable policy is one that brings about the most good overall. Generally speaking, organizations have a utilitarian value system designed to provide the greatest good for the greatest number. It follows that from an organization standpoint, considerations of respect for individual autonomy may be submerged in favor of such utilitarian considerations as efficiency of operations and economic stability. Simply stated, the organization that fulfills its function of providing a worthwhile service efficiently usually is believed to justify the means used to attain that end so long as the net result is a greater balance of benefits to humanity than would be realized if the organization did not exist.

Reflection

What more would you want to know before you accepted the Redfield Hospital administration's decision not to enact the group's recommendations because "they would cost too much"? In other words, what factors would sway you in agreeing that the costs would unduly outweigh the benefits?

The idea of cost-effectiveness often is cited as the appropriate goal of health plans. The definition of *cost-effectiveness* is that the greatest quality of care possible is provided at the lowest price. No one can argue with the underlying principle. The administrative arrangements, however, may succumb to the serious criticism that such efficiency can best be achieved through cutting costs by means that actually compromise quality.[3]

Because both mission statements and policies invariably are generalities, they cannot provide the optimum solution to every situation. They may be inappropriate or inadequate to handle every problem faced by a health professional. Therefore, they merely provide boundaries. We all find ourselves breaking rules when overriding them can be ethically justified—for example, parking in a No Parking zone to assist at the scene of an accident. That is, of course, why there is a prima facie but not an absolute duty to honor policies: What may be best for most people may not be best in a situation for a particular person.

SUMMARY

Policies may not provide guidance for all situations.

In the end, the decisions to resort to ignoring the spirit of a mission statement or breaking a policy on moral grounds must be implemented only after the greatest caution has been taken to ensure this is the only course of action remaining.

Obligations of Organizations to Individuals

A full understanding of the ethical norms that are relevant in Angelica's dilemma requires you to consider what she and her colleagues in the management group have a reasonable expectation, even right, to expect in this situation.

Policy in most organizations is established by those in powerful positions within the structure, although today multidisciplinary committees sometimes are assigned the task of designing, refining, and reviewing policy. In other words, more and more people from all echelons of the organization hierarchy are currently becoming involved in setting policy.

The Opportunity to Become Involved in Policy. Everyone should be given an opportunity to become involved in the policy process. The moral right of participation arises partly from the right to help determine those aspects of workplace practices that directly affect your well-being. Your involvement in policy development and review is the only way you can assure that you will not become caught in a situation in which you are forced to sacrifice important personal and professional values to the overriding organization value of efficiency. I have long argued that efficiency can be applauded when it can be brought in line with the professional values of faithfulness to patients, patients' and professionals' rights, and prevention of harm to anyone.[4] But only if concerned professionals are given—and take—the opportunity to become part of the policy development process will such coherence be the result.

Of course, Angelica and her colleagues in the management group are faced with a different challenge. They have been offered—and took—the opportunity to become involved in the refinement of policies related to patient care respect and access. Now they are not sure that they will have any voice after all because their recommendations seem to have been dismissed. Other alternatives are something they must consider; be that as it may, probably none of them would judge they would be better off not to have had any opportunity to think about the issues.

Reflection

A good place to start becoming involved in policy is your own place of employment or your professional association. If you have a job now, what is a policy you could recommend to improve the conditions or quality of productivity in your workplace?

Part of the ability to be involved in policy is to be able to ascertain where the policies are made and revised. Pertinent questions are:

1. What is the name of the committee for a given policy process?
2. Who sits on the committee and what are their qualifications?
3. What must you do to be nominated for or appointed to the committee?
4. To whom must you speak to express your interest?

Students often get their start in shaping an organization's structures by volunteering as student members of policy committees.

The Assurance of Relevant Policies. It also is reasonable to assume that your organization will have a range of policies and other administrative guidelines that give clear direction for your own practice.

The Joint Commission on Accreditation of Healthcare Organizations (JCAHO) has provided guidelines for the range of policies and practices that would meet their requirement for an ethical institution.[5] From their long list I conclude that one should be able to find the following types of policies related to direct patient care:

- Informed consent policy
- Withholding and withdrawing life-sustaining treatment policy
- Assisted suicide and euthanasia policy
- Advance directive policy
- Surrogate decision making, health care agents, durable power of attorney for health care, and guardianship process policies
- Do not resuscitate (DNR) policy
- Confidentiality and privacy policy
- Organ donation and procurement policy
- Human experimentation regulations (policies and procedures)
- Conflicts of interest policy (including patient care and research policies)
- Admission, discharge, and transfer policy
- Impaired providers policy (including reporting procedures for impaired providers and medical errors)
- Conscience clause policy and procedures
- Reproductive technology policies

Reflection

Can you think of other policies that would pertain to your professional responsibilities?

Administrative Commitment to Creating a Virtuous Organization

Sincere and intense commitment to creating humane organizations is essential if those involved in the organization and the larger community are to thrive. Because most organizations are similar to Redfield Hospital, governed by a small number of people who have the final say over what will happen to everyone, this commitment must begin with the individuals who have the most power and authority.

You already have learned that efficiency is one value of organizations because they are designed to meet multiple needs and render multiple services. From a social standpoint, many would say that a "good" or "well-run" institution is an efficient one. From the standpoint of your tasks within a health care organization, however, you would benefit from institutions and systems that reflect virtues in addition to efficiency.

John Rawls,[6] a philosopher you have met earlier in this textbook, maintains that if an institution is fair in its assignment of rights and duties and makes provision for a fair distribution of its resources, then individuals in those institutions will be able to live more moral lives.

Reflection

Can you imagine what a courageous organization would be like and what type of policies and administrative guidelines you would find there? What about a compassionate or merciful institution?

Philosophers, economists, and others maintain that institutions and other organizations do have "character" traits. They also acknowledge the power of organization structures to affect the lives of individuals in our highly bureaucratized society. The traits of health care organizations are one important focus of serious reflection today.[7]

SUMMARY

Underlying the ethical concern about institutional organizations is the awareness that they have the capacity to fragment lives, alienate individuals from their values and connectedness, and marginalize already oppressed groups. Organizations have an obligation to prevent such destructive conditions from occurring.

We have seen some problems at work in the Redfield Hospital setting. Because so many people spend more time each week in the organizations of work, government, education, health care, and religion than they do in their own homes, all organizations must assume an influential role in helping to foster high moral standards of institutions.

Step 4: Explore the Practical Alternatives

The management group at Redfield Hospital has to consider the practical alternatives open to them now that they have learned their recommendations are not being implemented. They are disappointed, of course, and some are angry. They gave considerable thought to the duties, relevant principles, and virtues they believe should govern such recommendations from the standpoint of their moral role as health professionals; they have taken into account that "the bottom line" does matter in institutions and that administrative decisions always must keep "the big picture" in focus, weighing the costs of one priority against another and honoring the importance of efficiency within the organization as a whole. Although they may not think this utilitarian balancing is appropriate for one-on-one decisions, all agree that it is necessary for institutional policies and practices. But they also have reckoned with the moral rights and reasonable expectations with which they undertook the responsibility of trying to help solve a major emerging problem in the hospital, including their right to relevant policies that will enable them to complete their jobs according to high ethical standards. They have taken their opportunity to help shape the institution's policies, and assumed that the hospital administration and trustees want to foster an environment consistent with the high moral and service standards of health care. They have appealed to the Redfield Hospital mission statement, which promises that the institution will treat its patients justly and compassionately. They are clear about what should be done. Now they have convened again to decide the course to take because, formally, their function as a management group is done and their advice has not been taken.

Reflection

List the practical alternatives Angelica and her management group have open to them. Surely one course of action would be to do nothing more. However, no one in the group wants to just let the matter drop. Would you?

The management group has several practical alternatives open to them, each requiring strategies that depend on working with the "powers that be." Angelica may well continue to talk privately to her boss and friend, Audrey Frankenthaler. Others may decide to ignore the top administration but begin to implement the ideas at their own levels of institutional responsibility. Still others may link arms with advocacy groups within the larger community to put external pressure on the hospital to be more responsive to the emerging problems.

Steps 5 and 6: Complete the Action and Evaluate the Process and Outcome

The management group itself must have the courage to take whatever steps the members decide on, individually or as a group. Short of this, their time, energies, and collective best judgment surely will give way to other priorities until a real crisis hits. Health professionals who are forced to provide care in a changing systemic environment where policies and practices seem at odds with the demands of their moral roles experience a feeling of loss of control, stress, discontent, and disheartenment.[8] The management group's goal (i.e., to help set policies that uphold the institution's high ethical standards and prevent harm to members of the new patient population) will be thwarted if they lag in their efforts now.

As with all important challenges, an agreement that they will have a debriefing from time to time to reflect on their successes and failures will strengthen them for additional such efforts. Moreover, they can find ways to share their successes with other groups attempting to deal with similar challenges regarding the increasingly rich mix of ethnicities and other aspects of diversity that most communities are facing.

Living with the Business Aspects of Health Care

Health care institutions are not just businesses. Bodenheimer and Grumbach[9] maintain that three major forces drive the organization of health care in the United States, and to some degree, in all economically developed nations: (1) the biomedical model, (2) financial incentives, and (3) professionalism. The institutions will, of course, reflect all three aspects. The service of health care is expressed through the biomedical and clinical skills of the professionals, the financial grounding through financial incentives, and the peculiar ethical standards through professionalism. Still, the financial incentives often are targeted in the literature as creating the biggest challenge to the professionals. In other words, the challenge for health professionals is the requirement of living with the "business" of health care but not letting it govern all the values and priorities of practice.

Business language often conjures up negative images of greedy health care institutions driven by profit at all costs. Although rare, such organizations do exist and, of course, create ethical dilemmas for any health care professional who works in them because they fail to meet reasonable expectations of patients and society. Not all health care institutions, however, are driven solely by a monetary bottom line. The business functions of any organization are designed to help meet the appropriate goals of that organization, whatever those goals may be. The business aspect of an organization primarily entails management related to advertising, hiring and firing of employees, establishment of policies and procedures, product or service management (design, production, and delivery), fiscal management, and operations.

Understandably, then, some major themes in business ethics are honesty in advertising and in dealings with partners and clients, fairness in the treatment of employees or others, criteria for quality control of the product or service, the meaning of fiscal accountability from the standpoint of taking everyone's legitimate interests into account, and the duty of respect for others in all the organization's interactions.

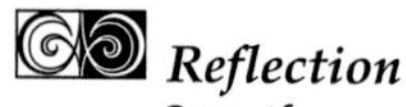

Reflection

Specify some ways a health care organization such as a hospital, a nursing home, a home health agency, or an HMO would have to gear its business goals, policies, and practices to meet high ethical standards of patient care.

To survive ethically within the organization where you work, you will need to identify the business realities and critique them. Although it goes beyond the parameters of this book to fully address the business dimensions of your practice, the next generation of health professionals, to which you will belong, will be forced to be more cognizant of them.

> **SUMMARY**
>
> A firm grounding in professional ethics combined with the tools for ethical analysis you are learning here provide a basic foundation for the task of living with the business aspects of organizations.

Summary

This chapter takes you, the moral agent, out of the clinic or other immediate work environment and into the committee room and administrator's offices. As the complexity of the health professions and health care environment continues to grow, so do the necessity and opportunity for becoming involved in the development of mission statements, policies, and administrative and business practices. Such involvement should enable you to maintain professional standards and a high level of ethical practice. The six-step process of ethical decision making can guide you in your role in this situation. Despite the help that the organization policies, practices, and environment can provide, they are not an automatic guarantee of high-quality patient care or fair practices toward employees, patients, or others. You still must exercise good moral judgment about ethical problems.

Questions for Thought and Discussion

1. List your own institutional obligations as a student or health professional and rank each one as having the following:
   a. No ethical significance
   b. Possible ethical significance
   c. Definite ethical significance

   Which ones are determined by policies? Which policies?

   ____
   ____
   ____
   ____

2. Can you describe a situation in which you would consider a strike as an ethical action for you to take?
   If so, list the pros and cons of the ethical issues.

   ____
   ____
   ____
   ____

If not, why not?

3. Eudora Cathay has been a unit clerk at the same community hospital for 2 years. The position of unit clerk is a demanding one that involves answering the phone, relaying messages, coordinating laboratory personnel in their rounds, responding to physicians' requests, and making sure that patients are in the right places at the right times. Eudora's striking appearance is enhanced by her native African dress style. Some of the more conservative members of the staff, particularly physicians and administrators, have been disturbed by her style of dress. Others find it attractive and an interesting change from the wall-to-wall white uniforms everywhere in the hospital. The dress policy does not require unit clerks to wear a uniform and stipulates only that they be neat and well groomed (which she is) and dressed "appropriately" (which is controversial). Someone in an administrative position asked Eudora to dress more conservatively. She refused on the grounds that she was neat and well groomed and any further demands were an invasion of her privacy. She was fired for her refusal to comply, amidst rampant rumors of racism. Discuss her situation in light of good policy. Should there be a dress policy? Is there anything ethical about such a policy? Why or why not?

References

1. Hall, R T. 2000. *An Introduction to Healthcare Organizational Ethics*. New York: Oxford University Press.
2. Glaser, J. 1997. Introduction. In Glaser, J., Hamel, R. (Eds.), *Three Realms of Managed Care: Societal, Individual, Institutional*. Kansas City, MO: Sheed and Ward, pp. vii–xiv.
3. Casilino, L., Gillies, R.R., Shortell, S.M., Schmittdiel, J.A., Bodenheimer, T., Robinson, J.C., Rundall, T., Oswald, N., Schauffler, H., Wang, M.C. 2003. External incentives, information technology and organized processes to improve health care quality for patients with chronic diseases. *JAMA* 289:434–441.
4. Purtilo, R. 1988. Saying "No" to patients for cost-related reasons. *Physical Therapy* 68(8):1243–1247.

5. Joint Commission, 1998. Ethical Issues and Patient Rights Across the Continuum of Care. Oakbrook Terrace, IL: Joint Commission on Accreditation of Healthcare Organizations.
6. Rawls, J. 1971. *A Theory of Justice*. Cambridge, MA: Harvard University Press.
7. Lawrence, D. 2003. *From Chaos to Care: The Promise of Team-Based Medicine*. Cambridge, MA: Da Capo Press.
8. Blau, R., Bolus, S., Carolan, T., Kramer, D., Mahoney E., Jette, D.U., Beal, J.A. 2002. The experience of providing physical therapy in a changing health care environment. *Physical Therapy* 82(7):648–657.
9. Bodeheimer, T.S., Grumbach, K. 2002. *Understanding Health Policy. A Clinical Approach* (3rd ed.). New York: McGraw-Hill, pp. 62–65.

8

Living Ethically as a Member of the Health Care Team

Objectives

The student should be able to:

- Describe some major areas of professional life that present ethical challenges as a member of a health care team.
- List five guidelines that are useful in assessing whether a prospective place of employment supports teamwork that is ethically and clinically of the highest quality.
- Discuss several reasonable expectations a health professional can have of professional peers.
- Define peer review and assess its usefulness as a mechanism to maintain the high moral standards of a profession.
- List several types of impairment that health professionals may experience that create ethical challenges for the whole team.
- Discuss some general guidelines on how to gather relevant information regarding an alleged incident of incompetent or unethical professional conduct.
- Outline the appropriate steps to be taken in a whistle-blowing situation.
- Develop several alternative strategies for dealing with a colleague who is engaging in incompetent or unethical conduct and describe probable outcomes of taking each line of action.

New terms and ideas you will encounter in this chapter

health care teams	whistle-blowing/whistle-blowers
supererogatory—beyond duty	impairment
due process (legal)	peer review

Topics in this chapter introduced in earlier chapters

Topic	*Introduced in chapter*
Taking care of yourself as a responsibility	6
Faithfulness or fidelity	3
Beneficence	3
Ethical dilemma	2
Justice or fairness	3
Six-step process of ethical decision making	4
Nonmaleficence	3
Deontology	3
Utilitarianism	3

Introduction

This chapter launches a new focus. Up until now you have been considering your moral agency role as an individual student or professional. But you are a moral agent in respect to other roles you assume, too, one of the most interesting being as a member of a health care team. There you work together with other professionals to provide optimally competent care to patients and to participate in other team activities. Moreover, your teammates deserve to be treated with respect. In one sense of the word the search for a caring response to them is as important for good patient care as is your commitment to finding a caring response toward each patient. Usually, the two focuses of your care are completely compatible with your ultimate goal of doing what is best for each patient. In fact, team-oriented care was *designed* to enhance the effectiveness of this goal. Occasionally, however, problems arise within teamwork that threaten to compromise the patient's good, the team's effectiveness, or both. You have an opportunity here to examine both some strengths and challenges in teamwork. The story of Maureen Sitler and Daniela Green is one example of how conflict or questions arise about the ethically right thing to do.

The Story of Maureen Sitler and Daniela Green

Maureen Sitler is the chief respiratory therapist in the respiratory intensive care unit (ICU) of a large university hospital. There are two staff therapists in the unit with her.

Maureen has been on vacation during the last 2 weeks and arrives home late Sunday night. When she reports to work on Monday morning she finds a note on her desk saying that Karen, one of the two staff therapists, has had to leave town to be with her mother, who has had a serious heart attack. Karen writes that she will be gone at least this week and maybe next.

The other therapist, Tom Morgane, arrives and brings Maureen up to date on the activities. He assures her that, as usual, the patient load soared immediately after she left and that the unit has been buzzing ever since.

They sort through the current patient load and are relieved that no new patients have come in over the weekend. They decide that between them they can just manage for the day. Suddenly Maureen feels weary, as if she had never been on vacation.

She is writing names of the patients on the schedule board in the office when a unit clerk brings a note to her detailing four patients in other parts of the hospital who need therapy. The note is from the hospital's other respiratory therapy department director, the one who serves the general inpatient population. Often the two directors make such requests of each other when their own loads are especially heavy. Maureen's first impulse is to refuse to accept any more patients, but she takes the note to her desk.

The first patient is an 81-year-old widow with inhalation burns. She accidentally started a fire that gutted her kitchen when a kitchen towel caught on fire. The second referral is a 3-year-old child with congenital lung and bronchial deformities. Another repair of the bronchial tubes had been performed. The third patient is a 31-year-old woman with severe asthma.

Maureen lays out the three referral sheets in front of her without bothering to read the fourth and studies the schedule again. At *most* they can accept only one more patient today. She decides to call the other chief therapist, Sandra Haynes, to ask her judgment regarding the relative urgency of these patients.

She is dialing, tapping idly with her forefinger on the one referral she has not yet read, when the name Daniela Green leaps off the page at her. She picks up the referral and reads it. Her heart begins to pound in her throat. She slams down the receiver and runs to the treatment area where Tom is working. "This can't be *our* Danie!" she exclaims. Tom puts a hand on her shoulder, "I'm sorry, I forgot to tell you with so much else to catch up on! As you can see she was hospitalized with severe pneumonia while you were gone. We should find a way to fit her in."

Maureen feels sick to her stomach. Daniela Green is the head nurse in the oncology unit. Daniela and Maureen often have the same patients so more often than not they find themselves on the same health care teams, whether it be in the oncology or respiratory ICU units or as members of the rehabilitation team. Daniela recently gave an excellent in-service workshop for the physical therapy, occupational therapy, and respiratory therapy departments. On a number of occasions Maureen and Daniela have attended plays and other social events together. Two years ago they initiated a drive to find support for improving or, as they put it, "humanizing" the environment of the waiting areas throughout the therapy areas. Of all her professional colleagues, Maureen feels she can trust Daniela the most. On several occasions Maureen has called on Daniela as a "sympathetic ear" and has found her insightful and understanding. During her vacation Maureen had been thinking that she should take the time to cultivate this budding friendship, knowing that it could take root and deepen.

Maureen's first reaction is to squeeze Daniela into the treatment schedule, no matter what. But something stops her. How can she be fair to all the patients on the list, she thinks, and still respond to the additional loyalties of kinship she feels toward her teammate Daniela?

You will have an opportunity to reflect on this case throughout the chapter because it highlights several strengths and types of ethical challenges that you could face—and probably will face—in your role as a team member. The first thing we'll consider is the importance of providing support to and accepting support from each other.

The Goal: A Caring Response

No one who works in the health care setting day in and day out escapes moments of self-doubt, anger, or utter frustration. As you read in Chapters 5, 6, and 7, a great deal is expected of you in regard to taking good care of yourself as a student or professional and in getting along in the institutions of health care. Even so, at times your involvement in the human suffering of illness and disease is intense, the responsibilities arduous, and the challenges monumental. The wear and tear of taxing schedules, patients whose problems seem overwhelming, or a day in which everything that could go wrong does can discourage even the most competent, optimistic person.

Maureen Sitler's situation illustrates well how easy (and how wonderful) it is to develop friendships in the work place. It is not surprising, considering that you will spend some of the best (and if not the best, at least the most) hours of your life in workplace settings! Friendships, a love relationship, and business partnerships with people you will meet first as a team member are all within the realm of possibility.

Many institutions currently recognize the need for team support. In some institutions there is an effort to hold departmental or interdepartmental meetings so that problems may be addressed in a nonthreatening, supportive setting. This type of arrangement usually improves and sustains good working relationships among team members and provides a refuge where individuals can receive needed support. In any department such arrangements can help to humanize the environment for workers and patients alike.[1] In this regard, it makes sense to think of teamwork as the institution's acknowledgment of such stresses and the implementation of actual mechanisms to address them as its caring response to the situation.

Many have found it wise when applying for a position in a new health care setting to find out whether there is a support network among team members. To make an assessment, you might want to keep the following suggestions in mind:

1. Inquire of your future employer whether there are team meetings or other sessions to freely discuss everyday stresses on the team.
2. Ask some of the people you will be working with what is the most stressful in that environment.
3. Ask them how each, as an individual, deals with stresses of his or her position as a team member and whether the environment as a whole is supportive or divisive.
4. Make a mental note of potential teammates who appear to be likely sources of support under stress, or if no one appears to be potentially supportive.
5. Perhaps most important, try to ascertain whether it will be possible to help try to decrease or eliminate sources of team stress and who will help accept responsibility for fostering such change. In other words, is there an attempt to identify institutional and policy-related problems?

Reflection

What *other* questions or concerns would you address when applying for a position and trying to assess the tone of the work environment?

Fortunately, it is extremely probable that you will be able to find a supportive work setting. Once you are employed, or if you already are, you can help create a greater support network among team members by being attentive to the blahs and blues that a colleague seems to be experiencing, by risking sharing your own "dark spaces" with people you judge to be trustworthy to help you through them, and by making suggestions regarding the need for mechanisms designed for working through problems. As Maureen's situation implies, friendships may take root in the shared experiences, concerns, and time spent with other members of the health care team. A friend you meet in a work situation may become the key figure in building a supportive network, and as friends the two of you can provide support to each other and others. The joy of discovering and cultivating such a friendship is among the most rewarding of the many fringe benefits of a health professional's career.

The ethical components guiding close, convivial working relationships are similar to those in the health professional–patient relationship.[2] Team members also should be the recipient of your caring response. Some ways to achieve it include telling the truth, honoring confidences, acting with compassion, and respecting the dignity of your colleagues.

Reflection

Because you are a moral agent with the responsibilities associated with it, what do you think you should be able to reasonably expect from your fellow teammates? Name some things that would indicate that you are the beneficiary of their respect and care.

From my own experience, I have developed a list of reasonable expectations—things I believe I should be able to count on in my workplace—based on the ethical principle of fidelity to each other. These expectations are:

1. Reassurance regarding my questions about good patient care or other matters of professional judgment;
2. An arrangement in which everyone carries a fair share of the workload;
3. Sympathetic understanding regarding my work-related stresses;
4. An environment conducive to a high level of functioning and one that fosters work satisfaction;
5. A commitment by everyone to respect differences and embrace each person's unique gifts;
6. Mechanisms for the protection of everyone's basic rights, including mine; and
7. Encouragement for me to develop both professionally and personally within the work environment.

As you think of other things you would expect and want to help protect and encourage, be bold in making suggestions to those with whom you work. Sometimes a word well placed can help to increase everyone's imagination about how the team can work together better.

SUMMARY

Good teamwork is based on respect. You can expect respect from others and also must show respect to them.

With the background established thus far in this chapter, I ask you to turn to the six-step process of ethical decision making to learn how well it also applies to team issues.

The Six-Step Process and Team Decisions

We will take Maureen's situation, with its potential for favoritism toward Daniela, to give you an opportunity to apply the six-step process of ethical decision making. So far you have applied this process to situations involving health professionals' decisions regarding direct patient care and institutional organizations. A team is designed to meet the same ethical goal of a caring response that individual professionals have as their goal, so that members of a team, working together, will accomplish collectively what individual professionals aim to do. At the same time, interprofessional issues also will arise among team members, and those issues lend themselves to analysis and (hopefully) resolution by use of the same process. Some ethical considerations you have not yet encountered must be taken into account in a team peer relationship. The last part of this chapter focuses on the challenges of peer review and the duty to report unacceptable conduct of a teammate.

Step 1: Gather Relevant Information for the Team Situation

Maureen has to gather all the relevant information about the patients on the waiting list that she would be morally obligated to do in any event. However, right away you can see that her discovery of Daniela as one of the potential patients complicates the situation in at least two ways: she has to decide whether her loyalty to her team member should have any bearing on her choice in the end, and she has to reckon with the fact that the two of them are now in a "dual role" with each other if and when Daniela becomes a patient.

Team Loyalty as Relevant Information

First of all, Maureen and Daniela are professional peers. We surmise it is influencing Maureen's decision, although she has not yet acted. No one would question how important it is to provide support to professional peers, and now here is a peer with a need to which Maureen is able to respond. It takes little imagination to understand why Maureen's emotional response is to immediately accept her as one of the patients. It would be easy to give Daniela the VIP ("very important person") treatment, slipping her in ahead of the others in the busy schedule, regardless of whether she will benefit the most. We don't know exactly why Tom urges Maureen to "fit her in." His statement may be based on something he knows about her physical situation relative to the others on the list. More likely, he is responding to the same urgings that Maureen is experiencing. He might also be imagining the backlash among their other teammates and professional colleagues throughout the institution if word gets out that Daniela was not given high priority. Maureen probably is well aware of these relevant "facts" of the situation.

The Ethical Challenge of Dual Roles

The two women are not only teammates but also enjoy a warm personal relationship. In other words, they are in a relationship both as peers and as friends. Now they are plunged into a third type of relationship: they are about to encounter each other as therapist and patient in a health professional–patient relationship.

The situation of a dual relationship is always one occasion for careful reflection about appropriate boundaries in the professional setting.[3] As Maureen tries to sort out her priorities in her role as a *health professional,* who will be treating the *patient,* Daniela, she becomes strikingly aware that she and Daniela are in new territory with each other. The health professional–patient relationship has ethical parameters that do not pertain to either their relationship as professional peers or as friends. In her professional role, if Maureen's favorable bias toward Daniela becomes an occasion for allowing an uncaring response to the other patients on the list, she will have acted unethically. Although Daniela may accept this situation with equanimity and understanding, anyone who has been very ill knows that it is difficult not to want attention immediately. The favoritism one would automatically hope for and reasonably expect from a friend is not alone sufficient reason for receiving top priority treatment.

SUMMARY

Loyalties to one's teammates and the situation of dual roles create occasions for ethical guidelines.

Steps 2 and 3: Identify the Type of Ethical Problem and the Ethics Approach to Analyze It

Maureen, the moral agent in this situation, is faced with an ethical problem.

Reflection

What do you judge the problem to be, and what kind of ethical problem is it?

When you have had sufficient time to think about it, read on and I will tell you how I would approach it. If your approach is different, discuss it with a colleague or in class to see how we may both be correct.

I believe Maureen has an ethical dilemma. First, other things being equal she would be justified in responding positively to her professional colleague. On the basis of providing good patient care, it is necessary for members of the team to pay due regard to each other. As you recall, earlier in this chapter I suggested a list of what I could "reasonably expect" from teammates in terms of their support and recommended you do the same. My list was based on the principle of faithfulness (fidelity), knowing that if a team does not stay together in its shared goal of providing good patient care, it will fail in meeting that goal. Therefore, it is not morally blameworthy of Maureen to have a deep affinity for the well-being of her colleague.

Maureen also has the duty to search for the most caring response to any one of the patients on that list. This peels off all the layers of other concerns and leaves the core of the patient–health professional relationship. If she believes any or all of those other patients have a more pressing need for her services, Maureen cannot both honor her fidelity to her teammate and her fidelity to the ethical core of her professional role.

In this type of dilemma the conflicting principles of fidelity to her peers and beneficence to the patients on the list summarizes her ethical quandary. However, her moral agency carries with it the power to allow harm or less than optimal benefit to ensue for the patients in relatively greater need if she is swayed by criteria inappropriate to a health professional's decision.

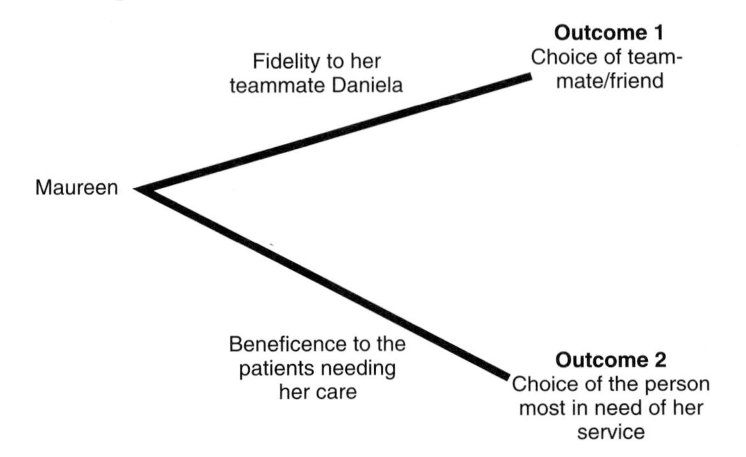

Given that these principles are markers to moral duties that Maureen is working with, one can conclude that she is sorting this out according to the framework a *deontologist* would use. As straightforward as this appears, Maureen may also be acutely aware that the *consequences* of not accepting Daniela, whatever the assessment of her relevant need, will be deleterious to the morale of the rest of the team. Therefore, she will have to further weigh in those utilitarian considerations before making her final decision.

Reflection

Having analyzed the situation this far, do you think her duties or utilitarian considerations should govern her decision? What character traits would you want Maureen to have when she is making this decision? Can you name some?

____

____

____

____

Step 4: Explore the Practical Alternatives

There are several options open to her, including:

1. Accepting Daniela Green for treatment because they are friends.
2. Accepting Daniela because she is well loved by many people in the hospital and not to give her priority will adversely affect the staff.
3. *Not* accepting Daniela because showing favoritism in such instances sends the wrong message.
4. *Not* accepting Daniela because she is in less immediate need of this particular health professional's services than the other three patients seem to be.
5. Choosing randomly who among the four patients will be treated today (draw straws).
6. Accepting the three other patients and treating Daniela after hours.

Can you add others?

First, let us consider the first option. As we discussed earlier, all things being equal, you would expect a friend or colleague to act favorably on your behalf and would be prepared to do likewise. One display of friendship and colleagueship is this type of commitment. But Maureen's ethical dilemma reveals that accepting Daniela for this reason oversimplifies the ethical problem she is facing because it ignores the reality of conflicting commitments.

The *second option* entails a type of utilitarian reasoning. Again, we speculated earlier that maybe if Daniela is not accepted for treatment, the morale of the whole hospital will be affected. The staff will think, "The same thing could happen to me. Would my colleagues overlook me for someone else, too?" Maureen might say, along this line of reasoning, "Particular loyalties and justice aside, it just doesn't pay in the long run to accept for treatment those who do not command the sympathies of the hospital the way that Daniela does."

Practically speaking, this type of reasoning often underlies decisions. But the moral point of view requires that the various duties experienced in the health professional–patient relationships not be ignored so facilely. Accepting Daniela for the reason stated in the second option again oversimplifies the ethical dilemma Maureen is facing.

The *third option* again emphasizes the difficulty of trying to proceed fairly or impartially when faced with a decision that involves someone the decision maker knows and cares about. Refusing Daniela treatment primarily because she and Maureen are teammates intuitively seems as unfair as automatically providing privileges because of it. And so, acting on the third option is not a morally adequate decision either. In contrast, Maureen's idea of telephoning her respiratory therapist colleague, who may know the other patients, is a good plan. The other therapist might provide insight and more balanced judgments regarding unfair biases Maureen would introduce by having such a vested interest in her friend's welfare.

We know the ethical priority in regard to Maureen's dilemma is the health professional–patient relationship rather than her relationship with another team member.[4] Why? Because Daniela is in *this* situation because of her clinical condition, and her need for Maureen in *this* instance specifically is the need that a patient experiences in relation to a health professional. Moreover, neither of them would want to allow suspicion that because they are both health professionals they had fallen suspect to a depersonalizing aspect of health professions practice—namely, the health professionals' propensities to cover for, show favoritism toward, and link arms with other health professionals.[5] Any appearance that this is happening must be avoided. Therefore, whether the bonds of friendship are generally more binding than the health professional–patient relationship may be an extremely interesting question, but the governing framework for *this* situation (and Maureen's position of moral agency in it) must be the health professional–patient relationship.

The *fourth option* comes much closer than the previous three to a decision that takes the following important ethical considerations into account:

1. The health professional–patient relationship as the proper relationship governing the decision
2. The principle of justice
3. An indication that degree of clinical need is the common element by which all four patients can be compared.

More detailed discussion regarding the criteria on which to base distributive justice decisions in health care will be postponed until Chapter 14. Here it is sufficient to point out that the degree of clinical need combined with Maureen's potential to be of benefit in each case is a reliable guide for the type of decision Maureen must make.[6] Because the patients' needs differ, Maureen does not have to resort to other criteria of selection (*the fifth option*).

If Maureen accepts this type of reasoning regarding the proper moral criteria for determining who should be accepted for treatment, it should in no way diminish her desire to expend her best energies for Daniela. The *sixth option* would enable her to do just that. By accepting the others on the basis of their greater medical need, she would meet the requirements of fairness to the other patients, who would receive treatment instead, but this does not prevent Maureen from taking an extra step to help her colleague. Philosophers call Maureen's conduct *supererogatory,* a type of morally praiseworthy conduct that goes beyond duty.[7] The problem for Maureen (and anyone who falls back on this solution), of course, is that although it might make her feel better about this particular situation, it cannot be used as a general practice to always "fix" conflicts involving how to deal with scarce resources.

Reflection

If you listed additional options, this is a good time to take a few minutes and analyze each, using a process similar to the one I used to analyze the others.

Step 5: Complete the Action

If Maureen decides not to show any favoritism toward her friend, we have helped her move in the direction of getting her priorities in order so that however much she may wish she did not face a dilemma, at least she knows why she will set priorities as she does.

Reflection

Now that you have walked through the options and know that she is at the decision point, what do you think she should do?

Step 6: Evaluate the Process and Outcome

Once the deed is done, Maureen would be wise to evaluate it. Hopefully, her action will have been such that a desire to give preferential treatment to a friend or close colleague will have been successfully weighed against the demands of her moral role as a professional. In her reflection, Maureen may wish to take this issue up with the other members of the team so that all of them will be better able to face a similar situation in the future with more confidence.

SUMMARY

One's loyalty to friendship does not preclude the moral necessity of honoring the tenets of ethical practice as a professional.

Peer Evaluation Issues

A second category of ethical challenge to team members arises around the concept of peer evaluation, or *peer review*. Increasingly, members of professional organizations, educational institutions, and treatment facilities are being asked to evaluate the quality of their colleague's work and moral character.[8]

Peer review is designed primarily to ensure that high standards of professional practice are upheld. The standards may be set by the professional body itself or may be imposed by governmental or other agencies. Health care institutions such as your place of employment may have mandatory peer review mechanisms, and you will be expected to participate in them.

Peer review often generates data that then become a basis for comparisons among similarly situated colleagues. It may be a source that is referred to when salary increases, honors, promotions, or other work-related distinctions are being determined. Reference letters and letters of recommendation for a new job are one form of peer review. A peer review also can become a source of evidence when a person is fired, demoted, denied tenure or licensure, or in other ways has negative sanctions imposed.

Therefore, although the main emphasis in peer review is on its value as a procedure to ensure that standards and practices remain of high quality in the health professions, it also functions secondarily as a personal profile of a person's progress (or lack of it) in attaining professional stature. With this understanding of peer review, let us go back to the character of Maureen Sitler, whom you met at the outset of this chapter. But now the focus will be on her relationship with her colleague, Tom Morgane. Maureen and Tom Morgane have not told anyone at work that they are in love and are planning to be married in autumn. They are both in their early 30s and wish to remain at their current place of employment because of the benefits they have built up by staying there, their favorable opportunities for advancement, and also because they enjoy the part of the country where they live.

Although both are about the same age, Maureen has worked longer as a respiratory therapist, and everyone agrees that she is exceptionally well qualified as director of the respiratory therapy unit in the ICU. She has written several articles, engaged in clinical studies, and learned some difficult diagnostic techniques through special training.

News has just come out that Sandra Haynes has decided to take a position elsewhere. The hospital administration has decided to unite Maureen's and Sandra's departments into one large hospital department, and a nationwide search will be conducted to find the best person to head this department. Within the hospital itself two people are obvious contenders. Maureen is one contender and the other is a woman who has been in the other department about as long as Maureen has been in the ICU and who seems well qualified.

After the first extensive search is made, four people are still in the running. Both Maureen and the other woman are among them. As part of the administration's attempt to make an informed choice, they now ask several people to submit peer evaluations of Maureen and the other candidate. Tom is among those asked to make this peer evaluation of each of the two candidates.

Maureen and Tom are elated at the possibility that Maureen may be appointed director of the new department. Tom believes not only that Maureen is well qualified, but also that she very much wants the position. They both are aware that her substantial increase in salary would be helpful for them financially and may even enable them to put a down payment on a house.

Reflection

Should he write a letter of recommendation for his fiancée? Why or why not?

Following is the way I reason out this situation. See if you agree and why or why not?

Tom may think that whatever he says is not going to make a difference anyway. But that is an avoidance of assuming the responsibility he has been asked to assume. From a moral standpoint, he should try to work out a method of acting responsibly by writing the assessments. At the same time, anyone who finds out about his "other" relationship with Maureen will certainly cast doubt on his objectivity and, likely, his intentions.

Because the primary purpose of peer evaluations should be to help maintain the high standards of professional practice, he must do some soul-searching to assure himself that the high esteem he has for Maureen professionally really is based on the high quality of her work and her skills. If he can give a positive response to that issue, he should go ahead, letting the administration know, however, that he and Maureen are engaged to be married. He should document his statement with examples of the work of each and try especially hard to recall areas he believes each can continue to grow. Disclosing that he has a vested interest as a friend or fiancée will allow the person reading his peer assessment to take into consideration the bias he may introduce. Hopefully, the person reading the review will know that it is difficult enough to evaluate one's peers and that additional difficulty is introduced by their personal relationship.

Even when the added component of friendship or a love relationship is not present, peer review by team members can be an emotionally taxing situation. Essentially you are being asked to engage in a process of affirming or discrediting your fellow team members in relation to their professional quality and skills. Why is it so difficult? In the first place, all health professionals have some doubt about their own judgments from time to time, simply because the nature of professional practice is fraught with ambiguities. As a result, it is not surprising if you are hesitant to pass negative judgment on someone else's activities, knowing well that everyone has an Achilles' heel. Second, there is the fear that if you are too rough on colleagues, the tables may one day be turned on you. Finally, sometimes loyalty to one's profession acts as a deterrent to saying anything negative about one of its members. Whatever the source of the difficulty, the health professional who assumes this responsibility with an honest, fair, and compassionate approach can help to uphold the high standards of professional practice. In the end it will benefit the peer, patients, and the professionals themselves.

SUMMARY

The aim of peer review is to uphold the high standards of professional practice. Your participation in such a process is one of your professional responsibilities.

In summary, the practice of involving several people in any review when it can be done without compromising confidentiality helps to mitigate biases and other difficulties. The person who reads peer evaluations (i.e., the administrator, search committee chairperson, or other evaluator) will look for areas of congruence among the several reviewers. If one evaluation is radically out of line with the others, further clarification may be sought.

Blowing the Whistle on Unethical or Incompetent Colleagues

A serious ethical challenge of another type arises when there is evidence that a team member is engaging in unethical or incompetent behavior. When such a person is reported, the person or persons making the report are called *whistle-blowers,* and their action is called *whistle-blowing.*

Currently, professional organizations, as well as government licensing and disciplinary boards, are acknowledging that unethical and incompetent behavior does occur by health professionals, clinical investigators, and health care administrators. The bases of such behaviors include severe substance abuse, the apparent inability to exercise sound professional judgment, severe depression, paranoia or other mental disorders, sexual abuse of patients, theft from patients or institutions, chronic lying, fee splitting, and practicing without a license or under other false pretenses. You need not watch soap operas to know that health professionals include all types of people.

To make matters more complicated, usually the knowledge of harm to patients or colleagues gradually comes to the attention of colleagues, and often in a form that creates many questions about the legitimacy of the rumor, the mental stability of the person in question, or other troubling factors. A rumor is heard that Miss Werthheimer, a nursing unit clerk, accused Patient A of threatening to kill her by poisoning her food, and she claims to have reported him to the CIA. Mr. Grabowski, a surgical technician, is said to have reported to work after an unexplained absence of 3 days with the smell of whisky on his breath and contaminated the surgical suite by not scrubbing in properly. Money has been reported missing from patients' homes after Mrs. Waltham has made a home visit to them. The mother of a young boy accuses Alan DeJong of sexually abusing him during a recent treatment. An old woman claims that Dr. Sakabuto tried to suffocate her with a pillow during the night. Word is out that Mr. Fried forged his papers and is not a graduate of an approved school.

These dramatic cases are the types that hit the newspapers if the wrongdoing is verified and made public. At the same time, more common problems arise that are not as dramatic but that potentially are just as dangerous to patients. For instance, take the case of a health professional who has family problems and copes by excessive drinking or abuse of over-the-counter or prescription medications.

These rumors are about people one works with, side by side, consults with, and has shared lunch or coffee with for months or years. Even the person who seems rather strange or is considered a loner is more easily dismissed as a curiosity than viewed as an enemy among the ranks. Unfortunately, rumors are more easily believed as carrying a kernel of truth when the person is disliked or suspected in the first place. But, even so, in almost all cases, this type of rumor is first met with disbelief by most people. Indeed, to base one's judgment solely on such a report would be morally indefensible behavior.

Reflection

What should guide you in your attempt to arrive at a caring response when faced with hearsay information?

As in most such situations, the information should not be totally denied or ignored, but no final judgment against the person should be made on this tenuous ground. The process of gathering relevant information must be taken seriously. The characteristics of the person who makes the complaint should be taken into consideration, but he or she should never be dismissed as senile, crazy, irrational, or otherwise unable to report accurately what has happened. At the very least the person making the complaint should be asked directly for details. A further step is to ask whether he or she is willing to put the complaint into writing. Although this in itself does not render the alleged offender guilty, it is a sign that the person observing the conduct is willing to describe his or her perceptions of the situation in writing and probably would be willing to defend it before a grievance committee or in a court of law if necessary. Hesitance to report someone in cases of a real offense often comes from fear of reprisal from the alleged offender or fear of stigma (e.g., in cases of rape).

In all but the most serious cases it is wise to hold final judgment in abeyance as long as the report remains at the level of one report by one person, especially if the person is not willing to put the incident into writing. However, if a pattern of alleged abuses or mistakes emerges, it definitely must be followed up immediately. Almost all institutions currently have appropriate processes for reporting suspicious or outright improper conduct. These processes are designed to protect the rights of everyone involved, to provide *due process* under the law, and should be followed rigorously. Of course, neither 2 nor 200 complaints *in themselves* render an alleged offender guilty. For example, in Nazi Germany, health professionals refusing to engage in inhumane medical research on prisoners were condemned as criminals by many other members of the German medical community (except, of course, the members of that community already in prison camps). You and I would hardly count them as guilty!

The moral decision to blow the whistle on a fellow team member can be among the most agonizing in your role as a health professional.[9] From a psychological viewpoint, there is tremendous potential for your own ego, beliefs, and hopes to take a battering. The loss of an errant colleague also can signal the loss of a friend or the loss of your belief in an ideal you thought was a shared ideal (Fig. 8–1). Understandably, it is a comfort to believe that you will not be faced with such a dilemma, especially if the offender is a close friend. But

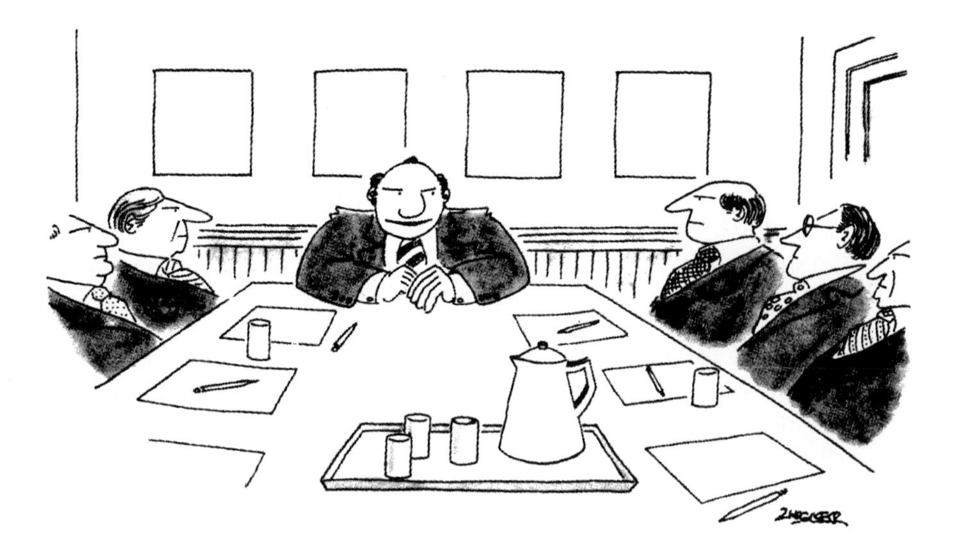

"Of course what we're doing is wrong, but that doesn't make it indefensible."

Figure 8–1. Drawing by Ziegler, ©1977 *The New Yorker* Collection. From cartoonbank.com. All rights reserved.

to hope for such good fortune does not excuse you from trying to prepare for it. Your moral character is always tested. It takes a full dose of courage, patience, fortitude, a striving toward justice, much compassion, and a capacity for sympathetic involvement to know when and how to proceed with incriminating evidence when a colleague or friend is implicated.

Reflection

Before reading ahead, list the alternate courses of action you could take if you increasingly believed that your colleague was seriously addicted to alcohol.

____

____

____

____

One alternative in some situations is to stave off a developing problem before a real offense is committed. Often, the breaking point between a professional's attempt to maintain self-esteem or professional responsibilities and total resignation to the destructive forces at work within is the realization that colleagues have turned their backs. Most people know when they are in trouble. At the point of greatest need and alienation a direct contact coming from someone who cares enough to confront the problem tactfully often can provide courage for one to seek help and can be the thin thread back to more sound functioning. Morag Coate, a British writer quoted in Kay Jamison's book *Night Falls Fast: Understanding Suicide,* was contemplating suicide but decided not to take her life when she became convinced that her doctor cared. She wrote afterward, "Because the doctors cared, and because one of them still believed in me when I believed in nothing, I have survived to tell the tale."[10] It is no different if the one "who believes in nothing," for whatever problem he or she is facing, is a patient or a teammate. Often, the one link is sufficient for the person who is spinning out of control to get her or his bearings.

Whenever possible, you should act to affirm such a person as someone in a struggle and offer your support. This may include suggesting that the person *not* continue to practice, at least until he or she is on more solid footing. The motivation for risking yourself enough to reach out to a fellow team member in distress often arises from a sense that it could be you in a similar situation and that, in some fundamental regard, we all are in the game together. Many years ago the poet John Donne captured our interdependence in this famous phrase:

> No man is an island, entire of itself; every man is a piece of the continent, a part of the main; if a clod be washed away by the sea, Europe is the less . . . any man's death diminishes me, because I am

involved in mankind; and therefore never send to know for whom the bell tolls; it tolls for thee.[11]

Of course, another possible course is to do nothing. The shortcoming of this position is that once you have identified the potential problem, doing nothing also is a course of action. When harm to patients is likely to ensue, your neglect has become complicity. The professional disciplinary committees of most states and the codes of ethics of most professions now count this as an offense as serious as committing wrongdoing yourself. Chapters 5 and 6 addressed this situation briefly in the discussion of your moral agency as a student and as a professional.

Reflection

If you have not already done so, check the code of ethics of your chosen profession to see if it includes a statement of responsibility to report unethical or incompetent colleagues.

A third course is to act decisively to remove the individual from a position in which he or she can do further harm. This is the appropriate course of action once the relevant information has been gathered and analyzed and is persuasive. A secure rule of thumb is to keep the information as contained as possible; use the usual channels of communication and institutional or other disciplinary mechanisms designed for this purpose. It is extremely important to honor the alleged violator's privacy, respect, and legal rights, no matter how grievous a "crime" you may think the person has committed.

Unquestionably, there are some difficult judgment calls involved in actually taking the final step of whistle-blowing. For instance, if possible, you should warn the person that you have reached the point where you plan to call attention to an alleged violation of ethical, competency, or legal standards. Also, you should decide whether to talk to anyone else before you act, knowing that sometimes there is strength in numbers and also that your own perceptions may be skewed. Finally, you should give careful attention to whether you have exhausted the other possibilities that may allow you to take a less radical step and still be responsible in your role as a moral agent.

Should you be faced with a whistle-blowing situation, your ability to strike a balance between your sensitivity to the situation and commitment to proceed will be one of the greatest challenges you face as a health professional. The attention you have given to it here will serve you well.

As always, any opportunity you have to help prevent such moments is time extremely well spent! Short of that, if your institution has developed guidelines about unethical or incompetent conduct, use them as aids. If not, you can contribute greatly to the constructive functioning of the institution by helping to develop policies that will implement whistle-blowing procedures with the following goals:

- to encourage thorough documentation
- to maintain due process judiciously
- to provide as much support all around as possible
- to require that the institution persevere to the completion of the review

Completion probably will involve the role of several others, such as administrators, regulatory board members, risk managers, or designated people in professional associations. The actual personnel and processes will vary. Your job in seeing the issue to completion is to work diligently within prescribed institutional mechanisms.

> **SUMMARY**
>
> Whistle-blowing may involve reporting impaired, unethical, or incompetent colleagues. You have a right to expect your institution to protect all parties involved in following up on your report.

It is in the heat of challenging situations that certain character traits disposing you to be thoughtful also will help you to know whether and how to proceed. An acute sensitivity to the various people affected, combined with the courage to act and the desire to act compassionately, are useful tools at such a moment.

Summary

This chapter focuses on several sources of support professionals have and can offer as members of a health care team. You have a right to expect support from your teammates and from your institution. The challenge of remaining ethical in peer evaluation situations was discussed, as well as serious challenges that arise when a colleague is engaging in unethical or illegal behavior. In the latter situation, the person may be ill, extremely stressed, addicted, or devious. Whatever the cause, your motive for whistle-blowing or other considered action is to protect patients, clients, or even society from the harm such a person may cause. Your moral agency positions you so that you can do no less than that.

Questions for Thought and Discussion

1. Uri is one of your colleagues. You and Uri enjoy a good working relationship, although you do not know much about his personal life outside of the work situation. You notice that during the past few days he has become increasingly irritable toward you. You wonder if it is something you have said or done that is making him angry.

a. What steps, if any, should you take to address this issue?

b. Would it make any difference in how you proceed if it appears that his attitude is interfering with the quality of his work? Why?

c. If he denies that it has anything to do with you, but his behavior begins to deteriorate to the point of his sharp responses to patient queries, what criteria would be useful for judging how far to pursue the issue?

2. You are asked to give a job recommendation for your friend Arthur. You have worked with Arthur for more than a year on the same health care team and feel qualified to provide such a recommendation. Arthur is an energetic, fun-loving person, and you enjoy his friendship. His manner with patients is sometimes disturbing to you, however. He seems careless at times, almost to the point of incompetence. Quite honestly you would have to recommend him with qualification for the position for which he is applying.
   a. Why would you agree or refuse to provide a recommendation?

   b. Do you have a responsibility to your colleague to tell him that you are giving him a "qualified" recommendation? Why or why not?

c. Do you have a responsibility to tell the party requesting the recommendation that you and Arthur are friends? Explain your position.

3. Dr. Heisler is a senior physician in the unit where Ms. McKenzie, a nurse, works. At about 7:00 PM, he is admitted to the unit as a patient complaining of chest pain and is seen by a colleague, Dr. Phillips. Several hours later, Dr. Heisler calls Ms. McKenzie, the head nurse on the unit, into his room and asks her for a sleeping pill. She says that Dr. Phillips did not order a sleeping pill, reportedly because Dr. Heisler said he did not need one. Dr. Heisler says that now he needs one. She puts in a call to Dr. Phillips but he does not return it. Dr. Heisler is getting more and more aggravated. Should she give it to him from the large supply of sleeping pills in her supply room? Defend why or why not, drawing on the duties, rights, and role issues discussed in your study of ethics so far.

4. Describe some areas of difference and similarity between the health professional–patient relationship and the relationship that exists between two friends.

5. You are told by a young patient, whose complications from child birth required her to remain hospitalized on the obstetrics ward, that Dr. Redmarck, a medical resident assigned to her case, is acting "inappropriately" toward her. She says she is scared, and she looks it. When you ask what she means, she says, "Twice this week he has stopped in during the late evening and has asked to examine my breasts. At first I didn't think anything about it, but then I started thinking that it didn't have anything to do with my condition. . . . He pulls the covers way back, and lifts up my gown. The way he looks at me and touches me down there. There's something strange. I dread seeing him." What steps would you take in response to this information?

6. You have been asked by the institution where you work to be on a policy committee dealing with whistle-blowing. Outline the steps that you think should be included in a policy document designed to protect all parties involved in a whistle-blowing situation.

References

1. Purtilo, R., Haddad, A. 2002. Enhancing self respect through good personal habits. In *Health Professional and Patient Interaction* (6th ed.). Philadelphia: WB Saunders, pp. 98–102.
2. Purtilo, R. 2000. Thirty-First Mary McMillan Lecture: A time to harvest, a time to sow: ethics for a shifting landscape. *Physical Therapy* 80:1112–1119.
3. Purtilo, R., Haddad, A. 2002. Professional boundaries guided by respect. In *Health Professional and Patient Interaction* (6th ed.). Philadelphia: WB Saunders, pp. 207–222.
4. Purtilo, R. 2004. Professional-patient relationship: Ethical issues. In Post, S. (Ed.), *Encyclopedia of Bioethics* (3rd ed., vol. 4). New York: Macmillan, pp. 2150–2157.
5. Ashley, B., O'Rourke, K. 1997. The health care profession. Section 4.1 Professions: depersonalizing trends. In *Health Care Ethics. A Theological Analysis* (4th ed.). Washington, DC: Georgetown University Press, pp. 69–71.
6. Sugarman, J. 2000. Conflicts of interest and obligation. In *20 Common Problems. Ethics in Primary Care*. New York: McGraw-Hill, pp. 98–99.
7. Beauchamp, T.L., Childress, J. 2001. The continuum from obligation to supererogation. In *Principles of Biomedical Ethics* (5th ed.). New York: Oxford University Press, pp. 41–43.
8. Purtilo, R. 2004. Teams-health care. In Post, S. (Ed.), *Encyclopedia of Bioethics* (3rd ed., vol. 5). New York: Macmillan, pp. 2495–2497.
9. Purtilo, R. 1994. Interdisciplinary health care teams and health care reform. *Journal of Law Medicine and Ethics* 22(2):121–126.
10. Jamison, K. 1999. *Night Falls Fast: Understanding Suicide*. New York: Knopf, p. 255.
11. Donne, J. 1623. *Devotions XVII*.

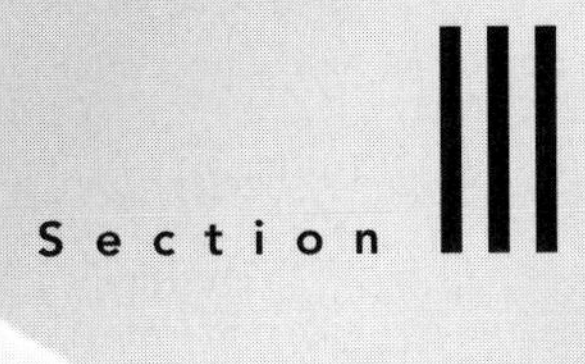

Ethical Dimensions of the Professional–Patient Relationship

9

Why Honor Confidentiality?

Objectives

The student should be able to:

- Define the terms *confidential information* and *confidentiality*.
- Identify the relationship of a patient's legal right to privacy with his reasonable expectations regarding confidential information.
- Describe how the telling and keeping of secrets is relevant to understanding the importance of confidentiality.
- Discuss the ethical norms involved in keeping and breaking professional confidences.
- Name five general legal exceptions to the professional standard of practice that confidences should not be broken.
- Consider practical options that a professional can take when faced with the possibility of breaking a confidence.
- Discuss some important aspects of documentation that affect confidentiality.
- Compare ethical issues of confidentiality traditionally conceived with those that have arisen because of computerized medical records and patient care information systems.
- Describe the key ethical strengths and challenges of the recent U.S. federal regulations related to privacy considerations (Health Insurance Portability and Accountability Act of 1996).

New terms and ideas you will encounter in this chapter

confidential information
trust
Health Insurance Portability and Accountability Act of 1996 (HIPAA)
secrets
right to privacy
protected health information
confidentiality
patient care information systems (PCIS)

Topics in this chapter introduced in earlier chapters

Topic	*Introduced in chapter*
Hippocratic Oath	1
Beneficence	3
Nonmaleficence	3
Fidelity	3
Autonomy	3
Character traits or virtues	3
Ethical dilemma	2
Paternalism	3

Introduction

In this and the next several chapters you will have an opportunity to think about specific ways in which patients or clients learn to put their trust in you. You already have met some patients through the case studies that have been presented to help focus your thinking, and in Chapter 7 you considered ways to make the health care environment as welcoming as humanly possible for such people. The idea of confidentiality in health care has ancient roots as a basic building block of trust between health professionals and patients. For instance, the Hippocratic Oath, written in the fourth century BC, says,

> And whatsoever I shall see or hear in the course of my profession, as well as outside my profession . . . if it be what should not be published abroad, I will never divulge, holding such things to be holy secrets.[1]

And so confidentiality is a splendid place to begin this focus on basic components of trust building. The story of Chaanda Jiwani, an occupational therapist, and Damian Doucet, a patient, helps set the stage for reflection on confidentiality.

The Story of Chaanda Jiwani and Damian Doucet

Chaanda Jiwani works as an occupational therapist in the student health center of a large university. Her patients are primarily outpatients who are students, but she also occasionally treats faculty or staff of the university. Although the student health center is in a building some distance from the university hospital, they are well connected electronically in one patient care information system. This arrangement allows Chaanda to enter her patient information into the hospital's database and also to receive instant, thorough information on any activity her patients may have in the larger health care system. This electronic record also contains patients' previous health history and treatment activity. She refers to it many times each day and enters her own data each evening. And so it is that the clinical record of her patient, Damian Doucet, is in "the system," and his progress after a fall from his parents' roof is being narrated. He has seen a surgeon, several nurses, and when he was preparing for discharge, a social worker. He is now being seen as an outpatient to regain function of his right hand, which was injured in the fall.

Chaanda has been taught to document all relevant information about a patient. Therefore, she is surprised about her own reluctance to record a conversation that occurred between Damian and herself today. During their treatment session, Damian blurts out that he is HIV-positive but that he was tested in another state and has decided to enter dental school in this university and to keep his secret from everyone.

He says to Chaanda, "I probably shouldn't have told you about this either. Now my secret is out. Please don't tell anyone. I am actually ashamed of it, you know. I don't want anybody to know about this. I am so afraid it might affect my career. A buddy of mine lost his health insurance when they found out he had AIDS. And I read that patients won't go to a doctor or dentist who is HIV-positive. Promise me you won't say anything!" She does not promise, but neither does she tell him that his secret is not safe. Instead, she tries to talk with him about the importance of seeking medical care and of being followed for troubling symptoms that may arise. But he says once again, "Please don't tell anyone."

Chaanda completes his treatment and goes to the computer. She opens his record and notes nothing about his being HIV-positive. She also realizes that if she does document this conversation, his secret will be out for everyone on the patient information system to read. Anyone who gains access to his clinical work for any purpose will know that he has told her he is HIV-positive. Suddenly she realizes that Damian has shared information with her that she really wishes she did not have. Now she wishes, too, that when he started talking about it she would have stopped him and said she could not promise to keep it confidential. But she didn't. Still, she feels that if she doesn't document their conversation, she could regret it later.

Reflection

What should she do next? Why? What should she ultimately do in regard to this situation? Why?

____

____

____

____

Many dimensions of her ethical quandary are identical to questions that have made confidentiality a compelling issue over the centuries. At the same time, the fact that this information is in regard to a virus that in many cases leads to full-blown AIDS, and that she lives in an era of computerized data entry, storage, and retrieval of patient information, her situation also is highly contemporary.

The Goal: A Caring Response

In light of all you have learned about Chaanda and Damian, you know that her ethical goal of finding a caring response requires her to address both traditional and contemporary dimensions of confidentiality and the specific type of confidential information that this patient has shared. She needs to be very clear about what confidentiality is and its appropriate use and limits. She needs to understand the related concept of privacy and to be savvy about new challenges regarding the use of computerized networks designed to manage information about patients.

Reflection

Can you define "confidential information"? Try to do so here before reading on.

____

____

____

____

The most commonly accepted idea of *confidential information* in the professions is that it is information about a patient or client that is harmful, shameful, or embarrassing. Does it necessarily have to come directly from that person? No. Information that is furnished by the patient directly, or comes to you in writing or through electronic data, or even from a third party might count as confidential.

Who is to be the judge of whether information is harmful, shameful, or embarrassing? The person himself or herself is the best judge, but any time you think a patient has a reasonable expectation that sensitive information will not be spread, it is best to err on the side of treating it as confidential. Of course, as Figure 9–1 illustrates, it is possible to go to extremes so that the best interests of the patient are lost in the process. A good general rule regarding potentially confidential information is to treat caution as a virtue.

Sometimes the notion of confidential information is discussed within the framework of the constitutional *right to privacy*.[2] It is not incorrect to do so because the right to privacy means that there are aspects of a person's being into which no one else should intrude. I will return to this idea of privacy later. At the same time, confidential information creates a situation a little different than privacy, taken alone.

Patients who share private information have chosen to relinquish their privacy because they have a reasonable expectation that sensitive information will be shared with certain people to further their welfare, but that it will be shared with no one else.[3] The patients think, "I may have to tell you something very private, perhaps some-

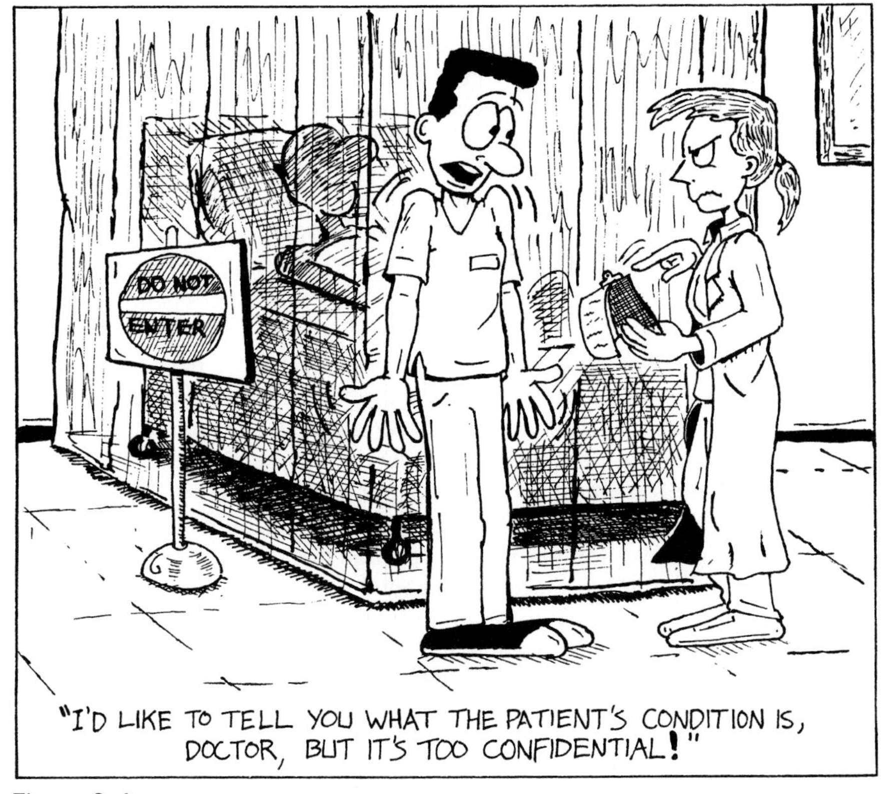

Figure 9–1.

thing I'm ashamed of, because I think you need to know it to plan what is best for me. But I do not want or expect you to spread the word around." There is an implicit understanding in the relationship that you, the professional, have a need to know certain things to perform your professional responsibilities.

When you have confidential information from patients, they have a right to expect that you will honor your professional promise of confidentiality.

Confidentiality is the practice of keeping harmful, shameful, or embarrassing patient information within proper bounds. Confidentiality always involves a relationship.

SUMMARY

Confidentiality is the most long-standing ethical dictum in health care codes of ethics.

Reflection

Go to the ethics code or other guidelines of your profession and write down what it says about confidentiality.

Developmental theorists tell us that concern about confidentiality begins when a child first is experiencing a desire to keep or tell *secrets*. Secrets manifest a developing sense of self as separate from others, and the desire to share secrets is an expression of reaching out for intimate relationships with others. How secrets are handled in those early stages of development can have long-lasting effects on an individual's sense of security, self-esteem, and success at developing intimacy.[4] The *power* of a secret, or of being in a position to tell a secret, is nowhere conveyed more clearly than when a 2-year-old child has a secret pertaining to someone's birthday present! When was the last time that you had a secret that was so potent it was difficult, maybe impossible, to keep it?

It is not considered a breach of confidentiality if you share "secret" information with other health professionals involved in the patient's care as long as the information has relevance to their role in the case. In fact, to share it is deemed essential for arriving at a caring response. A reliable general test for whom among team members should be given certain types of information is "the need to know" test. Do they need this information to help provide the most caring response to the patient?

SUMMARY

The immediate aims of confidential information are to:

1. Facilitate the sharing of sensitive information with the goal of helping the patient
2. Exclude unauthorized people from such information

It is a good idea to distinguish this type of information from that which a teammate might be interested to know, and especially from information that has no bearing on the teammate's ability to offer optimum care.

Keeping Confidences

In Chapters 2 and 3 you were introduced to the ideas of caring and the character traits that a health professional should cultivate. Keeping secret information that flows from patient to health professional is not valued as an end in itself but rather as an instrument that serves *trust*. And the ultimate value that both the keeping of confidences and the subsequent building of trust points to is human dignity.

SUMMARY

Keep confidences
to
Build trust into the relationship
to
Maintain patients' dignity

To decrease trust is to cause harm. Understandably, when there are no conflicts, the health professional will be motivated to keep the confidences entrusted to him or her because it has long been understood that a trusting health professional–patient relationship must be built. Confidentiality serves as one cornerstone for that solid foundation. However, that conflicts do arise in regard to keeping patient confidences is reflected in a number of codes of ethics. Many contain statements similar to this one from the American Medical Association (AMA) Principles of Medical Ethics:

> A physician shall respect the rights of patients, of colleagues and of other health professionals, and shall safeguard patient confidences within the constraints of the law.[5]

In such statements the conflict is presented as one in which the health professional's duty to benefit and refrain from harming a patient by keeping his secret is pitted against a duty to prevent harm to the patient himself, to someone else, or to society.

Breaking Confidences

In certain cases, the most caring response requires breaching the patient's confidence. Historically, such cases involved preventing harm to others, such as carriers of contagious diseases who wished to keep his or her condition a secret. The person did not have the prerogative of keeping her or his secret by requiring the professional to keep silent about the condition. Does this sound familiar? Currently, AIDS poses great challenges to confidentiality. Right away, that Damian declared himself to be HIV-positive raises some questions for Chaanda. She doesn't know if he is telling the truth, but his urgency in asking her to keep it confidential *suggests* he is. She doesn't know whether he has AIDS or has seroconverted to a positive HIV status without any of the clinical symptoms of AIDS. But she does know that certain behaviors he could engage in could harm others.

Legal exceptions to the standard of practice that confidences must be kept, except with the patient's consent or at the patient's request to break it, include the following[6]:

- An emergency in which keeping the confidence will harm the patient

- The patient is incompetent or incapacitated and a third party needs to be informed to be a surrogate decision-maker for the patient
- Third parties are at serious risk for harm (e.g., sexually transmitted diseases, child or other abuse)
- When requesting commitment or hospitalization of a psychiatrically ill patient
- When there is serious risk that many others may be harmed (a terrorist threat)

A good general rule of thumb is that you must not share confidential information unless it is authorized by the law or by the patient personally. The presumption is that health professionals will try to minimize the number of exceptions. Most patients do not know about the limits of confidentiality. It is a good practice to advise them before rather than after they have divulged sensitive information.

In conclusion, breaking confidences always entails at least one harm. Two questions I always ask when faced with such a decision are:

1. When is the harm of threatening the fragile trust in the relationship outweighed by the benefit?
2. How can the amount of harm be kept to a minimum when it becomes ethically appropriate to break a confidence?

The burden of proof is always on the health professional to minimize the harm.

The Six-Step Process in Confidentiality Situations

With the above description of what confidentiality is and when it may legally or ethically be breached, let us return to the story of Chaanda Jiwani and Damian Doucet to see how confidentiality works in everyday practice.

Step 1: Gather Relevant Information

One aspect of Chaanda's concern arises from the nature of Damian's comments. She always assumes that patients are telling the truth (until she has had it proven to the contrary). If so, she may want to talk to him more about his knowledge of his condition, because to do so will help her understand the situation better. Does he know that being HIV-positive means he can infect sexual partners? Does he know that some people who have an HIV-positive status (have "seroconverted") never go on to experience development of the clinical symptoms of AIDS? Has he sought treatment? Does he know that in this (and many) states a diagnosis of AIDS requires that the health professional making the diagnosis is legally required to report it to the health department? Has he told Chaanda because she is not in a position to diagnose the condition, but rather just to listen with a sympathetic ear?

Another avenue of discussion Chaanda may wish to pursue is *why* he does not want "anyone" to know. He has blurted out some reasons. In a probing analysis of what kinds of information people with AIDS share with those they care about, Klitzman and Bayer[7] show that often the patient has disclosed or withheld information on the basis of detailed moral, social, and psychological considerations involving deep emotional investment.

Steps 2 and 3: Identify the Type of Ethical Problem and the Ethics Approach to Analyze It

Chaanda knows that despite these caring responses, in the end it boils down to whether she should document their conversation in Damian's medical record, knowing that by doing so she is opening this information to others.

Reflection

What kind of ethical problem does Chaanda have? Is it ethical distress? An ethical dilemma? A locus of authority conflict? Take a minute to think about this before proceeding.

In some instances of confidentiality ethical distress may face the moral agent. However, Chaanda has not been prohibited from documenting the conversation. To the extent that she is experiencing such distress it is coming from her belief that she should, but knows when she does it may cause harm to Damian. At the very least it will shake his trust in her. In summary, she cannot achieve both the outcome of keeping the confidence and the one of doing her duty to document relevant information. She is facing a classical version of an ethical dilemma.

Reflection

From the standpoint of a health professional's goal of arriving at a caring response, name three ethical principles that will help guide your thinking about your conduct in regard to keeping confidences. Name some character traits that will help you in these challenging situations.

If you answered with the principles of beneficence, nonmaleficence, or fidelity and the right to autonomy, you are grasping the ethical principles or elements supporting confidentiality. A key character trait is trustworthiness (i.e., your part of the bargain if you are asking the patient to trust you). Other traits include kindness, compassion, and the courage to break confidences when it is ethically or legally necessary to do so.

Step 4: Explore the Practical Alternatives

What *options* does she have in trying to discern what to do?

One way that Chaanda can handle this situation is to keep the confidence by sharing it with another health professional on the team who would have a good reason to learn about this information. Often a health professional's inability to assess whether a person outside the immediate health care team should be given information leads the professional to discuss it with a trusted colleague first. For Chaanda, one person seems to be the obvious choice: a nurse practitioner who treated Damian at the hospital. Part of the motive of this discussion among professionals would be to clarify whether Damian has spoken to anyone else and also to confirm how she should proceed.

Often, an additional outcome of this type of in-house discussion is to determine whether further medical action on behalf of the patient should be taken. If so, and Damian remains unwilling to self-report, Chaanda will be in the type of situation that the AMA (and many other) codes have in mind when they suggest that breaking the confidence may "become necessary in order to protect the welfare of the individual." In Damian's case, Chaanda's colleague may agree wholeheartedly that his comments warrant documentation *and* follow-up. The nurse practitioner may suggest that Chaanda again recommend that Damian make an appointment to see one of the health center physicians. The suggestion could be put in such a way as to assure him that it is Chaanda's concern for him that prompts the suggestion. It may be exactly what Damian needs.

Another option for Chaanda would be to say nothing but still make note of the conversation on the patient's record.

Reflection

Do you think this is a good idea?

I don't. It breaks the confidence of the patient without taking any further direct action to let him know what she has decided to do and why. Although it may relieve the health professional's anxiety, at least momentarily, in this case it probably will serve little useful moral purpose in regard to helping Damian. In some cases, Chaanda may see this as her only alternative, but she has not yet tried to go back to Damian to warn him of what she has determined she must do.

It is quite possible that by going directly back to Damian and revealing to him in a supportive way that the conversation was deeply troubling to her, she will gain better insight into the seriousness of his comments. It is probable that if he is suffering from mental stress, she can be a help in getting him referred to someone who can assist him. But at least he will know that as he chose to proceed as he did (in telling her about his serious condition), Chaanda did not take his plight lightly.

Step 5: Complete the Action

This case, like many we discuss, does not admit of simple answers. It would seem, however, that given all the aspects of her role as a moral agent, Chaanda should go back to Damian immediately to discuss it further. She also should let him know that she is compelled to at least document the conversation because it is information highly relevant to his own care, as well as being a part of her moral duty to document such exchanges.

Step 6: Evaluate the Process and Outcome

Obviously, any caring professional would be concerned about the consequences of going against a patient's wishes in a situation where he thought he could count on the professional to keep a "deep, dark secret." Whatever Chaanda decides to do, she will benefit by taking time to review her actions and motives each step of the way.

Confidentiality, Records, and Patient Care Information Systems

Another aspect of confidentiality raised in this story is the process of information sharing and record keeping that goes on within the health care (and other institutional) systems. For example, Damian's report of being HIV-positive, if documented, will remain in his permanent file at the university health service, despite that he has not been treated for the condition there.

The issue of how far this information should and can go takes on greater importance when one considers modern, computerized systems of record keeping called *patient care information systems*. Virtually all major health care institutions and agencies currently use computerized data sheets that enable easy entry, storage, and retrieval of almost any information. This aspect of the patient's care has become so sophisticated that a group of professionals called *health information managers* are key members of the health care team. Their primary role is that they "are responsible for designing and maintaining the system that facilitates the collection, use and dissemination of health and medical information."[8] Depending on what is requested and the policies of the health care plan at this university, the information regarding Damian's self-report may be released to insurance agencies, registries of infectious and sexually transmitted disease, people conducting research, or future employers. In short, Damian is in danger of being *labeled* because of the diagnosis on his record. Chaanda must be aware that if she records their discussion, Damian may get stuck with a highly stigmatizing profile.

Although ethics as expressed in the codes of ethics of most health professions require that information about patients be kept confidential unless some strongly overriding argument for disclosure exists, the realities of modern health care make this almost impossible. As noted previously, these medical records are accessible to many different people and agencies, for many different reasons, and computerized data systems compound the problem. Thus, any information that may impair the patient's ability to function freely and confidently in society must be more carefully weighed than ever prior to it being recorded in the medical record.

The medical record is an extremely useful document for health professionals, however. If information about the patient is true and is relevant to his or her health care, then that information ought to be recorded there. At the same time harm can be done if faulty or vague information is included.

One example of this is the story of a middle-aged woman who was hospitalized at a university hospital where many invasive and dangerous procedures were carried out to evaluate a problem of incipient renal failure. Several doctors were writing the orders for these tests, and she judged that none of them bothered to explain fully what was being done or why, even though she signed consent forms. She became fearful, then hysterical, claiming that she could trust none of her doctors and that they were trying to kill her. She left the hospital against medical advice, and the intern writing her case summary included "acute paranoiac-type behavior" as one of the notations. Thus, her subsequent encounters with health professionals were strongly influenced by this incorrect "diagnosis."

In this case the patient was harmed by information in the record that was untrue. True information also can be harmful to a patient and, unless it is relevant to the health care of that person, should not be recorded. For example, a 62-year-old man hospitalized after a stroke was lying in bed and overheard two health professionals outside his room discussing how he had suffered his stroke while "getting it on" with his wife. He was embarrassed and angry and refused to accept their treatment attempts after that. It made him distrustful of all the other health professionals involved in his care, because he was sure that such gossip was not limited to the two whose conversation he had overheard. The information was written as part of his admitting history and physical: "The patient suddenly lost the function of his right arm and leg while having intercourse with his wife." This information is not relevant to his medical care and should not have been recorded on his chart. His privacy should have been respected in that regard, and the principle of confidentiality extended to excluding it from the medical record. Sexual activity or habits are sometimes relevant to medical care (e.g., in the case of sexually transmitted disease or sexual dysfunction), but if the information is not relevant, it need not and should not be recorded. In any case, such information should not be fodder for idle gossip in hospital corridors.

As you return to the story of Damian, it is important to recognize the great power of the information about your patients or others. Three guidelines are applicable:

1. Questionable information should be clearly labeled as questionable.
2. True information that is not relevant should not be recorded.
3. All information should be handled among health professionals with regard for the privacy and dignity of patients.

Information recorded in the medical record can be of great help or harm to the patient. For this reason the medical record needs to be treated with a great deal of respect. Health information managers and others involved with medical record information are usually highly aware of the power of these documents. They function as the gatekeepers for the records and rightfully take great pains to keep the records in order and to make sure that they are available to those professionals who need them and who have a right to see them. Conversely, they also need to be careful that the records are not abused or released to unauthorized persons. Sugarman notes:

> The increasing use of electronic medical records and the creation of computerized databases, while clearly beneficial for many aspects of patient care, raise important questions regarding privacy and confidentiality. The easy retrieval and transmission of such records make them tempting targets for those interested in unauthorized access.[9]

In the end *everyone* is responsible for the confidentiality of patient information, whether it be professional colleagues engaging in a conversation in the corridor, those handling the management of formal records, or the individual health professional being sure to properly dispose of work sheets and notes, taking care to log off the computer after use, and being vigilant in the use of fax or copy machines. The technology of health care information is only as effective as the professionals and others using the devices allow it to be.

SUMMARY

Confidentiality finally comes down to each professional being vigilant about the flow of patient information, guided by the goal of using information to help the patient. The medical record is the repository of this information.

Patient Privacy: Health Insurance Portability and Accountability Act of 1996

Earlier in this chapter the notion of privacy was mentioned as the right to keep information about oneself inaccessible to other people.

Traditionally, it has not been mentioned within codes of ethics in regards to confidentiality and, in fact, is a relatively new concept within health care. However, concerns about the use of sensitive information have led to much discussion by patients and the public in recent years, so that the notion of *private* information increasingly has been mentioned as relevant to considerations of confidentiality. For example, the following list of "confidential information" considerations from a recent textbook geared to palliative care teams includes the following:

- Identification: name, address, date of birth, sex, occupation, marital status, and so on, are all routinely collected by all health care organizations and are accessible to a wide range of administrative, clinical, and often ancillary staff such as those providing "hotel services" in hospitals.
- Medical information: diagnosis or diagnostic-related group, extent of the disease and disability, results of investigations, treatment details, and the medical history including alcohol or drug abuse. This is generally known to medical, nursing, and paramedical staff and also to administrative staff who process information.
- Social information: family and social relationships, housing, finances, and occupational history. This is accessible to the same group of staff as medical information.
- Psychological information: emotional state such as anxiety or depression; acceptance or denial of diagnostic information; marital, sexual, or family relationship problems; spiritual problems; and so on. This is accessible to medical, nursing, and paramedical staff, and to the extent that it is recorded in the notes or discussed verbally, it also is accessible to administrative staff who process the information.[10]

Reflection

Which of these items fit the older notion of "confidential information" as being that which is likely to be shameful or embarrassing to the person? As you can see, there is much more included than obviously "sensitive" information. Even a person's name or occupation is deemed sensitive.

One could argue that all information is sensitive, so in fact what is *private* versus what is *confidential* may become less of a distinction in years to come.

The United States has passed new regulations under the Health Insurance Portability and Accountability Act of 1996 (HIPAA), which impose considerable new constraints on the use and disclosure of a patient's personal and clinical information. These regulations went into effect in April 2003 and are in their first wave of use.

This set of regulations, called the New Federal Medical-Privacy Rule,[11] took 5 years to go into effect. The basic intent is to control the use or disclosure of "protected health information." One area that this rule strongly affects is the handling of information for purposes of research. It also has been interpreted to mean that information about patients (including family members) cannot be released.

"The rule concerns all 'individually identifiable' health information created or maintained by covered entity,* defined broadly as information about physical or mental health that either identifies an individual person or with respect to which there is a reasonable basis to believe the information can be used to identify the person."[12]

You are entering the health professions at a time when these new legal parameters about what can and cannot be shared will become a source of discussion, revision, and refinement, hopefully so that the intent of preventing undue invasion of a patient's privacy can be balanced against the legitimate incursions into privacy that have served patients' interests well over the centuries. In other words, the notion of privacy as a conceptual core for information that needs to be taken into account for patient care is an appropriate move. The details of how this will be best accomplished will continue to unfold.[13]

Summary

Keeping confidences is a general ethical guideline that the health professional can rely on to maintain trust and to foster dignity in the health professional–patient relationship. Sometimes, however, the interests of another person or of society or even the best interests of the patient seem to advise against keeping the confidence.

Current computerized methods of record keeping and information sharing raise additional, difficult ethical questions related to confidentiality. As a health professional you must rely on your considered judgment regarding the various moral obligations of professional practice, the rights of all involved, and the character traits that enable you to maintain a relationship of trust to arrive at a decision that is the most consistent with the goal of a caring response.

Questions for Thought and Discussion

1. The story of Mr. Shaw provides a good basis for thinking about some of the things you have just learned.

   Ann von Essen is a health professional, and David Shaw is a patient in the hospital where she works. He has been referred to her for discharge planning.

*A "covered entity" is defined as a health plan, data processing company, health care professional, or hospital.

Mr. Shaw is a pleasant man, 42 years old, whose family often is at his side during visiting hours. He was admitted to the hospital with numerous fractures and a contusion after an automobile accident in which his car "skidded out of control and hit a tree." He has no memory of the accident, but the person traveling behind him reported the scene.

The arrangement for his discharge is going smoothly. During one of Ann von Essen's visits, however, Mr. Shaw's mother, a wiry old woman of about 80 years, follows her down the corridor. At the elevator, Mrs. Shaw says, "I wish you'd tell sonny not to drive. It's those fits he has, you know. He's had 'em since he was a kid. Lordy, I'm scared to death he's going to kill himself and someone else too."

Ann is at a loss about what to say. She thanks Mrs. Shaw and jumps on the elevator. She goes down the elevator for one flight, gets off, and runs back up the stairs to the nurses' desk. She logs on to the computer to review Mr. Shaw's medical record and finds nothing about any type of seizures.

Put yourself in the place of Ann von Essen. Do you have confidential information? What should you do? Why?

___

___

___

___

Let us assume that in the state in which you work the law requires that people suffering from epileptic seizures be reported to the Department of Public Health, which in turn reports them to the Department of Motor Vehicles.

a. What do you think is the morally "right" action to take regarding Mr. Shaw once you have become the recipient of the information about his possible problem?

___

___

___

___

b. What duties and rights inform your decision about what to do?

___

___

___

___

2. Suppose you believe that it is morally right for the Department of Motor Vehicles to be advised of this situation. The obvious

course of action is for you to inform the physician, the physician to report to the Department of Public Health, and for them to report to the Department of Motor Vehicles. If any of the usual links in this process are broken by failure to communicate the information, do you have a responsibility to make sure the Department of Motor Vehicles has actually received this information? Defend your position regarding how far you believe you and anyone else in *your* profession should go in pursuing this matter.

References

1. Hippocrates. 1923. The Oath. In *Hippocrates I* (Jones, W.H.S., Trans., The Loeb Classic Library). Cambridge, MA: Harvard University Press, pp. 299–301.
2. *Griswold v Connecticut*. 1965. 381 U.S. 479. 85 S Ct. 1678.
3. Beauchamp, T.L., Childress, J. 2001. Professional-patient relationships. In *Principles of Biomedical Ethics* (5th ed.). New York: Oxford University Press, pp. 303–312.
4. Winslade, W. 2004. Confidentiality. In Post, S. (Ed.), *Encyclopedia of Bioethics* (3rd ed., vol. 4). New York: Macmillan, pp. 494–503.
5. American Medical Association. 2002. *Code of Medical Ethics*. Chicago: The Association.
6. Gutheil, T.G., Appelbaum, P.S. 1988. Confidentiality and privilege. In *Clinical Handbook of Psychiatry and the Law*. New York: McGraw-Hill, pp. 2–29.
7. Klitzman, R., Bayer, R. 2002. *Mortal Secrets. Truth and Lies in the Age of AIDS*. Baltimore: John Hopkins University Press.
8. Harman, L. 2001. *Ethical Challenges in the Management of Health Information*. Gaithersburg, MD: Aspen Publishers, Inc.
9. Sugarman, J. 2000. *20 Common Problems. Ethics in Primary Care*. New York: McGraw-Hill, pp. 158–159.
10. Randall, F., Downie, P. 1999. *Palliative Care Ethics. A Companion for all Specialties* (2nd ed.). New York: Oxford University Press, pp 152–153.
11. *Federal Register* 2002. 67:53182–53273.
12. Kulynych, J., Korn, D. 2002. The new federal medical privacy rule. *New England Journal of Medicine* 347(15):1133–1134.
13. Annas, G. 2003. HIPAA regulations—a new era of medical-record privacy? *New England Journal of Medicine* 348(15):1486–1490.

10

Why So Much Emphasis on Truth Telling?

Objectives

The student should be able to:

- Discuss the health professional's role as a person who should maintain a patient's hope.
- Identify one major argument that traditionally has been advanced regarding why patients should be protected from "bad news" and the ethical principles and reasoning that support this position.
- Identify major arguments that in recent years have been advanced as to why patients should be given information about their condition and the ethical principles and reasoning that support this position.
- Apply the six-step process of ethical analysis and decision making to truth-telling situations.
- Distinguish among the following notions: truth, deceit, lies, and truth telling.
- Define the terms *placebo* and *placebo effect*.
- Discuss possible benefits and harms of placebo use and the ethical principles that are important in analyzing placebo use from an ethics viewpoint.
- Identify three general guidelines for information disclosure that can be gleaned from the example of genetic information.

New terms and ideas you will encounter in this chapter

the professional's role to maintain hope
circularity
patient's right to information
genetic information
deceit
information disclosure
placebo effect
lies
benevolence
placebos
truth and falsehood
genetic counselor

Topics in this chapter introduced in earlier chapters

Topic	*Introduced in chapter*
Trust	2, 9
Honesty	2
Beneficence	3
Nonmaleficence	3
Veracity (truth telling)	3
Paternalism	3
Caring	2
Rights	3
Six-step process of ethical decision making	4
Ethical distress	2
Locus of authority problem	2
Deontology	3
Utilitarianism	3
Compassion	2
Ethics committees	1

Introduction

In Chapter 9 you were introduced to the value of trust and its role in confidentiality. In this chapter the focus is again on the idea of trust as it figures into truth-telling situations. In Chapter 11 trust is discussed in the context of informed consent.

In everyday life nothing is more central to a feeling of trust than assuming that others will be truthful in matters pertinent to our well-being. We assume that telling the truth is the right thing to do. Such action characterizes the honest person, and no one would question the moral value of honesty.

Therefore, it may come as a surprise that giving direct and honest answers to patients has long been a topic of controversy in the health professions, particularly when bad news must be conveyed. Questions of truth telling are complex because there are other moral considerations within the relationship that may appear to conflict with the idea that "honesty is the best policy." One of these norms is the disposition or character trait of benevolence—that one should be the type of person who behaves toward others in a way that is not menacing or harmful to them.

To help our discussion along, consider the story of Maria Priley and Kim Segard.

The Story of Maria Priley and Kim Segard

Maria Priley, an 87-year-old widow, had lived alone in her apartment for 12 years since her husband died, until 2 months ago when she slipped off the step stool in her kitchen and fell, fracturing her right hip. Her daughter

Diana, who lives across town, has checked in with her every other day or so ever since Mr. Priley died. When for 2 consecutive days her mother did not answer the phone, Diana became concerned. She rushed over to her mother's apartment. When she arrived she discovered that her mother had been lying on the floor for 2 days. She had pulled a comforter and pillow off the couch but had not been able to get to a phone.

The fracture has been healing slowly. Accordingly, Maria has been in a step-down unit in the local health care facility for 7 weeks. The social worker, Kim Segard, has been visiting her often to reassure her that all is well at the apartment, even though at times Kim has her doubts that Maria will be able to manage at home alone even if the fracture heals successfully. Maria is especially concerned about her canary and dog, although Diana reassures her that they are being well taken care of at Diana's home.

Kim has been working to help Mrs. Priley arrange her financial matters for securing the services of a home health aide when she returns home. However, at the beginning of the week Diana confided to Kim that she has decided her mother cannot go back to the apartment. Diana has begun to remove the furniture, take clothing to the Goodwill, and dispose of old belongings that her mother has refused to let go over the years. She also has begun looking for a nursing home for her mother and now asks for Kim's help.

Kim tells Diana that she believes Mrs. Priley should be brought in on the plans immediately. "Oh no!" Diana insists. "My mother would die right here and now if she knew she was not going back to her apartment. I have to have everything set up and simply bring her to her new home when she is discharged." She asks Kim to keep making plans with her mother for her mother's return home so that Maria "won't suspect anything." Kim argues that she is very uncomfortable doing this because she believes that in the end the deceit will harm Mrs. Priley. Diana says that she has already discussed this plan of action with Dr. Lee Hammill, the orthopedist who has been handling the case since the patient's surgery.

Kim calls Dr. Hammill, expressing her discomfort. Much to her surprise he says that he agrees with Diana's plan and urges Kim to buy into it, too. When Kim asks him why, he says that it is consistent with the way many families successfully have transitioned their elderly parents into a nursing home.

Maria continues to look forward to Kim's visits and talks excitedly about her return home. With each passing day Kim becomes more and more uncomfortable with having to carry on with this "charade" (as she has become accustomed to calling it).

This morning when Kim walks into Maria's room Maria is crying softly, a rosary draped across her hands. She says to Kim, "You know, dear, we have talked often and I have come to trust you. I'm grateful for the help you've given me and my daughter. But I have a feeling that something bad is going on. My daughter and Dr. Hammill are acting strange and yesterday my neighbor told me Diana and my grandson moved my old chest of drawers from my mother's home in Italy out the back door of my apartment! She hasn't said anything to you about moving me into a nursing home, has she?"

 ***Reflection***

What should Kim say? Should she tell Maria Priley what she knows? Not tell her? Take some other course of action? Defend your position.

The Goal: A Caring Response

In the history of health care there is a body of literature that would support not telling a patient bad news and one supporting the truthful course of action. Each course has been argued as being the most caring response. You will have an opportunity to think about your own conclusions on the matter as you read the arguments against and for disclosure.

Arguments Against Disclosure

The main argument advanced against disclosure of "bad news" is that the health professional role is to maintain the patient's hope, and hope may be shattered by bad news. That may be what Maria's daughter was concerned about, and often health professionals have the same thoughts.

Throughout most of the history of Western health care the patient has been defined as the one who needs to be cared for, who has little knowledge of medical science, who suffers passively from a disease, and who brings herself or himself to the health care system much in the same way that a car is brought to an automobile mechanic. As Edward said to Dr. Reilly in T. S. Eliot's *The Cocktail Party,*

> I can no longer act for myself.
> Coming to see you—That's the last decision
> I was capable of making. I am in your hands.
> I cannot take any further responsibility.[1]

Both character traits and duties are involved in this type of professional–patient encounter. A professional's *benevolent disposition* has been regarded as more important than an honest one, although both are extremely important. Duties involved in this type of situation include beneficence, nonmaleficence, and veracity.

> **SUMMARY**
>
> As you may recall from earlier discussions, sometimes the idea of beneficence involves acting independently of the patient's wishes. Such a way of acting is called paternalistic or parentalistic.

Arguments against disclosure of sensitive information have been based on paternalistic thinking. The health professional is privy to the awful truth of the inexorable progress of most diseases and decides what patients ought to be told based on an assessment of their welfare. Of course, such perceptions are heavily influenced by the professional's own concept of his or her role in the situation and attitudes about sickness and death.

This portrays a relationship that is unequal but well intentioned. Honesty is sacrificed to benevolence to maintain a patient's trust. As you can easily discern, Dr. Hammill is being benevolent insofar as he judges his course of action to be in Maria Priley's best interests. Now Kim Segard must make her own judgment about whether to act paternalistically or truthfully.

Arguments Favoring Disclosure

Today there is pressure on the health professions from within their own ranks (as well as from laypeople) to be candid and honest with patients. In the 1960s, Elisabeth Kübler-Ross,[2] a physician, spearheaded a revolutionary movement in health care by clarifying simple concepts about the dying process and making suggestions to improve care of the dying. She was convinced that patients with fatal illnesses could handle the truth about that awesome knowledge, and therefore information ought not be swept under the rug delicately but rather dealt with honestly, carefully, and realistically. She cited many cases of people having come to terms with the meaning of death and dying for themselves and their loved ones because they knew the truth about their own condition and its prognosis. Currently, thanks to Kübler-Ross and others like her, the topics of dying and death are not as taboo as they were a few years ago, but also there is a new openness in communication about many kinds of sensitive information. The idea that patients can handle difficult news, and may even benefit from knowing, has taken the health professionals down a new line of reasoning: the truth, rather than being a barrier to hope, may set the patient free. The AIDS epidemic has raised truth-telling questions and concerns to the forefront of health professionals' consciousness, because if the patient does not know, he or she cannot be responsible for preventing the spread of the disease.

In this interpretation an honest disposition is at least as important as, and is not necessarily in conflict with, a benevolent one. Acting truthfully is consistent with acting beneficently. You cannot discern what is "best" for the patient by making decisions independently on his or her behalf. Caring entails sharing pertinent information. The best way to maintain trust is to share relevant information with patients but to do so in ways that will be supportive of them.

Underlying this bias toward greater disclosure of information is the conviction that if you convey the message that you still care and have the intention and ability to comfort, then it is possible to tell the truth and still maintain the patient's trust and hope. Benevolence is expressed *through* honesty rather than played off *against* it.

Reflection

Give an example of when you think it is benevolent to share difficult information with a friend. What principles guide your thinking?

____

____

____

____

Today an additional factor supporting direct disclosure of information to patients is the understanding of patients' rights. It is believed that ***patients have a right to information*** about their conditions if they want this information.

SUMMARY

If a person has a right to X, then it is usually someone else's duty to give it to him or protect him in the possession of it.

Who shares the information depends on their relationship. In today's consumer-oriented health care system, patients sometimes are called "consumers." Accordingly, a U.S. Presidential Advisory Commission on Consumer Protection and Quality in the Health Care Industry developed a Consumer Bill of Rights and Responsibilities to capture the challenges confronting everyone.

There are several similarities and differences in these guidelines to others, including a new document entitled the "Patient Care Partnership," distributed by the American Hospital Association. References to the patients' right to know their condition and other details of their experience are included in the following phrases:

"You have the right to know the identity of doctors, nurses, and others involved in your care, and you have the right to know when they are students, residents or other trainees."

"If anything unexpected or significant (regarding your safety) happens during your hospital stay, you will be told what happened, and any resulting changes will be discussed with you."

"Please tell your caregivers if you need more information about treatment choices."

"Your doctor will explain the medical consequences of refusing recommended treatment."

"You will receive a Notice of Privacy Practices that describes the way we use, disclose, and safeguard patient information and that explains how you can obtain a copy of information from our records about your care."

"You also can expect to receive information and, where possible, training about the self-care you will need when you go home."

Finally,

"While you are here [in the hospital] you will receive more detailed notices about some of the rights you have as a hospital patient and how to exercise them."[3]

In such documents there is an assumption that a patient has a right to the truth about his or her condition, and it is reasonable to believe that you, the health professional, do not have the prerogative of withholding it. There is a duty to share the information if the patient wishes this information, and withholding it can be viewed as a type of injury to the patient's trust. If information is withheld, it must be on the basis of other moral considerations deemed more compelling than the patient's right and your corresponding duty to disclose in a given situation.

The Six-Step Process Regarding Truthful Disclosures

Dilemmas and the ethical distress problems that involve information disclosure lend themselves to a step-by-step analysis, just as other types of situations do. To illustrate, you have an opportunity to go, step by step, through the six-step process of decision making in the story of Maria Priley and Kim Segard.

Step 1: Gather Relevant Information

Kim's benevolence and honesty and her duties of beneficence and veracity support that she must attempt to assess Mrs. Priley's request accurately. It is possible that Mrs. Priley is asking Kim this question because she wants Kim to reassure her that she does not have to face losing the familiarity of her apartment. It also is possible that she wants reassurance that her daughter and grandson are not doing anything unacceptable behind her back.

It is important to be as sensitive as possible to the implicit, unspoken messages that are contained in language. This is true of all verbal communications between individuals. Here, Maria Priley is expressing a nameless fear with the statement that she has a "feeling that something bad is going on," fueled by her vulnerable situation at the moment. Often in such cases anxiety is heightened by the feelings of helplessness and insecurity that arise when an intelligent person who was strong and self-sufficient finds herself or himself in a situation in which there is reason to doubt the sincerity of those on whom the person depends. Here you can see one of the greatest risks of benevolence uncoupled from honesty: In assuming the responsibility for protecting a patient from knowledge we cannot protect her from the consequences and may, in fact, heighten her psychological torment by making her feel deceived by you, who also is charged with her care.

Mrs. Priley's real question may concern the extent of Kim's (and the health professions') commitment to her. She may be asking beyond "Am I going to a nursing home?" to "If I am, will you still care for me?" Mrs. Priley's anxiety illustrates well that fears of abandonment or other actions reflecting lack of respect toward the patient are not limited to people worried about their diagnosis! At such times, the therapeutic encounters in which the health professionals are involved must become the vehicle for such comfort. Regularly scheduled appointments, active gestures of caring, and just simply being there can assure the patient that the health professional, and by implication all the powers of the healing professions, will not abandon her or him.

In summary, the first important step in Kim's assessment of this situation is to *gather the relevant information* by gaining a better understanding of what Maria Priley is asking and what the sources of her discomfort are.

Reflection

I have listed some types of information I think are relevant. What other types of information would you want to have before proceeding in this situation?

____

____

____

____

Step 2: Identify the Type of Ethical Problem

In this situation Kim is faced with ethical distress. She thinks Maria Priley should have the information, but both Maria's daughter and her physician, Dr. Lee Hammill, disagree. Indeed, a central problem for Kim—and for health professionals other than physicians—specifically has to do with professional relationships. Nurses, therapists, chaplains, technologists, technicians, dietitians, pharmacists, social workers, and others may find themselves in the difficult position of being caught in the middle between the wishes of the physician and their own assessment of how a caring response consistent with the best interests of the patient can be realized. This situation was raised in Chapter 3 around the serious issue of whether a patient should be advised of a medical mistake if the health professional responsible for it does not take steps to disclose it.

The structure of the health care system, as it has developed throughout history, has been characterized by hierarchical relationships. All but physicians in this traditional hierarchy have been assigned the role to act in accordance with the best judgment of the physician. Recall that in Chapter 3 the radiologic technologist had information that the surgeon (and apparently also the radiologist) chose to conceal. The rationale in the traditional medical model was that the physician holds the greatest amount of concrete biomedical information; therefore, the physician was best qualified to coordinate necessary procedures and to make major therapy decisions, including what the patient needs to know. Currently, that model is being altered because more types of professionals serve as points of entry into the health care system and because of the greater sophistication of many team members. A well-coordinated team effort on behalf of the patient makes the most efficient use of resources, time, and energy and supports the patient's attitude of trust toward those entrusted with his or her care. But it appears in Kim's situation that both she and Dr. Hammill assume that the physician has the authority to decide whether and what information should be shared with Mrs. Priley.

Step 3: Use Ethics Theories or Approaches to Analyze the Problem

This step is designed to encourage you to reflect consciously on your basic ethical approach to complex problems, problems such as those illustrated by the story of Maria Priley.

SUMMARY

You probably have recognized that a heavy reliance on the duties and rights that come into conflict in this story places the analysis within the deontologic framework or approach to this issue.

It is not surprising that I am drawn to the deontologic approach, because much of the traditional health care approach to ethical problems relies on an understanding of our various duties, commitments, rights, or loyalties. Do you also find yourself thinking as a deontologist about this problem?

If you depend solely on neither duties nor rights, your approach may look more to the consequences that will be brought about by Kim's actions toward Maria Priley. In this case, you are reasoning as a *utilitarian*.

Reflection

Which consequences are relevant for your consideration in the story of Maria Priley and Kim Segard? Which ones would weigh the most heavily? Why?

Once you have identified relevant duties, rights, and consequences and have determined the approach you will use, you are in a position to determine an ***ideal*** course of action for Kim to take. This ideal course also should be guided by character traits of compassion and integrity.

As we live in a less than perfect world, however, Kim must now begin the arduous task of identifying the several practical alternatives.

Step 4: Explore the Practical Alternatives

Seemingly good rapport exists between the physician and social worker. Dr. Hammill expresses concern regarding Maria Priley's psychological state and apparently has given it much thought before making the decision not to talk with her about her daughter's decision. This decision has been reached "for her own good," and the information for its support has come not only from his past experience but from the patient's daughter. Still, Kim has now been asked directly by the patient, therefore this is new knowledge that both Diana and the physician should have. In other words, the door is open for Kim to again contact Dr. Hammill, reporting Maria Priley's question. Thus, the fourth step in Kim's process of moral judgment and action may well be to telephone the physician at once. In this action, Kim is fulfilling her professional loyalty to the physician in a way that is likely to benefit the patient as well. But this solution works only in a setting of good communication and mutual respect among the various members of the health care team.

Kim is still faced with the decision about what to say to Maria Priley in response to the question that was first posed. She could say, "I don't know all the details of your daughter's plans for you, but I can see you are really worried about it. Why don't you ask her and also the doctor about it when they come by later today?" Or, "Shall I speak to Dr. Hammill and tell him that you are concerned about this?"

Thinking prospectively, Kim's response at the time of the telephone conversation with Lee Hammill could have gone differently. Supposing you are Kim, you could:

- Advise the physician you will tell Mrs. Priley what you do know if she should ask directly. You will then know what to expect from the physician when it happens, or the conversation may give you some further insights into how you two professionals can best work together to make the most caring response possible.

- Tell the physician you would like to meet with Maria's daughter and him together so that everyone's judgment, feelings, and possible responses are shared information.
- Tell the physician you will not tell Maria what you know but will inform the physician of any pertinent questions or comments made by her.
- Suggest that Dr. Hammill talk to the nurse or to any other person who you know to be close to Mrs. Priley or who may have insight into how to proceed.
- Actively support the physician in his attempt to discover Maria Priley's wishes. This may lead to further discussion between you, putting you more on a basis of mutual trust and respect.

Or, before seeing Mrs. Priley again, you could:

- Think through possible conditions under which you will tell her the truth about the plans to have her move permanently to a nursing home.
- Talk to Diana Priley.
- Talk to the nurse or others who may have ideas about how Maria Priley will react.

If the situation were different and you (or any health professional) believed the physician was unresponsive to the patient's needs or was not open to communication of this sort from others, then the problem is much more difficult. If the physician is not acting in a way that seems to be furthering the patient's well-being, you could ask the ethics committee or ethics consultant in the institution to help. This is less likely to be appropriate for resolving the type of situation Kim is in than, for example, a decision not to reveal a serious diagnosis or to make a life-or-death decision regarding treatment if the patient is competent to participate in the decision. The important point is that such resources increasingly are available and have as their goal the resolution of ethical problems.

If all these alternatives fail, a last resort alternative is that you may decide to tell the patient yourself and risk the personal consequences. In many settings these consequences could range from a simple reprimand all the way to the loss of your job.

Reflection

Now that you have read *my* list of ideas about the practical options open to Kim, add some more of your own if you have them.

Step 5: Complete the Action

Whatever Kim decides to do, she now needs the courage to do it. The hardest case scenario will be if she decides she has to break faith with the physician. This should be considered only if:

- Kim is convinced the patient is requesting a direct answer *from her alone,*
- Kim believes that the patient's request can be honored *only* by Kim personally delivering that information, and
- Kim feels obligated to be the one to share the information despite the physician's and daughter's request that it not be shared.

Step 6: Evaluate the Process and Outcome

When Kim has completed the action, has she carried out her professional responsibility? If on reviewing her action she realizes it followed the most thorough and careful ethical analysis that she was able to exercise in this situation, she can rest assured that she has given everyone involved her best effort. Checking out your thinking with colleagues can further help you make an accurate assessment.

Truth, Truth Telling, and Deceit

We have been discussing Mrs. Priley's predicament as a truth-telling issue, but we have not really discussed the basic concepts involved: truth, falsehood, deceit, lies, and truth telling. To do so was not crucial for your thinking to this point, but it will be important for the next section on placebos. In philosophy there are whole theories of truth—a coherence theory, a correspondence theory, a performative one, and a pragmatic theory, among others—each of which tries to place truth within the world of our concepts. To think about truthfulness we should consider the question, "What is a *falsehood*?"

Summary

Truth is one of those wonderfully rich concepts in philosophy that is easiest to understand by talking about it in relation to its opposite.

If you answered, "an untruth," you are correct. How does untruth or falsehood function in our everyday life? When someone speaks a falsehood, it is either out of not having accurate information or out of intent to deceive the listener. When a moral agent has information but does not have accurate information, we judge the person to be ignorant. If it is information that another has a reasonable expectation of the person in question to have, we judge the person to be negligent. If the intent is to deceive, we say that the person is deceitful and his act is one of *lying*.

Summary

A lie is a falsehood based on intent to deceive.

Reflection

In Mrs. Priley's situation, she was not getting information about her future situation from her physician or social worker. Were they intending to deceive? Upon what do you base your opinion?

From what we know I believe they intended to deceive by failing to talk with the patient about the plans once it became clear that Maria's lack of information is causing her great distress. Although we usually do not talk about the withholding of information as lying, the neglect to provide accurate information when one is morally obligated to do so is a form of lying. This is called "an act of omission." In an earlier section of this chapter I described how today the ethical guidelines of the health professions treat information disclosure as a duty based on a patient's right to it. Whether telling an outright falsehood (i.e., "you have nothing to worry about, you will be going back to your apartment") or intentionally omitting key information the professional has that would allow the truth to be confirmed, the same deceitful end is achieved.

This brings us to our next practical point regarding these concepts. Information-sharing discussions in the health professions context are about making true statements or, as we usually call it, truth telling, on the basis that this best serves the patient well. And so we must explore the situation further to know how to judge Dr. Hammill's and, if she remains silent, Kim Segard's falsehood. As we have seen, Lee Hammill decided to deceive Maria Priley on the basis of a paternalistic posture toward this patient. We can conclude that the physician's intent is indeed to protect Mrs. Priley from suffering. Kim Segard is not at all convinced that the patient is actually benefiting from this deception. One should think of information as power to be used or abused by the moral agent. The very fact that Mrs. Priley has deep suspicions will cause most people considering the issue to conclude that she must be told about her situation in the most caring way possible. This may require the health professionals, working as a team with Diana, to develop a plan for how to share the information, why the initial course was taken and what kinds of support each is able to provide as this patient tries to come to grips with her future. In the end, the intent to deceive did not serve the positive purpose they had in mind, and this, combined with the wrong imposed by deceit in the first place, leaves him with no compelling moral argument for withholding the information from the patient.

I hope that this brief explanation of truth and falsehood will help you to examine your own conduct if you are confronted with challenging situations regarding information disclosure.

Placebos: A Special Case of Information Disclosure

The issue of *placebo* use has received some attention from psychiatrists and ethicists, but most of the literature on placebos has been directed toward physicians. Little research has been done concerning the role of other health professionals and the use of placebo medications and procedures, and yet nurses and pharmacists, in particular, play a direct and essential part in this particular form of deception in health care practice. To think clearly about the ethical problems that may arise in such a situation it is important to understand the physician's role in prescribing a placebo and some of the history and psychology of the placebo response.

Placebo comes from a Latin word meaning "I shall please." It can be defined as any therapeutic procedure (or component of one) that is given for a condition on which it has no known pharmacologic effect. A pure placebo is a preparation of an inert substance that is not known to have any pharmacologic effect. An impure placebo is an active drug given for its psychological effect even though it has no known effect on the disorder in question, such as an antibiotic for a common cold or other viral infection. Administering the latter type of placebo carries the risk for real side effects, as well as the interpersonal and professional risks we will discuss in regard to pure placebos.

Physicians rarely give pure placebos, such as sugar pills or saline injections, but when they do, serious ethical issues need to be considered. One important aspect of the practice of giving placebos is what is called the placebo effect. Virtually all treatments (and also some diagnostic studies) have positive effects for some patients over and above the specific effects of their pharmacologic mechanisms. Beecher[4] published the classic study in 1955 showing that placebos are effective in treating pain in 35% of patients, regardless of the source of pain or clinical condition of the patient. Later studies have done little to alter these percentages. Modern neuropharmacology research has discovered that the brain produces its own chemicals, which can act as analgesics and relaxants. These chemicals, called endorphins, seem to work better for some people than for others, which may explain scientifically why some people react to placebos and others do not. A common error made by health professionals has been the assumption that a symptom (e.g., pain) successfully treated by a placebo is therefore not real or is "only psychological."

SUMMARY

The discovery of endorphins gives us a scientific way of understanding some of the powerful physiologic effects of placebos.

The placebo effect may be partly responsible for the success of ancient remedies given by shamans or medicine men. Some of these remedies contained pharmacologically active agents, but others did not, and much of the healer's work consisted of rituals and symbols. That the medicine men often were successful is a tribute to the power of the therapeutic partnership.

Modern examples of the placebo effect are the effects of suggestion in decreasing stomach acid in patients with ulcers, alleviating bronchospasm in asthma, and decreasing blood pressure. The phenomenon of the placebo effect is widespread and powerful enough so that no research trials of new medications or even surgical procedures are considered truly rigorous unless the element of suggestion has been effectively eliminated, as in randomized, double-blind, clinical trials.

Some ethicists and others oppose the use of placebos in health care because they see it as an example of deception or outright lying. We have considered the problem of lying to patients in regard to the disclosure of situations that have serious consequences for the patient.

Reflection

Do you think there are times when placebo use would justify the deception? If no, why? If yes, what are they?

A utilitarian approach to thinking about the use of placebos would suggest that one must weigh positive effects against the possible negative ones that could result from placebo therapy.

Reflection

Thinking as a utilitarian, what do you think are some of the potential harmful consequences?

____

____

____

____

Now that you have listed some, following are two that often are suggested.

Loss of trust in the therapeutic relationship is viewed as one harmful consequence. Such deception preempts the patient's capacity to share in the responsibility for his or her health. Allowing deception in our professional and private relationships tends to diminish the overall quality of those relationships.

Inadequate diagnosis is another dangerous consequence.[5] If a physician is too quick to use a placebo for treating a patient's aches and pains, a potentially serious and treatable medical disorder may be overlooked. Thus, it is important that a thorough medical and psychological evaluation be made if the use of placebo therapy is to be considered.

Much of the harm attributed to placebo use comes when it is given without respect for the patient as a person. Physicians may prescribe placebos inappropriately: They may use them to prove patients wrong when they feel too angry to give the patient real medication, to punish problem patients, or to release staff frustrations.[6] Health professionals find it difficult to respect patients who respond to placebos because of our emphasis on mechanistic physiologic explanations. Many health professionals feel that a patient's positive response to a placebo indicates that the symptom is not real, even though this has been disproved by many studies, such as Beecher's study, and by the recent discovery of endorphins. A good response to placebos does not indicate that the patient is a hypochondriac. Patients in perfect mental health with real pain and illness may respond to placebos.[7] In fact, cooperative patients who have stable relationships with their caregivers are more likely to respond well to placebos than are the more difficult or less cooperative patients. Thus, these are significant risks that ought always to be kept in mind, but it seems unwise to rule out the possibility of placebo use completely. We are beginning to learn more about the therapeutic powers (psychological and chemical) of the mind, but we must also remember that we live in a society that has become dependent on pills and potions—symbolically and actually. Compassion allows us to use placebos in situations where a patient may be respectfully benefited and where that patient is likely to be unable to produce the desired effect without the symbol of the medication or other medical procedure.

Disclosure of Genetic Information

Two years ago, Meg Perkins was diagnosed with ovarian cancer. Recently, she was diagnosed with breast cancer. While scanning the Web to learn more about her condition she learns about ovarian–breast cancer syndrome, a genetically linked condition that manifests itself in ovarian and breast cancer. This is sobering news to her because she has two daughters of child-bearing age and wants to share any information she can with them about her condition if she has this syndrome, and, also, what it may mean for them. She also learns that some women who have this syndrome undergo prophylactic mastectomy or removal of their ovaries, although this is still controversial. She tells her daughters about what she has learned from her research on the Internet and that she plans to be tested. One daughter is anxious to learn everything she can; the other says she "wants nothing to do with this nonsense" and that she does not want to know the outcome of her mother's genetic testing.

Helen Williams is the genetic counselor that Meg visits after her test. Helen is faced with the difficult task of telling Meg that because her tests reveal the genetic conditions that put her at a 85% risk for having this syndrome, she is correct in thinking about how this involves the whole family. She also tells her that at least one of her two daughters is at a very high risk for experiencing development of cancer. The genetic counselor offers to provide Meg's husband and daughters with accurate information in language they can understand so that they will be able to make informed decisions. She explains to Meg that this is the job of the genetic counselor and that Meg is not different from many patients who, because of the expansion of genetic information, have found the need to seek professional counsel on this issue.[8]

Because disclosure of genetic information almost always is sensitive, rules of thumb for sharing such information provides the professional with some good insights regarding all types of disclosure.

How the information is conveyed matters. If Helen had said, "You have an 85% risk for a serious defect," it would convey a different story than, "You do have an 85% chance of a condition that has the following characteristics, generally speaking, but you also have a 15% chance that you do not have it." This illustrates that the profession of genetic counseling has as one of its ethical tenets to try to convey information in as neutral and encouraging language as possible. The goal is to optimize the autonomy and respect of all family members in their decisions. This is a posture that all health professionals guided by the goal of a caring response can exercise, no matter the type of information.

The extent of information also is important. Today, unexpected findings often accompany a genetic screening or laboratory test, therefore health professionals are faced with the challenge of deciding how much of the unexpected information should be included. The desire to determine the appropriate limits of sharing this additional information is not restricted to genetic information. Due regard for the patient and the significance of the additional information for the patient's health are warranted in any communication with the patient.

Genetic information sometimes creates a particularly unique social situation because of the multigenerational dimension of the findings and their deeply relational implications for the offspring.[9] The person with the genetic condition may not want other family members to feel guilty, may have fear about his or her possible contribution to the syndrome, or may fear that the news will cause psychological harm if the condition will lead to more challenges or suffering for loved ones. Because of the potent nature of genetic information, it also raises the question of whether a patient and his or her family members have a right *not to know*.

The Right Not to Know

Genetic information has enhanced the questions about the possibilities that individuals have a right not to know about information that could be harmful, shameful, or embarrassing about themselves and that they would choose not to know.

Suppose that Meg's daughters are identical twins. If one is tested and found to have the gene composition that gives her a high probability for the development of breast and ovarian cancer, and she decides to take the drastic measure of a prophylactic radical mastectomy before the appearance of cancer, her sister (who has the identical genetic makeup as her twin) who did not want to know inevitably *will* know that she has the gene.

The two sisters meet with Helen and discuss their conflict. Twin A says she will consider it abandonment if she is not tested and allowed to make this choice. Twin B says that she will be betrayed if, having been offered the opportunity and refused, Twin A is given the opportunity for testing then takes steps that will in fact reveal the status to Twin B. Is there any moral claim on the genetic team not to proceed with the genetic testing of Twin A?

The possibility of "the right not to know" certainly supports the idea that the professional ought not to force information on a client, compromising her psychological defenses and well-being. In our current story, however, the psychological well-being of one twin (A) appears in direct conflict with the other (B), and the resolution between them probably cannot be solved satisfactorily by the health professionals refusing to offer testing, counseling, and treatment to Twin A.

In summary, genetic information is especially powerful because of its ability to involve whole kinships. The extra precautions of care that physicians, geneticists, and genetic counselors use in disclosing genetic information provide useful cautions for all health professionals in the disclosure of any sensitive information.

Summary

The story of Mrs. Priley and Kim Segard, discussion of placebos, and the sketch about Meg and her daughters are examples of the ethical challenges involved in the issue of truth telling. Our discussion is intended to stimulate your thoughts on the subject and not to cover all the possible situations you are likely to encounter as you search for a caring response in truth-telling challenges. Here, as in the other issues in this section of the book, the decision about what to do must be influenced by what is deemed necessary for maintaining the patient's trust and for acknowledging his or her dignity as a human being. The six-step process will assist you in proceeding to a decision and acting on it. But the situation may require action in the face of seemingly unresolvable conflict or may carry the potential of dire personal consequences. At such moments the dispositions of honesty, benevolence, and courage support you in persevering in what you judge to be the most appropriate of the options available. The special case of placebo use and the challenges posed by genetic information illustrate how complex the disclosure of information can become. As you develop in your professional role, you will have ample opportunity for reflection and thoughtful action around these issues.

Questions for Thought and Discussion

1. Immanuel Kant, an influential philosopher of the formalist school who lived in the 1700s, declared, "The duty of being truthful . . . is unconditional. To be truthful in all declarations . . . is a sacred and absolutely commanding decree of reason, limited by no expediency."[10] In contrast, Nicolai Hartmann, a more contemporary philosopher, has maintained that in health care practice the health professional is sometimes required to tell the "necessary lie" to avoid inflicting great harm on the patient.[11] Describe where you are on this continuum and why. Give examples from health care to support your position.

2. You have been receiving placebos.
   a. What would be your initial response to your physician if she informed you the medication that was relieving your severe stomach pains was a sugar capsule?

   b. Suppose that your physician feels obliged to tell you about the placebo used to relieve your stomach problems. How might she disclose this information in a way that affirms the caring aspects of her relationship with you?

3. It has been maintained that patients have a right to complete information about their conditions. But what happens when the diagnosis reveals a *genetic* disorder that can have harmful effects on the children? Should the spouse automatically be told? The children? Other relatives? Who is "the patient" in such situations?

4. Is there a right *not* to know the truth? Under what, if any, conditions might such a right be argued?

References

1. Eliot, T.S. 1950. *The Cocktail Party.* London: Harcourt, Brace Jovanovich.
2. Kübler-Ross, E. 1969. *On Death and Dying.* New York: Macmillan.
3. American Hospital Association. 2003. The Patient Care Partnership. Chicago: The Association.
4. Beecher, H.K. 1955. The powerful placebo. *Journal of the American Medical Association* 159:1602–1606.
5. Garrett, T., Baillie, H., Garrett, R. 2001. Principles of confidentiality and truthfulness. In *Health Care Ethics. Principles and Problems* (4th ed.). Upper Saddle River, NJ: Prentice Hall, pp. 111–135.
6. Martinez, R. 2001. Losing empathy. Commentary. In Kuschner, T., Thomasma, D. (Eds.), *Ward Ethics: Dilemmas for Medical Students and Doctors in Training.* Cambridge, UK: Cambridge University Press, pp. 104–108.
7. Katz, J. 2002. The placebo effect of the physician. *The Silent World of Doctor and Patient.* Baltimore: The Johns Hopkins University Press, pp. 189–195.
8. Cummings, S. 2000. The genetics testing process: how much counseling is needed? *Journal of Clinical Oncology* 18(Suppl. 1):60s–64s.
9. Clayton, E. 2003. Review article. Ethical, legal, and social implications of genomic medicine. *New England Journal of Medicine* 349(6):562–569.
10. Kant, I. 1963. In *Lectures on Ethics* (Infield, L., Trans.). New York: Harper & Row, pp. 147–154.
11. Hartmann, N. 1932. *Ethics.* New York: Humanities Press, p. 282.

11

Why Care about Informed Consent?

Objectives

The student should be able to:

- Describe three basic legal concepts that led to the doctrine of informed consent.
- Describe three approaches to determining the disclosure standard for judging that a patient or client has been informed.
- Discuss three major aspects of the process of obtaining informed consent.
- Distinguish "general consent" from "special consent" documents.
- Differentiate between the never-competent and once-competent patient or client and the challenges posed by each in regard to informed consent.
- Compare informed consent as it is used in health care practice and in human studies research.
- Describe some considerations one must always take into account to be sure one is being culturally competent and honoring cultural difference when informed consent is the standard.

New terms and ideas you will encounter in this chapter

informed consent
battery (legal)
disclosure (legal)
fiduciary relationship (legal)
contract (legal)
disclosure standards
general consent
special consent
guardian (legal)
institutional review board (IRB)
voluntariness
mental competence or incompetence
mental capacitation or incapacitation
never competent
once competent
surrogate proxy consent
best interests standard
substituted judgment standard
advance directives

Topics in this chapter introduced in earlier chapters

Topic	*Introduced in chapter*
A caring response	2
Virtue	3
Autonomy	3
Beneficence	3
Nonmaleficence	3
Trust	2

Introduction

One important avenue to your success as a professional who has learned how to arrive at a caring response is to perfect the communication, listening, and interpretive skills required to honor *informed consent,* one of the cornerstones of the current U.S. and Canadian health care systems. Although the doctrine is the most formalized in these countries, it is an important concept in most Western health care systems. Whether engaging with patients, clients, or research subjects, basic principles of respect for the person undergird informed consent. By going step by step through the ethical decision-making process, the importance of several aspects of informed consent in achieving your goals as a moral agent should become apparent. To inform your thinking, consider the story of Jason Fruhling and Faye Nesbitt.

The Story of Jason Fruhling and Faye Nesbitt

Jason Fruhling, a 34-year-old cross-country truck driver, came to the emergency department of his hometown hospital because of "kidney problems" and dehydration. The health care team quickly decided that he should be admitted for further tests. He balked, saying he was "allergic" to hospitals but after talking to the doctor in the emergency department agreed to "stay overnight—that's all." Faye Nesbitt, a nurse practitioner from the renal unit, came down to the emergency department and accompanied him to the admissions area because he seemed very weak and a little disoriented. When the intake clerk presented him with the general hospital admissions informed consent form he retorted, "You got a noose around my neck. I know I gotta sign this thing to get treated." Faye encouraged him to read it and went over the main points with him.

Jason was admitted to the general medical unit because no beds were available in the renal unit. The next day he was presented with another consent form by the medical unit nurse, this one for the tests themselves, and he became belligerent. He asked for "that nurse that helped me last night." Faye was called from the renal unit and came into his room. He said he couldn't understand what they were trying to get him to do. She patiently explained the procedure he would undergo, referring to the informed consent form each step of the way. Although she herself thought it seemed quite well written, it took almost 20 minutes of talking with him before he decided to sign it. But when the imaging team took him to prep him with dye, he again became agitated, claiming he had never been told that they were going to "inject poison" into him. The imaging team leader took out the form and showed him the place where it had been discussed. He still seemed disgruntled but just shrugged his shoulders and said, "Okay. But I hope that woman who explained it to me knows she did a terrible job because I would have never signed it."

The imaging team gave some consideration to postponing his test, but when they asked him if this is what he wanted he grunted, "Go ahead! Do the test!" The team also thought about whether to tell Faye about his comment and decided to do so. At first she was annoyed, but later she found herself thinking about what to do to avoid this kind of thing happening to a patient again. Maybe he really *didn't* understand!

Reflection

Before you continue, take a minute to jot down your own response to this situation in regard to Faye's and the other health professionals' role in explaining the procedure. Can you think of anything else they could have done to help Jason?

You will have an opportunity to revisit their situation as you study this chapter. You can begin to assess it by comparing it with any experience you may have had in which you were asked to give your "informed consent" for a treatment or diagnostic intervention, or for participation as a research subject.

Reflection

If you have ever been asked to sign an informed consent form, could you understand it easily? Did you have to sign your name? Was there someone on hand to answer questions you may have had at the time or a telephone number where you could reach someone later? Did reading and signing the form make you feel more reassured about what you were about to experience? Why or why not?

Now that you have a story to refer to and have considered your own experience, if any, you are ready to read on about informed consent.

The Goal: A Caring Response

Informed consent is founded on basic legal–ethical principles, entails a process of decision making, and is a procedure. The idea is that you can perform your professional tasks better and in a morally praiseworthy way by bringing the person's informed preferences into your plans. In summary, it is another tool to assist you in your skillful search for what a caring response entails.

An example of an informed consent document is provided for you in Figure 11–1.

You can see from this example that an informed consent document spells out how the health professionals intend to use specific diagnostic or treatment interventions for the purpose of improving a patient's condition. If designed appropriately, the document enables the person to become well informed before entering into the decision-making process. Informed consent, then, becomes a vehicle

MEDICAL RECORD | **REQUEST FOR ADMINISTRATION OF ANESTHESIA AND FOR PERFORMANCE OF OPERATIONS AND OTHER PROCEDURES**

A. IDENTIFICATION

1. OPERATION OR PROCEDURE

B. STATEMENT OF REQUEST

1. The nature and purpose of the operation or procedure, possible alternative methods of treatment, the risks involved, and the possibility of complications have been fully explained to me. I acknowledge that no guarantees have been made to me concerning the results of the operation or procedure. I understand the nature of the operation or procedure to be ____________
(Description of operation or procedure in layman's language)

2. I request the performance of the above-named operation or procedure and of such additional operations or procedures as are found to be necessary or desirable, in the judgment of the professional staff of the below-named medical facility, during the course of the above-named operation or procedure.

3. I request the administration of such anesthesia as may be considered necessary or advisable in the judgment of the professional staff of the below-named medical facility.

4. Exceptions to surgery or anesthesia, if any, are: ____________
(If "none", so state)

5. I request the disposal by authorities of the below-named medical facility of any tissues or parts which it may be necessary to remove.

6. I understand that photographs and movies may be taken of this operation, and that they may be viewed by various personnel undergoing training or indoctrination at this or other facilities. I consent to the taking of such pictures and observation of the operation by authorized personnel, subject to the following conditions:

a. The name of the patient and his/her family is not used to identify said pictures.

b. Said pictures be used only for purposes of medical study or research.

(Cross out any parts above which are not appropriate)

C. SIGNATURES *(Appropriate items in Parts A and B must be completed before signing)*

1. COUNSELING PHYSICIAN: I have counseled this patient as to the nature of the proposed procedure(s), attendant risks involved, and expected results, as described above.

(Signature of Counseling Physician)

2. PATIENT: I understand the nature of the proposed procedure(s), attendant risks involved, and expected results, as described above, and hereby request such procedure(s) be performed.

(Signature of Witness, excluding members of operating team) (Signature of Patient) (Date & Time)

3. SPONSOR OR GUARDIAN: (When patient is a minor or unable to give consent) I, ____________ sponsor/guardian of ____________ understand the nature of the proposed procedure(s), attendant risks involved, and expected results, as described above, and hereby request such procedure(s) be performed.

(Signature of Witness, excluding members of operating team) (Signature of Sponsor/Legal Guardian) (Date & Time)

PATIENT'S IDENTIFICATION *(For typed or written entries give: Name—last, first, middle; grade; date; hospital or medical facility)*

REGISTER NO. | WARD NO.

STANDARD FORM 522
January 1973 (Rev.)
General Services Administration & Interagency Comm. on Medical Records
FPMR 101–11.809–3
522–107

U. S. GOVERNMENT PRINTING OFFICE : 1976 O - 211-869

Figure 11–1. Informed consent document.

for protecting a patient's dignity in the health care environment, the fundamental belief being that such consent should foster and engender trust between the health professional and the person receiving the services.

Reflection

What strengths and weaknesses do you see in using the informed consent document in Figure 11–1 to foster the ideal of engendering trust?

To help you better understand how informed consent became so central to the health professional–patient relationship, I invite you to engage in the six-step process of ethical decision making with your focus on informed consent.

The Six-Step Process in Informed Consent Situations

The most important thing to bear in mind as you analyze the specific informed consent-related challenges facing Jason Fruhling and Faye Nesbitt is that the informed consent document, process, and procedures can support important ethical dimensions of the relationship. Its importance can be better understood better by examining some aspects of the development of the idea.

Step 1: Gather Relevant Information

As you may recall when the six-step process was introduced in Chapter 4, I provided a long list of types of information that you would need to help you arrive at a caring response. I also warned you that there may be other types of information that could help as well, information not related to the patient's specific situation. Information about the legal principles underlying informed consent is one example; elements of the process related to disclosure in informed consent is another. Let us examine each before going on to identify the type of ethical problem facing Faye Nesbitt.

Relevant Legal Concepts Supporting Informed Consent

Among the most important legal concepts that have given rise to our thinking about informed consent are battery, disclosure, and the fiduciary relationship. The common law legal right of self-determination and constitutional right to privacy also are instrumental in legal thinking. You will consider self-determination for its *ethical* implications in another section of this chapter.

Battery, based on common law in the United States and other Western countries, is the act of offensive touching done without the consent of the person being touched, however benign the motive or effects of the touching.[1]

Disclosure guarantees the legal right of a person to be informed of what will happen to him or her. Several landmark legal cases have set precedents for current thinking on the importance of disclosure. Some practical challenges encountered regarding the appropriate standard of disclosure to use are discussed in the next section.

One of the earliest U.S. legal cases related to disclosure is *Schloendorff v. Society of New York Hospital.* This case emphasized the relationship of disclosure to autonomy. This 1914 ruling stated that every human being of adult years and sound mind has a right to determine what shall be done with his or her body. For example, a surgeon who performs an operation without the patient's consent is liable.[2]

In the 1918 *Hunter v. Burroughs* case, the courts ruled that a physician has a duty to warn a patient of dangers associated with prescribed remedies. Both rulings were early attempts by the courts to bring the patient's preferences into the decision regarding what would happen to his or her own body.[3]

A third related legal concept is the idea of a *fiduciary relationship.* In such a relationship a person in whom another person has placed a special trust or confidence is required to watch out for the best interests of the other party. Most health professional–patient (or client) relationships are considered to be this type. The physician–patient relationship in the United States was ruled a fiduciary relationship in a 1974 case, *Miller v. Kennedy,* on the basis of the "ignorance and helplessness of the patient regarding his own physical condition."[4] This is, of course, an outdated understanding of the patient as "ignorant and helpless," but that does not negate the basic idea of the need for faithfulness on the part of all health professionals.

The legal case that gave to posterity the term *informed consent* is *Salgo v. Leland Stanford Board of Trustees* (1957). It stated that the physician violates his or her legal duty by withholding information necessary for a patient to make a rational decision regarding care. In addition, the physician must disclose "all the facts which materially affect the patient's rights and interests and the risks, hazard and danger, if any."[5] With this ruling the U.S. courts firmly wedded the notion of a patient's self-determination with that of a health professional's duty to warn of known danger or harm. In other words, the courts recognized that a caring response couldn't be achieved without those aspects of the interaction.

Relevant Facts Regarding the Process of Obtaining Consent

Let us go on to some practical matters. Currently, the law supports that a client or patient should gain information about the proposed procedure and should have a voice in the decision. However, it also recognizes that there may be several challenges in attempting to implement the procedure in a meaningful manner. Some challenges are related to the standard and amount of disclosure, whereas others are related to the person's ability to grasp the situation (Fig. 11–2).

The Disclosure Standard. The standard of disclosure is a key consideration. You have seen that a major legal concern is that a patient be *informed.* What *disclosure standard* can be used to judge that the level of information was sufficiently clear to be understood? One suggestion has been that "customary medical language" be the standard of disclosure. Others, emphasizing the likelihood that patients will misunderstand technical terms used by the health professional, suggest that the standard be determined by what a "reasonable" person would need to make an informed decision. Finding one standard appropriate for everyone continues to perplex many. In fact, the courts have not settled on one standard, either. Some have concluded that the only alternative is to adopt an *individualized* standard for each patient.

Reflection

What are some practical barriers to institutionalizing any of the three suggested standards for an individual patient?

A related disclosure issue focuses on the appropriate *amount* of information shared. In many health care settings patients are directed

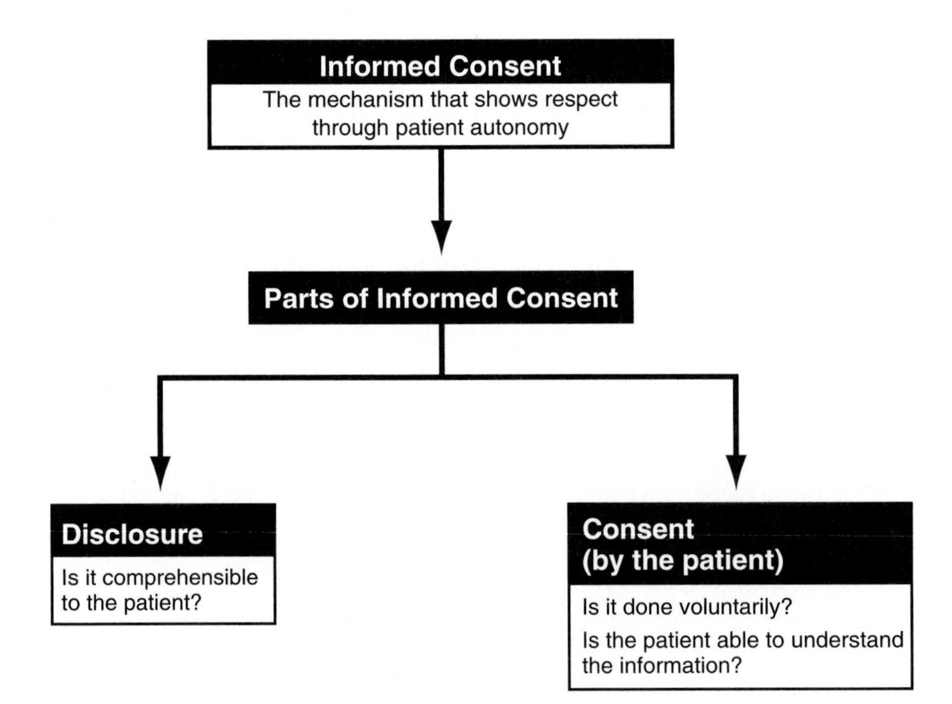

Figure 11–2. The two dimensions of informed consent.

to sign a standardized *general consent* form when they are admitted. You will recall that this happened to Jason and was the trigger for his first outburst of concern. The wording appearing on a typical document states that a patient is consenting to routine services and treatment, the goal being the best care possible. In a teaching hospital, the person also is told that on entering the hospital she or he consents to become a participant in the hospital's educational programs. Then, when certain invasive procedures are being considered, the consent is valid only when the person signs a *special consent* form (such as the one in Fig. 11–1). Recall that Jason also was asked to sign a special consent form for his renal function tests, and that became the source of his second outburst of frustration. The amount and type of information deemed adequate and appropriate in the special consent form may vary tremendously from one institution to another.

The goal is to take the patient's background into consideration and determine the relative advantages and disadvantages of each decision choice for that patient's future well-being. A 1995 study of patients at two public hospitals in an urban area showed that of 2659 predominantly indigent and minority patients presenting for acute care, 59.5% (more than 1500) of patients could not read a standard informed consent document. The investigators came to the stunning conclusion that "many patients in our institutions cannot perform the basic reading tasks required to function in the health care environment."[6] This in itself is a barrier to such patients' receiving high-quality care unless great attention is directed to providing a level and amount of disclosure that is consistent with patients' literacy and numeracy skills.

Anxiety and fear created by the unknown or general distrust of the health care system leave many with the sense that unfair advantage is being taken of them. When presenting informed consent documents, you should be found on the side of "taking too much time" with each patient, all the while being attentive to the patient's cues regarding his or her level of comprehension.

SUMMARY

The standard and amount of information disclosed combined with psychological factors influencing the patient's experience must all be taken into account in assessing if disclosure is consistent with a caring response.

Voluntariness Must Be Assured. Informed consent assumes that a person voluntarily agrees to the procedure or process he or she is about to undergo. A person speaks or acts voluntarily when no coercion compels her to do so against her own best interests and wishes.

For this reason, individuals judged to be in vulnerable situations in which their ability to say "no" or "this is what I want" is compromised should be treated with special regard. As you may recall, Jason told Faye, the nurse practitioner, that he felt pressured to sign the consent form. A good informed consent *process* (in contrast to just an informed consent *form*) will allow him either to increase his comfort level to the point of being willing to sign the form or to go away being very clear why he chose to refuse treatment.

Reflection

What steps did Faye Nesbitt and others take each step of the way to try to meet the criterion of voluntariness? Do you feel confident that they succeeded? Why or why not?

One instance testing the limits of voluntariness as a standard of respect for a person is the psychiatric practice of involuntary commitment for mental illness. This practice long has been condoned by the medical profession and often by society as well. The increasing awareness of the importance of voluntariness, however, has created an environment in which such patients are able to maintain control over large parts of their treatment regimen, sometimes including whether to accept or reject medications.

SUMMARY

A conviction that the patient's consent voluntarily is given must be added to the condition of adequate disclosure for the ethical goals of *informed consent* to be realized.

Competence as a Consideration. Health professionals have a moral obligation to ascertain the level of a patient's ability to grasp the situation. The ability to grasp it is called *mental competence* or *capacitation.* The criterion for competence in the informed consent idea assumes that individuals possess certain crucial knowledge without which they are unable to engage willfully in an act. Take, for example, the act of making a will. The person who does not know the general value of his estate or who does not have the mental capacity to recognize the existence of a rightful heir is not in a position to sign a valid will no matter what he or she may know about himself or herself or the world in general. These two pieces of information are so essential to the making of a will that unless one is in possession of them, one cannot properly dispose of one's estate. In the same fashion a person must be knowledgeable about certain crucial aspects of his or her health and the condition creating the problem to offer truly informed consent. This formulation of competency is too narrow, however, when taken alone. It still tends to focus a clinical evaluation in terms of how much a person is told and how much he or she can repeat back to you. This surely is not all you will wish to know concerning a patient's capacity. A fundamental concern is whether the patient truly understands the nature of his or her illness and the basis for consenting or refusing intervention. For example, Jason may be having difficulty comprehending because of mental changes associated with uremia. This is something to which Faye must pay close attention.

In 1988, Appelbaum and Grisso[7] proposed the following four levels of competence, a paradigm still used today:

1. The first level is the ability to communicate choices. Beyond that, there is the ability to maintain and communicate these choices consistently over time.
2. The second, a qualitatively different level, is the ability to understand relevant information on which the choice is based.
3. The third level is the ability to appreciate the situation according to one's own values.
4. The fourth level is the ability to weigh various values to arrive at a decision.[7]

Ideally, a person should have all four levels of competence. For instance, nothing we know about Jason would suggest that previously he was incompetent or incapacitated. At the same time, Faye has knowledge about the effects of uremia that may give her pause about his mental acuity at this moment in time. As a part of her caring for him, she must take every precaution to assure that he is competent, a topic that is pursued in more depth later in this chapter.

Step 2: Identify the Type of Ethical Problem

Faye and the other health professionals seem to have little doubt about the importance of assuring that Jason be comfortable in giving his consent for general and special intervention purposes. They recognize themselves as moral agents *(A)* responsible for a caring response to his concerns. They believe the appropriate outcome *(O)* is for him to be fully informed and willingly able to give (or refuse) consent. The challenge seems to be HOW to get to that outcome. They are experiencing barriers in the course of action *(C)* designed by the institution to reach the result of informed consent.

Reflection

What kind of ethical problem focuses on barriers to an ethically optimal outcome?

If you responded "ethical distress" you have remembered well what you learned earlier. In this case, Faye Nesbitt (who has become the person Jason seems to trust the most) has to overcome the barriers to achieving her intended ethical goal. Because she can speculate what the range of barriers are, her distress falls into ethical distress type A. Schematically, her problem looks like this:

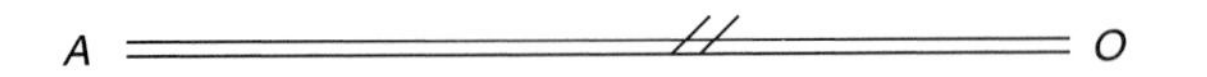

Ethical Distress

What kind of possible barriers are there?

First, there may be a problem with the wording of the informed consent form itself. You have already been introduced in this chapter to the challenges that the basic idea of informed consent raises regarding standards and amount of disclosure needed for different patients. Or maybe the form is so badly worded that no one is really benefited by this mechanism, and Jason is just one of the people to bring it to the attention of the health professionals.

Second, the barrier she might be facing is that Jason may have life experiences that make him extremely anxious about giving away his autonomy. Has he been a prisoner of war or had other traumatic experiences? We don't know. We certainly can observe that anxiety played a part in his reactions to the requests for him to sign the documents.

Third, he might be afraid of what he, or the health professionals, will find out if they go ahead with the tests. In other words, his reluctance may not be centered on the consent itself, but rather what it represents. His reaction at the time he is about to have the dye injected and the diagnostic test performed may be indicative of his fear of what the tests will reveal.

Fourth, although Faye thinks she is doing a good job, the barrier to her achieving her goal may come from that the patient is not able to comprehend what is really happening, even though he pretends to in the end. He may be mentally incompetent, or have a reading or learning disability, or in some other way be deeply confused about this whole thing.

Reflection

Can you think of other possibilities? If so, jot them down.

Once the type of ethical problem is identified, Faye can use the tools of ethics to analyze (and hopefully move toward resolution of) it.

Step 3: Use Ethical Theories or Approaches to Analyze the Problem

Faye, the unit nurse, and the medical imaging team are working well together to address this problem. Faye, in particular, has a challenge; obviously she has other things to do, as well as be concerned about Mr. Fruhling, who is not one of "her" patients in the strict sense of the word.

The resolution of her ethical distress requires her to call on both virtues and the help of ethical principles to guide her.

Virtues Associated with Caring

In Chapter 3 you were introduced to the idea of virtue, the expression of which is in the form of character traits or dispositions. Character traits help a health professional stand firmly in her or his commitment to find a "caring response" in a great variety of situations. When I reflect on the challenge facing Faye Nesbitt, the common health care virtues like honesty, compassion, or courage don't seem entirely fitting for her situation. What dispositions can help her remove the barriers that are keeping her from her desired outcome—that is, confidence that she has supported Jason's right to give (or refuse) informed consent? Character traits that come to mind in observing her at work toward the achievement of this goal include kindness, thoroughness, patience, and sympathy. We also can assume she knows that if she sloughs off on this task, the self-respect needed for maintaining her own integrity as a professional will receive a blow. Hers is an apt example of how different character traits are needed for different types of ethically challenging situations.

She also will want to move toward further action, and for that she can find some guidance in the principles of patient autonomy, beneficence, and nonmaleficence.

The Principle of Patient Autonomy

Beauchamp and Faden[8] note that, "As the idea of informed consent evolved, discussion of appropriate (ethical) guidelines moved increasingly from a narrow focus on the physician's or researcher's obligation to disclose information to the quality of a patient's or subject's understanding of information and right to authorize or refuse biomedical intervention." The governing ethical principle in informed consent is the *right to self-determination* or *autonomy.* It also is reflected in a legal right today.

The health professional can think of informed consent as a claim on him or her to provide a communication process that allows the person to make an informed choice. One could go further and say it is a claim to honor all the conditions, including a communications process, that allows the person to make an informed choice.

Because Jason Fruhling still seems upset after he has signed the second form, we can conclude that communication may have broken down somewhere.

Reflection

Do you think Faye Nesbitt met the conditions that would foster good communication between herself and Jason? From what you know, what, if anything, could she have done differently at the outset during their initial exchange to avoid his negative response?

You begin to see that information disclosure, taken alone, is not adequate. The key is that the information be useful to the person in making the best decision.

The Principles of Beneficence and Nonmaleficence

Two additional principles, *beneficence* and *nonmaleficence,* also are basic foundations in the idea of informed consent. These two, taken together, morally require you to do everything possible to refrain from harming the patient and also meet your positive obligation to help him become adequately informed to make the best possible choice. This aspect of the health professional and patient or client relationship can be thought of as a contract. A *contract* implies that each person involved in the contract has full knowledge of the situation and willingly has "contracted." When you provide information to the patient or client, you are acknowledging an initial imbalance of information between the two of you. Because of this imbalance, the patient's self-determination is compromised. Therefore, you are responsible for informing the person of the conditions under which a contract will be struck. Only then can both parties enter into dialogue and agreement as equals. Failure to provide the information constitutes a type of harm: You fail to conform to the principle of nonmaleficence ("do no harm").

SUMMARY

Both character traits and principles can help informed consent be realized as an integral aspect of a caring response. The patient's autonomy and the health professional's duties of nonmaleficence and beneficence are important markers toward achieving that goal.

Step 4: Explore the Practical Alternatives

We are catching Faye "downstream" in her ethical distress, since we know from the story that Jason signed the form and had the diagnostic procedure. We also know that he seemed unhappy at the end and that she, too, is now concerned. However, whether we look at her predicament at the time she was first discussing the informed consent form with him, or the second time, or even now, after the fact, her concern is that there was/is a barrier to her arriving at the outcome of a caring response.

Reflection

What do you think she should do once she learns that this patient—who was not her patient in the first place—seems to be struggling with the issue of informed consent?

Let us pick up her story at the current time, with her pondering what to do because no matter what she did in the past he seemed "dissatisfied."

One option is to talk with him again herself. Let him know what she heard from the imaging team and ask him what happened that led him to be so unsatisfied with the outcome of their exchange. Perhaps through that action she will be able to understand better where she let him down (if she did) or if his lingering reluctance had nothing to do with her exchanges with him.

A second option is to go directly to the medical unit where he is a patient and discuss the whole situation with them so that they can have insight into their own future care of him.

A third option is to take the informed consent forms to the appropriate committees within her institution, probably the committees that designed the forms, and ask them to review the documents for clarity, accuracy, and completeness.

Finally, a fourth option is to let the matter drop. It is over and done.

Steps 5 and 6: Complete the Action and Evaluate the Process and Outcome

Given Faye's continued concern and Jason's apparent continued unease, the first through third options combined with further reflection on her experience are warranted. Each may provide insight not only into the possible failures of the informed consent process but also into what the health professionals can do in the future to help assure a more positive outcome.

One area for reflection will be taken care of by the institution's committees: Faye's experience provides them with an opportunity to review the documents, processes, and procedures of informed consent.

Another area for reflection is that Faye and her colleagues should try to better understand the various sources of anxiety and fear that the form, the discussion about the procedures, or other aspects of the informed consent procedure might generate in patients.

A third is that the challenge of arriving at a caring response through the use of informed consent requires diligence regarding how to show respect, taking into account differences among individuals and groups of patients. For instance, the story of Jason and Faye probably evokes for you the picture of two Northern European white people. In fact, Jason grew up in a small village in Northern Thailand with a mother of Thai descent and a father who is half Thai and half German. He immigrated to the United States only 2 years ago. He was sent to an English-speaking school in Bangkok when he was 10 years old, therefore language is not much of a barrier for him in his adopted land. Faye is a fifth generation "Yankee" who married her high school sweetheart. Both she and her husband grew up in Stoningham, Connecticut.

Reflection

List some cultural or ethnic groups who would not find the idea of informed consent for each individual member of their group consistent with their moral norms. If you know of none, you have an important task to do in acquainting yourself with the rich diversity of patients and clients you are bound to see.

Much of informed consent presupposes that a patient desires to be independent and in control of his or her own individual destiny. Your professional goal and privilege of arriving at a caring response goes beyond assuming this. The differences can cause such profound mistakes that a later section of this chapter is devoted entirely to the topic.

SUMMARY

The health professional providing the patient with pertinent information for informed consent inevitably must personalize the amount and the type of information provided despite the difficulty in doing so. Even then the process has but begun of arriving at a caring response.

When Faye engages in Step 6 of the ethical decision-making process (i.e., evaluating the process and outcome), she may conclude that she "missed the mark" somewhere. If not, she will have at least been diligent in her commitment to finding a caring response in this dimension of her professional role. I ask you to turn now to additional important considerations relevant to your skillful use of informed consent as an ethical tool.

The Special Challenge of Incompetence or Incapacity

Incompetence and incapacity are two terms used to describe the condition of patients for whom the process of truly informed decision making and consent to such decisions are not possible. *Capacity* is a legal term. *Competence* is a clinical judgment made by a professional of a patient's ability to give informed consent. Most writing and reflection on the subject urges extreme caution and diligence in discerning how far to proceed with evaluation and treatment if a patient is incapable of making a competent decision to accept procedures. There are two types of incompetent patients, those who were *never competent* and those who were *once competent*. Some examples of patients who were never competent include newborns, small children, and individuals who have been severely mentally disabled from birth. In such instances, *surrogate* or *proxy consent* usually is sought.

When never-competent persons become patients, a *legal guardian* is appointed. Obviously, such a person also has had a guardian for other purposes, and in most instances the same person is appointed. The next of kin usually but not always is considered the most qualified to be the guardian. The goal here is to determine who can speak for the best interests of this person who has never been in a position to voice her or his informed wishes. (This is called the *best interests standard*.) In contrast, for individuals who were once competent (e.g., those who have organic brain damage that developed in later life, or adult psychoses), a guardian also may be appointed. You must then attempt to make your decision on the basis of what a person would have wanted when competent. (This is called a *substituted judgment standard*.) Sometimes a next of kin or other person makes statements that reflect what the guardian believes the patient said when he or she was competent. Often, this is helpful evidence of what a now incapacitated person would want. Other signs are letters, past conversations, comments about other incapacitated people, or the person's general lifestyle.

In recent years, proxy consent for once-competent persons has been further formalized by the advent of *advance directives*. The general idea is to allow each person while still competent to make his or her wishes known regarding decisions that will be made at a time when he or she becomes incapacitated, especially in illnesses that will end in death. Some types of advance directives include living wills, durable power of attorney documents, medical directive documents, and values histories. They are discussed further in Chapter 13. Because these documents vary in focus, you are encouraged to check with your place of employment and also with any state laws that may guide the legal use of such documents where you live.

In most regards, the bottom line remains the same regardless of whether a patient is competent—they have a right to informed input and the final say in what happens. The concern over what happens when that input capacity is diminished or missing is greater because informed consent is not always taken as seriously in the health care setting as it should be. Patients often are asked to sign such forms with little more than a perfunctory explanation: "You have to sign this so we can do the operation." In all cases a professional should be present who is able to explain the procedure and its risks to the patient (or, if incompetent, the surrogate) and to answer any questions. Many people have the misconception that if a patient or surrogate signs the form, consent is legally binding no matter what. The form alone is only evidence that they have signed a piece of paper.

But in a busy health care setting, where patients' lack of willingness to move quickly may be getting in the way of the efficient operation of the institution, there is a great risk that the consent form becomes an empty substitute for truly informed consent.

SUMMARY

Informed consent forms are the beginning of a conversation about the patient's informed preferences. They cannot be substituted for good communication with the patient.

Informed Consent in Research

To help focus your attention on this important aspect of informed consent, consider an informed consent form used for research, as shown in Figure 11–3.

Reflection

Would you sign this form? What is clearly stated? What should be written differently?

Almost every experimental procedure within the health care setting necessitates some infringement on a person's physical or psychological independence. If the dignity of a person being subjected to an experimental procedure is to be preserved and his or her personal freedom recognized, he or she must be allowed to grant consent to the procedure. In summary, individuals must not be involuntarily submitted to experimental procedures. Rather, they must freely and willingly give their consent to the procedure, even though there may be little personal risk involved. By granting consent the patient agrees to the means used to bring about the investigator's desired end and expresses willingness to participate in bringing about that end.

Following are the basic ethical and legal stipulations involved:

- An investigator cannot perform a research procedure, even of no or minimal risk, without the subject's consent.
- Consent is meaningful only if it is based on relevant information and is not coerced.

RESPONSIBLE INVESTIGATOR:

TITLE OF PROTOCOL:

TITLE OF CONSENT FORM *(if different from protocol):*

I have been asked to participate in a research study that is investigating *(describe purpose of study).* In participating in this study I agree to *(describe briefly and in lay terms procedures to which subject is consenting).*

I understand that

a) The possible risks of this procedure include *(list known risks or side effects; if none, so state).* Alternative treatments include *(list alternative treatments and briefly describe advantages and disadvantages of each; if none, so state).*

b) The possible benefits of this study to me are *(enumerate; if none, so state).*

c) Any questions I have concerning my participation in this study will be answered by *(list names and degrees of people who will be available to answer questions).*

d) I may withdraw from the study at any time without prejudice.

e) The results of this study may be published, but my name or identity will not be revealed and my records will remain confidential unless disclosure of my identity is required by law.

f) My consent is given voluntarily without being coerced or forced.

g) In the event of physical injury resulting from the study, medical care and treatment will be available at this institution.

For eligible veterans, compensation (damages) may be payable under 38USC 351 or, in some circumstances, under the Federal Tort claims Act.

For non-eligible veterans and non-veterans, compensation would be limited to situations where negligence occurred and would be controlled by the provisions of the Federal Tort Claims Act.

For clarification of these laws, contact the District Counsel (213) 824-7379.

________________ DATE

________________ PATIENT OR RESPONSIBLE PARTY

________________ PATIENT'S SOCIAL SECURITY NUMBER

________________ AUDITOR/WITNESS

________________ INVESTIGATOR/PHYSICIAN REPRESENTATIVE

Figure 11–3. Human studies consent form.

Continued

Protocol C.A.V.: A pilot study to evaluate short-course irradiation to small cell bronchogenic carcinoma with combination chemotherapy including the drugs Cytoxan, Adriamycin, and vincristine, and prophylactic brain irradiation. The drugs are to be started on Day 1 with the irradiation and repeated on Day 29 and thereafter every 21 days for 6 cycles.

You have been found to have a tumor of the lung which is best treated by drugs because of the extent of disease, metastases, involvement of the lymph glands or ____.

Antitumor drugs (chemotherapy) have been found to be effective in slowing tumor growth, but are not curative as of now. New drugs and various combinations of new and current antitumor drugs are being tried in the hope of finding better drugs and more effective combinations. The aim of the treatment is to slow or to halt the spread of disease and permit you a longer period of relative well-being.

Radiation therapy is also a proven effective method of killing tumor cells. In this treatment plan for lung cancer, the affected lung will be irradiated for three weeks to maximize the potential reduction of your tumor. Your brain will also be treated with a modest dose of irradiation in order to ward off the spread of disease to this area. A temporary loss of hair may be expected within the field of irradiation.

You will also be given chemotherapy drugs (Cytoxan, Adriamycin, and vincristine) in combination with the irradiation. These drugs will be given to you intravenously on Day 1 and 29 of treatment and thereafter every 21 days for 6 cycles.

Antitumor drugs, such as the ones used in this plan, and radiation therapy may produce some damage to normal cells in the body, even though the treatments are designed to attack primarily the tumor cells. Care will be used to try to minimize the effect of the damage to your normal cells. The particular forms of damage include: nausea, vomiting, diarrhea, lowered white blood cell count, mouth ulcers, and loss of hair. The drug Adriamycin might make worse any cardiac problems you have. During the treatment you will be monitored carefully with blood tests, urine examination, x-ray examination, ECG, chemical tests, and other studies. Should any of these untoward effects occur, your treatment plan will be reevaluated and, if necessary, modified.

If you have any questions, these will be answered prior to starting the treatment program. You are under no obligation to join this study. You will continue to be treated if you refuse. You are free to withdraw your consent to participate in the study at any time without any prejudice to your continued medical care. The confidential nature of your case will be maintained.

I have read the information contained on this page and all my questions have been answered to my satisfaction. I consent to participate in this medical study.

____
Patient's Signature   Date

____
Witness (Investigator)   Date

____
Witness   Date

Figure 11–3, cont'd.

- Consent may be a necessary, but not sufficient, condition for the investigator to proceed. (For example, homicide is not justified despite a subject's consent.)[9]

The procedure by which consent is brought about is to inform the patient of the range of benefits and risks related to the procedures. The consent form must be signed by the patient, rendering him or her also a research subject.

What about people who for some reason cannot give consent for experimentation? Can consent be given on their behalf by someone who is judged to have the person's interests in mind? Because of the possibilities for abuse of such persons, considerable attention has been devoted in recent years to trying to set up reasonable guidelines for ensuring their protection. There is still much disagreement about the morally acceptable way to proceed. Most discussion has taken place within the context of research on children and mentally retarded persons, as well as prisoners, students, or others who are in a compromised position or in no position to refuse. Sometimes they are referred to collectively as "vulnerable populations." At one extreme is the position that people in vulnerable populations should not be subjected to research unless it is related to their own illness (i.e., it must be therapeutic research). This implies that a parent or other guardian cannot second guess what the person would do if given the opportunity to consent to a research project that did not also offer some direct therapeutic benefit to the person.

Others argue that this position is too conservative regarding experimentation in children and mentally retarded persons. For instance, it excludes the possibility of obtaining values for various bodily fluids in healthy newborns. Without this information newborns with life-threatening conditions may die because there are insufficient data to judge the degree of their problem. This may be an instance in which the minimal risks involved (taking bodily fluids from healthy newborns without their consent) are overridden by the great benefits gained by the research. The above discussion points to the difficulty of arriving at a policy position to meet at least the basic requirements of morality for a wide range of investigators.

SUMMARY

As in most areas of ethical reflection in the health professions, dilemmas around clinical research on patients require that professionals engage in continual weighing and decision making in their attempt to honor the subject's values.

One institutional mechanism that has become a regular means of monitoring the quality of informed consent in research is the *institutional review board* (IRB). The IRB was implemented in the 1980s to help assure not only that persons consenting to research understood what they were getting into but also that the research project itself was ethical in its design and inception. In addition to informed consent considerations, the IRB of the institution must assess the necessity of the project, the type of findings that will result, and the way that the subjects will be treated during the study. It also assesses whether the study involves any inhumane treatment of individuals or groups. If you are asked to do a human subjects study as a part of your professional preparation, you probably will have to fill out the forms required by your local IRB.

Like the informed consent form itself, completing the necessary forms for the IRB does not assure that humane practices in human subject research will be followed. It does, however, at least submit the investigator to the rigors of review by a panel of concerned professionals and laypeople.

Sensitivity to Cultural and Other Differences

I asked you to take into account the possibility that Jason's and Faye's difficulty regarding a mutually agreeable positive outcome may have some diversity challenges buried in it. An ethical challenge as a health professional is to be as sensitive as possible to informed consent issues in the context of different cultures, whether it be for treatment or experimentation. The emphasis on individual autonomy and the right of the patient to receive information about his or her illness is a Western European notion. Even within the United States and Western Europe there will be many different ethnic, cultural, and religious groups whose beliefs vary from the standard Northern European emphasis on individual autonomy and the right to information.[10]

Ramsden[11] tells a story of a patient with lung cancer who lived in the middle of the United States, but who had been born in a small rural community in South America. He and his wife continued to live according to a belief system that pervaded their culture, retaining their national customs and traditions, as well as the language. This patient did not ask about the nature of his illness, and the family insisted that he not be told. After considerable effort the health professional learned that in this patient's native country it is considered inhumane to burden the person with information about the illness. Even so, Ramsden notes, one must be careful not to stereotype South Americans as a group. There are more than 1500 language groups on this continent and numerous religious and ethnic groups.[11] The type of experience that Ramsden describes and her reflections about the variations within groups should be reminders that individual preferences do not stand outside of cultural, religious, and other values.

There is a growing body of inquiry about the customs and culture of numerous immigrant groups within the United States and Canada. Surprisingly, however, little research has been done overall on the variability of patients' wishes and values within minority subgroups. A particularly helpful study entitled "Western Bioethics on the Navajo Reservation: Benefit or Harm?" highlights the idea that informed consent and advanced directives may have a harmful effect on Navajo patients. The investigators learned that discussing bad news conflicts with the Navajo concept of Hózhó and is viewed as potentially harmful by these Navajo subjects. Policies complying with the Patient Self-Determination Act, intended to expose all hospitalized Navajo patients to advanced care planning, are ethically troublesome and warrant evaluation. In this culture, then, the helpfulness is related to Hózhó, which combines "concepts of beauty, goodness, or harmony, and everything that is positive or ideal."[12]

SUMMARY

The well-intentioned but autonomy-dominated principles of informed consent are not universally beneficial to patients.

There are many ways in which language and related cultural barriers can diminish positive effects.[13] At the same time it may be too presumptuous to assume that it cannot be applied at all in cultures that appear to be more communal in their approach to issues affecting an individual.[14] Each case warrants the professional's most vigilant attention if a caring response is to be achieved.

Summary

Informed consent in health care and human subjects' research has become a standard part of Western health care practice and policy. Addressing the shortcomings and adopting varying approaches in different situations are challenges that must be met. Schematically, the idea of informed consent in both the healthy care and human subjects' research setting has two dimensions: the information disclosed and the voluntariness of the respondent. The advent of advance directives and surrogate decision making is an apt reminder of your responsibility for understanding and abiding by the patient's considered wishes.

Informed consent in health care should be yet another means of facilitating communication between patient and health professional. The document is supposed to be tangible evidence that informed consent was, in fact, given. But health care professionals generally place too much emphasis on the form and too little on the informed consent process. Even when the process is emphasized appropriately, the dominant ethical principle of individual autonomy that sometimes dominates must be placed within the larger context of respect for individuals. At times respect requires that the participation of the patient be conducted with cultural or other norms that do not place individual autonomy in such a prime position.

Questions for Thought and Discussion

1. The wife of an Asian immigrant requested that her husband not be told that his kidney cancer was fatal. She explained that in her homeland it would be considered inappropriate to burden a patient with such unfortunate news. The U.S. surgeon felt uncomfortable withholding this information from her patient. What should she do?

2. Describe a clinical research project that you might conduct within your health profession. Try to evaluate it according to the potential risks and benefits to the patients or subjects. Make an outline of what you believe ought to be included in the informed consent form so that the person knows what is involved in the research project.

3. Suppose you are asked to serve on a national commission for the protection of human subjects. What positions regarding research on children and mentally incompetent people would you adopt? State reasons for your choice.

References

1. *Black's Law Dictionary* (7th ed.). 1999. St. Paul, MN: West Group, p. 146.
2. *Schloendorff v. Society of New York Hospital.* 1914. 211 N.Y. 125, 105 N.E. 92.
3. *Hunter v. Burroughs.* 1918. 123 Va 113, 96 SE. 360.
4. *Richard R. Miller, Appellant v. John A. Kennedy, Respondent.* 1974. Court of Appeals of Washington, Division One 11 Wash. App. 27222 P.2d 852.
5. *Salgo v. Leland Stanford Board of Trustees.* 1957. 154 Cal. App 2nd 560, 317 P. 2d 170, 177.
6. Williams, M.V., Parker, R.M., Baker, D.W., Parikh, N.S., Pitkin, K., Coates, W.C., Nurss, J.R. 1995. Inadequate functional health literacy among patients at two public hospitals. *JAMA* 274(21):1677–1686.
7. Appelbaum, P.S., Grisso, T. 1988. Assessing patients' capacities to consent to treatment. *New England Journal of Medicine* 319(25):1635–1638.
8. Beauchamp, T.L., Faden, R. 2004. Informed consent: The history of informed consent. In Post, S. (Ed.), *Encyclopedia of Bioethics* (3rd ed., vol. 3). New York: Macmillan, pp. 1271–1276.
9. Shamoo, A.E., Resnik, D.B. 2003. *Responsible Conduct of Research.* New York: Oxford University Press.
10. Hyon, I. 2001. Authentic values and individual autonomy. *Journal of Value Inquiry* 35(2):195–208.
11. Ramsden, E. 1993. In the context of culture and faith. *PT Magazine* 2(4):68–69.
12. Carrese, J., Rhodes, L. 1995. Western bioethics on the Navajo reservation: Benefit or harm? *JAMA* 274(10):826–829.
13. Vaught, W. 2003. Patient expectations of benefit from Phase I clinical trials: Linguistic considerations in diagnosing a therapeutic misconception. *Theoretical Medicine and Bioethics* 24(4):301–328.
14. Hyon, I. 2002. Waiver of informed consent, cultural sensitivity and the problem of unjust families and traditions. *Hastings Center Report* 32(5):14–22.

Section IV

Ethical Dimensions of Chronic and End-of-Life Care

12

The Growing Ethical Challenges of Chronic and Long-Term Care

Objectives

The student should be able to:

- List several common medical conditions that are chronic illnesses requiring long-term care interventions over months or years.
- Describe four considerations a professional usually must take into account in arriving at a caring response in a chronic illness situation compared with an acute illness situation.
- Discuss how and why quality of life considerations become a major feature of care for individuals with chronic symptoms.
- Identify several ways in which the patient–family caregiver unit is an essential focus of decision making in situations involving chronic illness.

New terms and ideas you will encounter in this chapter

chronic care
long-term care

Topics in this chapter introduced in earlier chapters

Topic	*Introduced in chapter*
A caring response	2
Quality of life	3
The health care team	8
Utilitarianism	3
Principle of nonmaleficence	3
Principle of beneficence	3
Locus of authority problem	2
Ethical dilemma	2
Ethics committee and ethics consults	1

Introduction

Chronic care and long-term care are demanding the attention of the health care system more than ever before.[1] Many factors contribute to the increase in the number of chronic illnesses and symptoms that currently plague patients—advances in newborn intensive care, the increasing incidence of long-term survival after traumatic brain injury occurring anywhere across the life span, an increase in longevity with its unintended side effects such as Alzheimer disease and other dementias or joint breakdowns. These examples are just some sources of this growing population of patients nationally and globally.

The terms chronic (from *kronos,* which means "time" in Latin) and long-term care do not denote that the person will die of the condition, although some fall into this category. In fact, Chapter 13 discusses a patient in that category, and other examples include amyotrophic lateral sclerosis, muscular dystrophy, multiple sclerosis, Parkinson's disease, Huntington's disease, and severe chronic obstructive pulmonary disease. But the common denominator is that the symptoms persist over time. Many chronic and long-term care conditions last for months, years, or a lifetime, with the symptoms persisting but not directly leading to the individual's death. Arthritis is a good example, as are some forms of leukemia, clinical depression, schizophrenia, and dyslexias or other communication disorders. The presence of all these forms lend support to the idea that in the generation of the health professionals you represent, most of you will be deeply involved in the treatment of chronic symptoms and the disability that often accompanies them.[2] This chapter focuses directly on the ethical challenges this population presents and how you can respond to them appropriately. The insights in this chapter allow you also to draw on dimensions of their care discussed in other chapters, using chronic illness as a patient's condition.

Reflection

Do you have a friend, family member, or colleague who has a chronic condition that requires ongoing clinical interventions? What are the major challenges you think, or know, this person faces that others do not need to think about? Are there disruptions in everyday activity? Jot down a few notes about this so that as you go through the chapter you can relate that person's situation back to the opportunities health professionals have to help the person thrive while living with the chronic condition.

As you have experienced in previous chapters, to further help set your thinking you have an opportunity to examine a narrative, this one of a family who is interacting with the health care system because one family member is in a situation that requires an ongoing interaction with health professionals and the health care system.

The Story of the McDonalds, the Experimental Drug, and the Doubters

The pregnancy had been without complication and the delivery was much easier than Megan had imagined it would be. She and Jerry beheld the screaming newborn with the pride that only new parents can feel. Mary Elizabeth McDonald had entered this world with all the gusto her parents presumed she would need as a second-generation immigrant in their adopted land.

And so it came as a shock to parents and clinical staff alike when shortly after her birth Mary Elizabeth developed serious respiratory distress. She was placed in the neonatal intensive care unit, and after several tests the clinicians told her parents that Mary Elizabeth had cystic fibrosis. The parents asked many questions about this condition and nothing they heard sounded encouraging. Jerry went online to find out all he could from the Internet and that plunged them into despair. The health care team in the perinatal unit, the genetic counselor, social workers, and others tried to console and encourage them, highlighting the great strides in treatment and longevity that individuals with this incurable chronic condition have enjoyed in the past several years. But Megan and Jerry feared that they had brought this long-awaited and beloved child into the world to endure a life of suffering if, indeed, Mary Elizabeth lived at all.

That was 11 years ago. Mary Elizabeth is a bright, beautiful child, small for her age physically, but with a happy spirit. Her inner vitality is a joy to all that meet her. Only a few in her acquaintance know that her life includes long periods of hospitalization and home schooling (and treatment) because of the seriousness of her symptoms, that she begins and ends each day with bouts of severe coughing, sometimes for an hour at a time, and that several times she has had pneumonia so serious that the family's parish priest has administered the sacrament of Last Rites, which is provided only for persons who are believed to be dying. Her school schedule is arranged so that only a few of her classmates surmise where she goes when she leaves daily for the school clinic for the vigorous percussion needed to loosen the thick brown mucus that continuously gathers in her lungs. The entire family agrees that it was worth the expense to move to a larger city where they have access to the ongoing availability of an excellent cystic fibrosis team. Among the most helpful is team member Betty Mortimer, whose own family has a history of cystic fibrosis.

Mary Elizabeth excels in school and is seen as a leader among her peers. Over the years all three McDonalds have learned to live a day at a time to see what it holds for them as a family. Some days Megan's activities are completely given over to tending to Mary Elizabeth, other times she almost forgets that there is any difference between her daughter and other children. Jerry has taken a second job to help defray expenses. Currently, both parents are concerned that Mary Elizabeth is entering puberty and fear that the teen years will present her with new challenges exacerbated by her chronic symptoms. They have long belonged to a parent support group and know that some young people with cystic fibrosis have less difficulty than others making the transition into the teen and adult years, succeeding in their social life and studies, having satisfying careers, and finding a life partner. They also have learned more about the genetic component of cystic fibrosis and know that soon they will have to discuss with her the probabilities of her own children having the condition or being carriers of it. Given their strong religious position on abortion, Megan was shocked to overhear Mary Elizabeth say to a friend recently, "If I became pregnant, I'd have an abortion so that child wouldn't have to go through what I'm goin' through." Megan wept all day.

Meanwhile, unbeknown to the McDonalds, the cystic fibrosis team is having a crisis of its own. The head pulmonary specialist on this team, a world-renowned expert in the field who has managed Mary Elizabeth for 8 years, announces to the team that once again he plans to put a patient on an experimental medication that they have used in two other instances rather than offer the alternative of a lung transplant to this family. He believes Mary Elizabeth would qualify to be on this drug and that her results should be excellent. A visible pall falls over the room, although three of the eight-member team quickly affirm the physician's decision. The second most experienced physician on the team begins to argue with the first about his decision. What all of them know is that although this experimental intervention has been heralded in reputable journals and medical circles as a "miracle drug," decreasing the rate of breakdown of the respiratory system, the first time it was attempted at this institution the patient died of a severe asthma attack. Since then, two additional serious asthma attacks in response to the initiation of the drug have appeared in the literature, although neither of those patients has died. The second patient who has been placed on it at their institution appears to be doing no better or worse than the team assumes she would be doing without the drug. Now the specialist is going to recommend the drug to the McDonalds, emphasizing the benefits and that the major caution is the very small percentage of people who experience "a severe, life-threatening asthma attack" while on the drug. He also is not going to mention a lung transplant, believing that this intervention carries too great a risk for this particular patient, a point that the second physician also loudly questions. The physician advocating for the medication reassures the team that he will have the "crash cart" and resuscitation team ready if there are any initial respiratory problems.

The next day the chief pulmonary specialist (who is also the team leader) announces to the team that he raised the issue with the McDonalds. Mary Elizabeth was there and she was very excited. "Maybe I can play soccer like my friends!" she is reported as saying. Although more cautious, the McDonalds, he reported, decided to go ahead, hoping that she might be among the first to benefit from this new intervention. Looking around the room and seeing their questioning eyes, he says, "Come on, you doubters. We all have the same goals in mind and we have to pull together!"

After the rounds end that day, all but the physician among the five members who disagreed with the team leader's decision lag behind in the lounge. They are sensitive to the fact that their team leader has referred to them as "the doubters" and decide that this is what they will call themselves in regard to this decision. More importantly, they are distressed. They know that the drug has been approved for human use in serious situations, such as Mary Elizabeth's case, and that the alternatives for Mary Elizabeth are few. They know all too well that a lung transplant is a high-risk surgery and that for some patients the symptoms of cystic fibrosis grow more serious during puberty and adulthood. Finally, they hit on a plan. Each will do his or her best to make sure the McDonalds actually know the doubters' reservations and will report back to each other about what they said and also how the McDonalds responded. Then, if they are not satisfied that the course of action is the morally correct one, Betty Mortimer, one of the team members, will take their deep reservations back to the team leader and the rest of the team. If they get nowhere, they will request an ethics consultation before any action is taken. They are aware that the team leader has little time for what he calls the "armchair philosophers" on the ethics committee, and he prides the team in being able to work out their differences in a reasonable and respectful manner. So he will be upset with them if his decision goes to the ethics committee, but at least "the doubters" will feel confident their deep concerns will have been heard.

While the doubters were discussing their plan of action, Betty did agree to assume the role as spokesperson back to the whole team, knowing that she is well respected by everyone and has a longer history on this unit than any of the others. In fact, she is old enough to be the team leader's mother. But when she heads home after her shift she finds herself wondering why she allowed herself to get into this position. She also is trying to decide what to say to the McDonalds, knowing how much they respect her and suspecting that if she shares her doubts about the drug and their lack of information about a lung transplant alternative they may decide against enrolling their daughter in the experimental protocol. If that is the outcome, she knows that the team leader will accuse her of acting inappropriately, sincerely believing she has robbed the McDonalds of an opportunity for a better quality of life for the whole family.

This team, the patient, and the family are in a relationship that is not unusual in instances of chronic and long-term care. Their shared concern is for the patient, they have known each other for a long period, the family caregivers are very much affected by the patient's condition, and the care being provided is by a multidisciplinary team. We turn now to the challenges they face together.

The Goal: A Caring Response

The means by which the goal of a caring response in this situation can be realized is, in many regards, similar to those in any other type of situation. For instance, the care must be personalized to the needs of the patient's specific situation. However, a key consideration that distinguishes this situation from many others is that collectively the interventions extend over a long period, sometimes from the patient's birth to her or his adulthood and beyond.[3] Figure 12–1 outlines several dimensions of the range and possible lifelong duration of chronic illnesses.

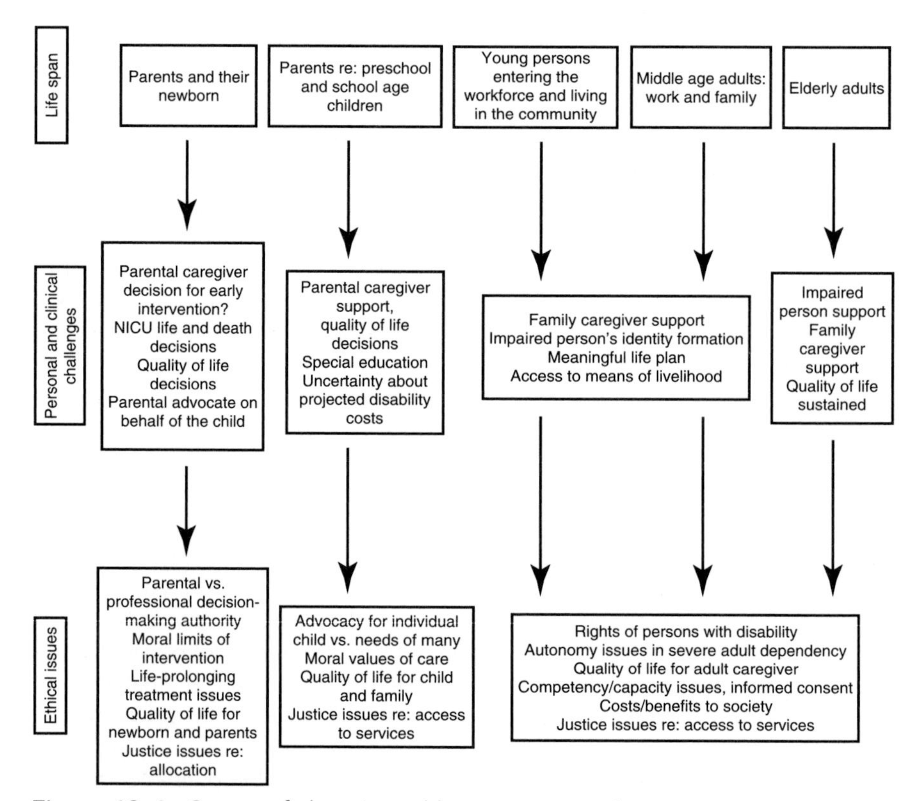

Figure 12–1. Scope of chronic and long-term care issues.

We can predict that in Mary Elizabeth's case she (and until she reaches adulthood, her parents) will be in relationships with health professionals on a regular basis. For her, this will continue throughout her entire life.[4]

There also are several generic considerations applying to all individuals with chronic conditions. First, for most patients, the health professional's *goal is not to effect a cure*. Neither, in most instances, will the patient's condition result in death within a short period; therefore the goal is not to help the person and his or her family in the dying process. Unlike many fatal illnesses, the team's goal of a caring response first must take into account the long duration of the patient's need for intervention and their (or other professionals') ongoing relationship with the patient and family.

Second, the point of interventions is the patient's *quality of life*, whether they be prevention of secondary symptoms, pain control and other comfort measures, or rehabilitation designed to help the patient build or sustain important functions, relationships, and roles. Well, you reply, that is no different from a caring response for any group of patients. In many fundamental regards you are right. However, the health fostering and health maintenance interventions for the patient with one underlying condition (complete with its constant or predictably evolving symptoms over months or years) do cast the challenge in a somewhat different light than acute symptoms.

Third, and related to the second, health professionals must design treatment programs with the idea that *the family (or other significant other) caregiver is crucial* to the treatment plan. More than in most other types of treatment planning, the health professionals must take the family caregivers' well-being into account (see later for further discussion of this point). There are not only ethical but also economic and other practical reasons for making decisions that are appropriate for the family caregivers' needs, as well as the patient's.[5]

Fourth, clinically and socially, the patient viewed as "chronically ill" may have *difficulty harnessing appropriate long-term care services*. A caring response on the part of the professional must include concerted advocacy efforts designed to counteract and denounce such discrimination and dehumanizing experiences. An example that discrimination does exist is illustrated in a study reporting the shortcomings of policies geared to patients with noncancer chronic symptoms. Of the 988 patients in the study, 41% had substantial unmet needs for assistance with their daily needs over time, 23% had problems related to being left unattended, and 20% had to rely on out-of-pocket caregivers. The differences between policies governing their care and the care of cancer patients with similar symptoms was most pronounced in noncancer patients who had a roller coaster pattern of exacerbations and remissions over several years.[6]

 *Reflection*

Can you think of other considerations that should inform health professionals who are working with chronic conditions, but might not be as important in acute care settings?

SUMMARY

In chronic illness situations, some factors affecting treatment decisions are that cure often is not the goal, whereas quality of life is; the family caregivers are deeply involved in the follow-up; and resources to pay for services may become a special challenge when compared with other types of interventions.

As in other types of situations facing health professionals, the six-step process again can be called on for assessing and deciding a course of action in the face of an ethical problem.

The Six-Step Process in Chronic and Long-Term Care Situations

Let us return to the McDonalds and the cystic fibrosis team, picking up the story at the juncture where the team has become divided about the decision made by the team leader and "the doubters" are plotting their course of action. The first step is to gather relevant information.

Step 1: Gather Relevant Information

The team is paying attention to information that has caused them concern. Betty needs to pay attention to several types of relevant information to play her role in Mary Elizabeth's team as they work to arrive at a truly caring response. She has been volunteered to be the spokesperson who will summarize the doubters' information and advocate for an ethics consult if they think it is necessary. She herself must bring reliable information back to the table of negotiation.

She has been working with the McDonalds for several years; therefore she has a reasonable understanding of Mary Elizabeth's current clinical status. It can be characterized as stable. We also can assume she can compare it with other similarly situated patients, because Betty's clinical expertise is in cystic fibrosis and respiratory disease. Naturally, she also needs to find out as much as possible about the exact effects and side effects of the experimental substance being proposed for Mary Elizabeth's treatment. Her firsthand experience with it to date is limited to the serious negative outcome it had for their one other patient on the unit. She will have to do her homework regarding this drug, and also regarding the state of the art of lung transplantation. She is moving ahead with her task, knowing that overall she is privileged to work with a group of outstanding colleagues in this field of medicine, at one of the world's top academic medical centers specializing in respiratory and pulmonary disease. The team is a "dream team" (most of the time!), hitting the rough spots with their common goals to guide them, and with deep respect for each other's competence.

At this "rough spot," Betty can organize her own information gathering around the four generic considerations outlined in the previous section.

First, the team is in it (as are the McDonald family) for the long haul. Betty knows that so far the team has been able to help the McDonalds manage Mary Elizabeth's symptoms. Unfortunately, at this pivotal moment in the team's relationship they themselves are divided. A part of her relevant information simply is that the McDonalds have a deep trust in the team as a unit and that anything she, or anyone else, does should be pursued in a manner that allows their trust to be sustained over the long road ahead.

Second, what can she say about Mary Elizabeth's quality of life? We can reasonably assume that Betty is totally convinced, on the evidence she has, that this young woman and her family are not keenly enough aware of the risks associated with the new treatment protocol and do not know how the risks might compare with those of a lung transplant. This whole family's quality of life may be compromised by their not being fully informed agents in the important decisions they are making.

In taking quality of life considerations into account, Betty also has to look beyond the specific symptoms of cystic fibrosis to consider the positive aspects of Mary Elizabeth's current social situation. Examined in this more general context, Betty might conclude that Mary Elizabeth's quality of life is quite good: this girl appears to be successful academically, is well accepted at school, and has the benefit of a devoted and capable health care team with back-up clinical support in her school system. However, she also is approaching an age when her paroxysms of coughing, the exhaustion it can cause, and other signs of pulmonary compromise may make it difficult for her to participate in the rigorous everyday activities that teens enjoy. She may start to feel the negative effects of one who is viewed as "disabled" in some regards. In other words, as she becomes a teenager, she may experience the disdain of others in her peer group because of her physical difference, and may be discriminated against, openly or subtly, in the social activities appropriate for her age group. She may begin to experience discrimination in the workplace if she looks for an after school job. None of these negative effects would be surprising because there is a tendency for society overall to show such disrespect to persons with disabilities.[7] Is there any way that this information, too, can help the team support the right decision?

Third, Betty needs to get a better idea, if she can, about the basis of the McDonald *family's* enthusiasm regarding the proposed implementation of the experimental drug. These caregiver parents are reported to have decided to implement the experimental regimen. Even if Mary Elizabeth fails to benefit appreciably in terms of her physical symptoms, the whole family may feel better in the long run about contributing to the ongoing search for a means by which the debilitating effects of the disease could be decreased, if not for her, perhaps for others.[8] The whole team must reckon with the knowledge that this patient's immediate family is an excellent support system. Mary Elizabeth can count on both parents to be there for her. Knowing that, the team should use every means to discern the decision that will best keep this tightly knit family unit strong and optimally functional. Theirs is a long and arduous road ahead, and the opportunity for the patient to take the experimental medication is but a moment in their lifelong relationship. Not only is respect for the parents' wishes warranted, they also must be protected against any outside influences (Betty and her doubting colleagues among them) that will create needless guilt, unnecessary resignation, burnout, or other debilitating events in their life. In summary, the way Betty and her team members approach the McDonalds is extremely important.

Fourth, Betty needs to gain a better idea of the various financial supports available to this pre-teen and her family. Sometimes insurance or other coverage that pays for treatments for a given period run out, either because the patient reaches a certain age, or school level, or the source of insurance caps out at a certain dollar amount that has now been expended. Moreover, a confusing variable in insurance coverage for different chronic conditions is that a diagnosis may slip from one coverage category to another. For example, elsewhere I have raised a worry that chronic conditions that have a genetic component requiring long-term care may become "lost" between the two categories of coverage.[9] What is the McDonald's situation regarding insurance coverage? Were any of these considerations being taken into account, influencing both the physician's and parents' decision? The team must have this information, too.

Reflection

Can you think of other information that Betty Mortimer and the other members of the team should have in their assessment of their team leader's decision? If so, jot them down for further discussion.

____

____

____

____

Step 2: Identify the Type of Ethical Problem

This story presents you with an interesting question about the moral agent. Obviously, there are several agents, namely the physician who is the team leader, the team as a whole, Betty Mortimer as a spokesperson back to the team, and, of course, the patient's parents. Therefore, on the one hand, this issue could be viewed strictly as a locus of authority ethical problem. On the other hand, I propose that we encountered these key players at a point where we must follow Betty's progress as a moral agent (acting as an individual health professional but also acting as a representative of the team members who are the doubters). How she and the doubter group proceed and what the team decides to do on the basis of the group's report back to the whole team may deeply influence the next step in Mary Elizabeth's long-term treatment regimen. Betty and her group of teammates who are questioning the current decision are faced with an ethical problem that I believe best can be characterized as an *ethical dilemma.*

I invite you to go back to the schematic view of an ethical dilemma, where one morally correct course of action is taken at the price of another morally correct course of action.

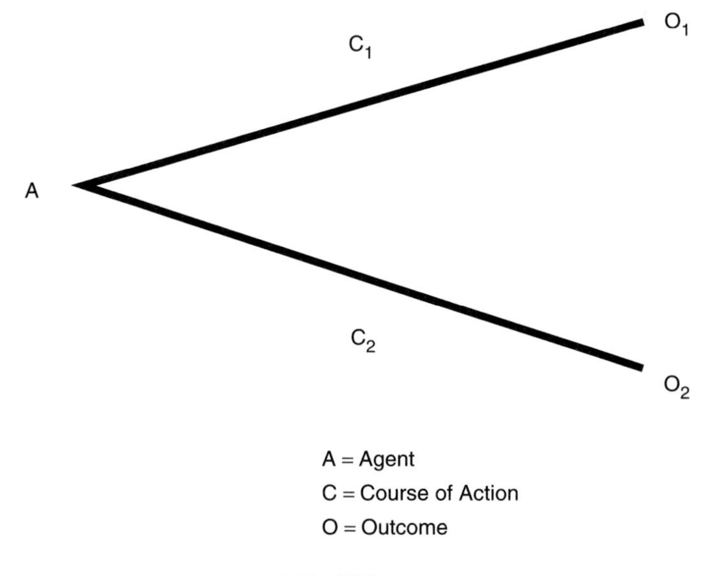

Ethical Dilemma

Reflection

If you accept my premise that the problem is an ethical dilemma, take a moment to identify two desirable outcomes they might achieve. This is the root of their problem because taking a course of action on the basis of one loyalty will result in a positive outcome but also will risk compromising another positive outcome.

This is the way I see Betty's predicament. The family wants to go ahead. So what is the problem? The problem is that the doubters share a deep level of discomfort about the outcome for that patient and family, somewhat based on their experience with another patient and also on their as-yet-unconfirmed concern that the McDonald family was not given all the options, even though none are self-evidently "the best." They also are proceeding with the belief that in this case the decision is not easily going to be opened for discussion again unless they insist it goes to the ethics committee. However, here's the other part of the predicament. Betty and her colleagues who question what has been decided do not believe their team leader has acted in bad faith. In fact, they respect him (as do others in their field) and know he is convinced that the decision is the right one. So one good outcome is to keep this team working as well as it usually does, under the leadership of their "captain."

Betty's agency *(A)* as a representative on behalf of the group may take a course of action *(C_1)* that includes pushing the envelope of the original decision, even to the point of calling in an ethics consultant. The outcome *(O_1)* may be to go back to this patient's family and, subsequently, again involve them in a process that leads them to a different decision regarding their preferred treatment for Mary Elizabeth. All of this will be done with the goal of achieving what is best for the patient, and no one can argue against that course of action or outcome.

A second course of action *(C_2)* will ensue if after thinking it over Betty and more of the doubting team members decide that their conduct will have such a disabling effect on their normally harmonious team that they should leave well enough alone. In other words, they will be moved to inaction, which also counts as an action because it causes a different outcome. In this second course of action, the outcome *(O_2)* is to preserve the integrity of the team or at least not risk causing the members to function under circumstances of greatly heightened stress or discord. One can hardly argue with this course of action and outcome either, especially if the team members are uncertain exactly what effect the discord on the team might have on the patient.

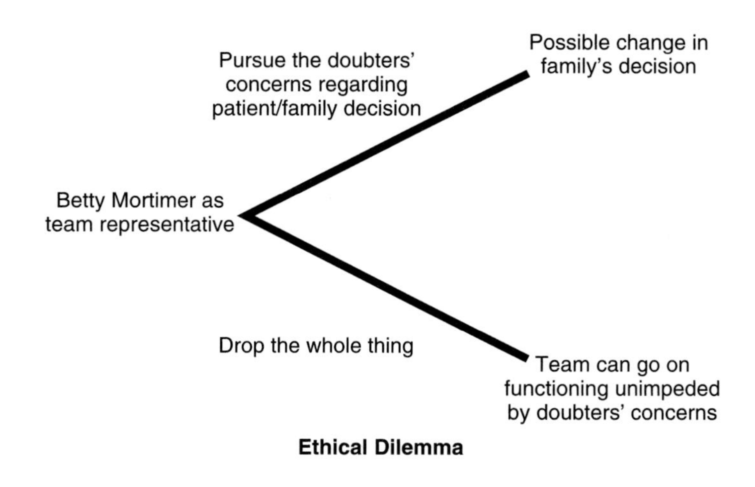

Reflection

Suppose the discord in this particular team is kept so well under wraps (they must have hit such a moment at some time previously in their considerable history together) that the patient's parents never know. Do the doubters still have an ethical dilemma?

I conclude that even if the discord never trickles into the awareness of the parents, the doubting team members have an ethical dilemma, because to look out for the best interests of the patient requires conduct that might compromise the stability and effectiveness of the team. They simply cannot have it both ways without the risk for compromise of one set of values they have good reason to want to protect and to nurture.

Step 3: Use Ethics Theories or Approaches to Analyze the Problem

Betty and the group of doubters could appeal to their knowledge about the consequences they believe will be brought about by various courses of action, and try to conclude which will bring about the most good. In so doing, they would be acting as utilitarians, trying to optimize the balance of benefits for everyone involved over the burdens brought about. Which consequences do you think should take precedent? Whatever your response, there is a problem with using this theoretic approach because there are several unknowns about the consequences of their action, reliance on this weighing alone seems insufficient to bring about the most morally supportable outcome. At the very least, Betty and the team members have the additional tool of ethical principles to help them in their assessment.

 ***Reflection***

Name at least two principles you think Betty should rely on in guiding the others during their deliberation about a course of action.

I suggest the principles of nonmaleficence and beneficence provide additional guidance for them. You may think of others that are appropriate as well, but I'll focus my comments on these two.

The Principle of Nonmaleficence

As you may recall, the principle of nonmaleficence means that the health professional (including the team) must "do no harm." The obligation to do no harm requires professionals to look closely at the means they are using, not just the ends (i.e., overall balance of good over harm) they might achieve. It includes *not causing harm directly, removing it* when it is present, and *preventing it* from happening. Each of these aspects of nonmaleficence are briefly examined below.

Some harms the doubters must guard against causing have been alluded to in the earlier discussion. For example, their actions must not cause the family, who needs the team over a long haul, to experience the direct harm of distrust—the McDonalds have to be able to trust the motivation and actions of the team leader and members. Therefore, nonmaleficence includes *how* Betty and the doubters approach the family regarding the decision they have already made about the experimental treatment regimen. Nonmaleficence also includes *how* the team leader and the team members who supported his decision handle the information that Betty and her doubter group bring back to them. You can see that both of these "how" scenarios become morally significant in not causing harm in this stressful situation.

At the same time, we believe Betty and the doubters are worried that harm already has been done by virtue of the McDonalds acting on information that may be incomplete. They aren't sure; therefore they have to examine their concern skillfully and with the compassion this family deserves. It is true that the principle to "do no harm" involves removing harm that has been done; therefore if Mary Elizabeth's parents have made a decision without all the relevant knowledge, Betty and the doubters should be agents in helping the whole team rectify the shortcoming.

In addition, harm must be prevented. In most chronic illness and long-term care situations, the health of the whole family is so intricately connected to the patient's well-being that the caregivers (in Mary Elizabeth's case, her parents) must never be put in a position to believe they have done anything but the best for the patient. This dimension of nonmaleficence supports the idea that the team collectively must be sure the parents have all the pertinent facts and give assurances that the McDonald family will be supported in their decision.

The Principle of Beneficence

The principle of beneficence requires the professional to not only do no harm but seek the very best outcome possible for the patient. That must be the goal of the entire team. Again the patient–family caregiver unit comes into central focus. The best possible outcome for the patient also must take seriously into account what constitutes the well-being of the family caregivers. This is true not only for instances such as the McDonalds, where the patient is a minor, but for all situations of serious chronic and long-term care situations. Obviously, some people with chronic conditions can live independently, but many require assistance with some aspects of their daily functioning. To give you an idea of the magnitude of this concern, at the time this book is being written, it is estimated that in one of four households (22.4 million people) in the United States alone, chronically ill or disabled persons older than 50 years are being cared for by family members.[10] Caregiving in the home traditionally has fallen to women, and in the great majority of cases still does, although currently an increasing number of men also are becoming family caregivers.[11] Thus, the "best decision" for the patient cannot be made in isolation from what will sustain and nourish the relationship of the caregiver as an individual and in relationship with the patient, whether the caregiver be a family member, friend, or other layperson.[12]

SUMMARY
In chronic illness situations every ethical consideration must consider the long-term course of decisions and how it will affect the family or other caregiver network.

In summary, benefits and burdens weighed in a purely utilitarian fashion must be informed by at least the considerations that come to light by identifying specific harms and benefits this patient, this family, and this team face by various courses of action the doubters may take with Betty as their spokesperson.

Step 4: Explore the Practical Alternatives

By now you know that one difficulty professionals face in a dilemma is stress. And when there is stress the range of alternatives often seems small. For that reason, in each chapter of this book I have encouraged you to think about specific stories in terms of the practical alternatives open to the moral agent(s).

Reflection

Before moving on, consider some alternatives you think Betty and the doubters have to help assure the most appropriate caring response is provided to the McDonalds.

The *first option* is to do nothing but support the team leader and the McDonalds. What is done is done, and the concern of the doubters may be unfounded anyway. The McDonalds may very well be best served by this approach.

A *second option* is to go directly to them, as the doubter members of the team already had decided to do. This assures that the McDonalds have an opportunity to directly provide some feedback to help inform the doubters what this family knows and why they arrived at their decision.

A *third option* is for Betty and the doubters not to go to the McDonalds but to go back to the other members of the team again and make their concerns once again known. That may be enough of a prod to persuade the team leader to at least take their concerns more seriously than he may have done to date. Of course, in acting on this alternative the doubters must take care not to become so strident in their preconceived conclusion that they unnecessarily further divide the team rather than helping it to come to a consensus.

A *fourth option* is to add an ethics consultation to the third alternative so that some objective third parties can help the whole team reexamine the doubters causes for concern, listen carefully to the team leader's reasons for his decision and help decide, from an ethics point of view, which course would most fully support the basic principles of nonmaleficence and beneficence toward the patient. This consult also could provide some insights into how the team might coalesce around a mutually arrived at next step with the least fallout among the team members.

Step 5: Complete the Action

Betty Mortimer and the doubters now have a lot of information to guide them and several alternatives from which to choose. Once the principles of nonmaleficence and beneficence are included in the mix of considerations, they will see that their course of action must fall on the side of the patient's (and her family's) best interests over the course of action that will be the least stressful for the team. When push comes to shove, the team's comfort cannot be honored over the patient's well-being. On that basis alone, the second through fourth alternatives are the most morally supportable. At the same time, the team is divided and the more it becomes so the more likely some other negative side effects of that division will spill over to the McDonalds. Therefore, Betty and the doubters must make a considered judgment about which of the options two through four to take.

What do you think about getting either the family or the ethics consult team involved before the whole team again addresses this issue among themselves? I think it is morally a riskier approach than going back to the other team members directly for another discussion first. My support for the third alternative comes from some things we know about this situation. First, the team is a longstanding and well working team. They have their history of trust and mutual respect going for them so the doubters must screw up their courage enough to bring that trust into this difficult moment. Second, we have no reason to believe that the team leader (or any member of the team) had ulterior motives in mind when recommending the experimental drug regimen, therefore the doubters should give the group who support the team leader an opportunity to explain their position. In turn, the doubters have a right to be heard, too. Third, we know the feeling of the team leader about getting an ethics consultation, therefore he should have an opportunity to at least hear Betty and her colleagues' reasoning in the more familiar context of the usual team meeting before the next step is taken (i.e., Betty calls an ethics consultation meeting). All in all, the third alternative is the best one, at least as the next step for Betty Mortimer to take in her role both as advocate for the patient and spokesperson for the doubter group of team members.

Step 6: Evaluate the Process and Outcome

As in every difficult ethical situation, the subgroup of team members should take time to reflect back on whatever does happen next and how their own dispositions, reasoning, and conduct played in the final decision. They also should also use the opportunity, if possible, to reflect with the whole team on why and how the division occurred in the first place. We know the circumstances that triggered a negative response in some to the team leader's decision initially. Once they have gone through the six-step process of decision making, they will have accumulated a lot more information and probably a lot more insight into the variables at stake.

Because they will again have been reminded that in the end the team's role is first and foremost to get behind the patient's best interests, they will have an opportunity to glean from their experience how those interests can be honored.

SUMMARY

In chronic conditions team approaches dominate, and therefore an effective team is essential to good care.

The McDonalds as a family unit not only will have benefited (we hope), but also will have been teachers, demonstrating once again that especially in long-term illness and chronic conditions the patient–family caregiver unit must be considered at all times.

Summary

The increase in scope and number of patients presenting to the health care system with chronic symptoms and illnesses, together with the increasing range of interventions available to them, create an opportunity for you to meet the goal of a caring response for this population. Actual interventions include prevention of new symptoms or decrease in their severity when they do appear, rehabilitation and health maintenance within the constraints of the disease, and vigilance not to assume every new symptom is part of the constellation of symptoms associated with the original chronic condition. Some key factors to take into consideration while arriving at a caring response are the persistence of the patient's symptoms or the generally predictable evolution of a specific chronic condition. The importance of nurturing the family or other caregiver relationships cannot be underscored enough. In Chapter 13 you will have an opportunity to carry some of these considerations over into the area of end-of-life care.

Questions for Thought and Discussion

1. Saul is 47 years old and has recently been diagnosed with Parkinson's disease. A movie producer in Hollywood, he knows he has all the benefits of modern medicine at his disposal. Still, he slowly is acknowledging that nothing he has read or learned from his numerous sources of information promise him anything but increasing loss of physical and cognitive faculties over time.

   You are a therapist working in a sports center where a number of movie stars, producers, and other notables of the film industry work out. Saul has grown quite fond of you and often stays after his workout to chat. But today he is very sad and depressed. He tells you about the diagnosis, which you had not known, and asks you "as a member of the medical world" if you think there is any hope for him, or whether he should just give up now. How will you respond to this man who is reaching out to you in your role as a health professional, but who is not your patient per se? How will you define "hope" as you think about how to respond to him?

2. The leading cause of disability in the United States is arthritis, affecting one of every six people. You are asked to serve on a national commission because of the role your profession plays in the clinical management of arthritis. The charge to each commissioner is to identify how your profession can contribute to a greater quality of life for individuals with the painful and dysfunction symptoms of arthritis. Each profession will be advocating for policies that allow them to be reimbursed for beneficial services rendered by its members. You have a moral obligation to advocate for patients as the representative of your profession. List how your profession factors into the overall picture of symptom management. What arguments will you bring to the commission on behalf of your profession?

___

___

___

___

3. Chronic illness and disability often are treated as one and the same. Still, many individuals with disabilities do not have illnesses or symptoms that require health care interventions. One downside of this conflation of the two ideas is that persons with disability often are treated as if they are "sick." Discuss the problem from the flip side of the coin: namely, the ethical issues that arise when a person with a chronic illness is treated as if he or she has a disability, not an illness or clinical symptom. Name some chronic illnesses in which there is likely also to be disability.

___

___

___

___

References

1. Tu, H.T., Reed, M.C. 2002. Options for expanding health insurance for people with chronic conditions. *Issue Brief: Findings from Health System Change* 50:1–4.
2. Cutler, D.M. 2003. Disability and the future of Medicare. *New England Journal of Medicine* 349(11):1084–1085.
3. U.S. Department of Health and Human Services. 2000. *Healthy People 2010: Understanding and Improving Health* (2nd ed.). Washington, DC: U.S. Government Printing Office.
4. Rothenberg, L. 2003. *Breathing for a Living: A Memoir*. New York: Hyperion.
5. Norton, E.C. 2000. Long term care. In Culyer, A.J., Newhouse, J.P. (Eds.), *Handbook of Health Economics* (vol. 1B.). Amsterdam: Elsevier, pp. 955–988.
6. Emanuel, E. 1999. Assistance from the family members, friends, paid care givers and volunteers in the care of terminally ill patients. *New England Journal of Medicine* 341(13):956–963.
7. Purtilo, R. 2003. *When Disabilities Get Genetic Labels: Ethical Issues*. Presentation at the MGH Institute of Health Professions Annual Henry Knox Sherrill Lecture in Ethics, Boston, Massachusetts, May 12, 2003.
8. Botkin, J. 2003 Preventing exploitation in pediatric research. *American Journal of Bioethics* 3(4):31–33.
9. Purtilo, R. 2004. Genetic labels and long-term care policies: A winning or losing proposition for patients? In Magill, G. (Ed.), *Genetics and Ethics: An Interdisciplinary Study*. St. Louis: St. Louis University Press, pp. 153–163.
10. U.S. Department of Labor Women's Resource Division. 2000. Reported in Martha Nussbaum, 2001. Disabled Lives: Who cares? *New York Review of Books,* 11 January, pp. 34–37.
11. Kittay, E.F. 2001. *Loves Labor: Essays on Women, Equality and Dependency*. New York: Rutledge.
12. Levine, C. 1999. The loneliness of the long-term care giver. *New England Journal of Medicine* 340(15):87–88.

13

Ethical Issues in End-of-Life Care

Objectives

The student should be able to:

- List six ways that a caring response can be achieved in end-of-life care.
- Define *palliative care* and give at least three examples of how it is expressed.
- Identify some practical means by which a dying patient's trust can be fostered and reasonable expectations can be met by health professionals.
- Discuss how abandonment affects people with life-threatening conditions.
- Describe four guidelines that can help you continue to "abide with" a patient who is dying.
- Identify some basic ethical concepts that have special importance in the treatment of patients who have life-threatening conditions.
- Identify three "faces" of the virtue of compassion.
- Discuss the professional's duty of nonmaleficence for its relevance in end-of-life care.
- Distinguish ordinary and extraordinary or heroic interventions and list two criteria for deciding that an intervention is extraordinary.
- Describe the idea of medical futility and its role in the ethical debate about appropriate end-of-life interventions.
- Describe the ethical principle of double effect and its usefulness.
- List three mechanisms to assist patients and professionals in discerning the proper moral limits of intervention.
- List and discuss the merits of advance directives.
- Summarize the ethical debate about clinically assisted suicide and medical euthanasia.

New terms and ideas you will encounter in this chapter

end-of-life care	personalized care	palliative care
hospice	physical abandonment	psychological abandonment

compassion
withdrawal of treatment
U.S. Patient Self-Determination Act (PSDA)
usual and customary treatment
principle of double effect
advance care planning
clinically assisted suicide
abiding with patients
withholding of treatment
acts of commission
burdens and benefits
ratio test
ordinary vs. extraordinary care
living will
life-prolonging interventions
supererogation
life supports
acts of omission
medical futility
advance directive
durable power of attorney
voluntary vs. involuntary medical euthanasia

Topics in this chapter introduced in earlier chapters

Topic	*Introduced in chapter*
Care and a caring response	2
Ethics of care approach	3
Virtue	3
Benevolence	3
Fidelity	3
Nonmaleficence	3
Quality of life	2
Informed consent	11
Surrogate decision maker	11
Autonomy or self-determination	3
Health care teams	8
Ethics committees	1
Ethics consultation	1
Six-step process of ethical decision making	4

Introduction

Working with patients and their loved ones when the person has a condition that carries a medical prognosis of being incurable poses special ethical challenges. How should you, the health professional, treat such persons with the dignity they deserve? The terminology encountered in the medical literature (e.g., terminal, fatal, irreversible, incurable) adds to many persons' anxiety when health professionals use it in conversation with the patient and his or her family. At the same time, your work with these patients can be the perfect opportunity to be a positive influence in their lives. For this and other reasons I will address ethical issues that come sharply into focus when a person is going to die because of his or her medical condition.

Throughout this textbook you have been reminded of the importance of care in the ethics of the health professional–patient relationship. There is no situation where this applies more than in the treatment of persons who are coming to the end of their life. Most health professionals want to convey to patients who have incurable illnesses, "I care," and the examples in this chapter illustrate ways in which that message can be meaningfully conveyed. It requires a clear understanding of special ethical considerations that emerge in this type of situation, rigorous application of your technical competence, and personal adaptability to each patient. To help focus your thinking, consider the following story.

The Story of Almena Lykes, Jarda Roubal, and Roy Moser

Mrs. Almena Lykes is 42 years old and was diagnosed with amyotrophic lateral sclerosis (ALS) about 18 months ago. When she was admitted to the hospital with severe pneumonia and shortness of breath, she had some movement in her legs and could get around in the wheelchair. Despite physical and respiratory therapy and good nursing care, she has become weaker since being institutionalized. Tests indicate that her pneumonia probably developed because of weakness of the swallowing muscles (which allowed aspiration of mouth contents into the lungs). She is discouraged knowing that her condition is going to get progressively worse and that she will eventually die. She also believes that her husband is not willing to care for her at home any longer, a fact that the staff cannot confirm because he has not called or appeared since she was admitted.

After a 2-week course she takes a decisive turn for the worse. Dr. Jarda Roubal, her physician, believes that she is not going to be able to bounce back from this pneumonia even if there is vigorous treatment with antibiotics and respiratory therapy because of rapid deterioration of her swallowing and breathing muscles. Dr. Roubal discusses the seriousness of her prognosis, the options open to her for interventions regarding her pneumonia (medications, respiratory therapy), and predicts that she is near to the time when she will have to be on a ventilator permanently. He answers all questions directly about the seriousness of her prognosis. He asks her nurse, Roy Moser, to place a respirator in her room for quick initiation of ventilator support should it be needed.

Yesterday evening Mrs. Lykes asked Roy to sit down with her by her bed. Tearfully, she told him that she really was ready to die. She requested that her treatments in physical, occupational, and respiratory therapy be discontinued and that she not be placed on a respirator unless it would mean she would suffer less while she was dying. She said she had seen a movie in which a woman was given morphine to speed up the dying process and make it painless and explained that was what she wanted. She also has requested a Do Not Resuscitate status.

"Dr. Roubal means well, but he will make a vegetable out of me," she says, breaking down. Roy said he would be sure to talk to Dr. Roubal about her wishes but that the final decision would be made by the doctor and her. Then Roy documented the conversation in her clinical record.

That afternoon when Dr. Roubal came through to check on the patients Roy Moser took him aside and conveyed the whole conversation as best he could recall it, word for word. Dr. Roubal listened intently and said, "What do YOU think?"

"I think we should do what she suggests. She isn't going to get better."

After a moment Dr. Roubal said, "Well you are right about her not getting better, but I think she is depressed and once she gets on a respirator and over the pneumonia she will see it differently. She still has a lot of life in her." He said to Almena, "The nurse has told me about your concerns. I would like you to think it over. There's still a lot we can do for you."

Later that evening Roy went back to Almena Lykes's room. Almena looked extremely sad and alone, her eyes puffy from crying. Now she was dry eyed and made an attempt to lift her limp hand. "I don't know what to do." she said.

Before continuing, take a minute to think about Dr. Jarda Roubal's and Roy Moser's response to Almena Lykes.

Reflection

What is each doing to show a caring response to her problems? Do you think one or the other is more correct in their judgment about whether to continue treatment? On what do you base your opinion?

In this story you can quickly discern by now that several important ethical dimensions of professional practice come into full view. As in previous chapters I will guide you through the six-step process to highlight some of them, knowing that you may identify others.

The Goal: A Caring Response

Suppose that you are Dr. Jarda Roubal or Roy Moser. It goes without saying that Mrs. Lykes deserves all the respectful consideration from you that you would give to any patient. She needs to feel confident that you are competent, because her life literally may be in your hands. In a word, she expects you to give her your best attention consistent with a caring response.

Caring is a balancing act. As the very purpose of your professional role is to administer effectively to clinical need, you cannot ever *substitute* fluffing pillows or flashing encouraging smiles in these circumstances, as reassuring as they may be to Mrs. Lykes. However, currently more often the criticism is expressed that health professionals working with people who have incurable medical conditions may be technically competent but fail to show personalized nurturing also required for true care.

The health professional who is committed to providing personalized care will do at least the following:

Maintain vigilant attention to clinical interventions appropriate for the person's condition whether preventive, rehabilitative, or comfort enhancing. The diagnosis of an incurable condition does not mean that the whole range of interventions may be prematurely dropped from the clinician's resources for optimal treatment.

Take enough time to communicate with the patient (and loved ones) to get a "feel" for the person's values, strongly held beliefs, habits, cultural and ethnic characteristics, and personality.

Think about how to address a patient or client (i.e., decide whether to use the first or last name of each new person, knowing the casual use of the first name may be offensive to some people).

Show interest in the patient or client but do not encourage a relationship that will lead to overdependence or interfere with the patient's personal relationships.

Listen carefully to what the person has to say.

Maintain a balance between providing sound health care services and fostering friendly exchanges.

A focus on the patient's quality of life governs you in your attempt to create a warm, personal environment. Only the patient's (or if the patient is incapable of indicating her preferences, the surrogate's) interpretation of what makes life worthwhile counts, not yours or anyone else's. Sometimes concerns that are important to the patient seem insignificant to a health professional.

Reflection

What might you expect would weigh heavy on Mrs. Lykes's mind right now? How can you respond in a warm and supportive manner to her concerns?

SUMMARY

A caring response in end-of-life situations requires apt attention to quality of life issues for the patient and family.

Palliative Care

As we come to realize that health care includes the provision of comfort measures to people who are dying, as well as trying curative and restorative treatments until they are shown to be futile, the notion of *palliative care* becomes integral to a caring response. *Palliation* means to relieve or lessen without curing, to moderate or alleviate its intensity.[1] It is not limited to individuals with incurable conditions that will lead to death, although that will be the focus of our discussion.

Some objectives of palliative care include the following general guidelines:

- People with advanced, potentially fatal conditions and those close to them should expect and receive skillful and supportive care not focused on curing the patient.
- Health professionals must commit themselves to using their professional knowledge effectively to prevent and relieve pain and other disturbing symptoms.
- Health professionals should regain an awareness and humility about what modern medicine can and cannot do so that patients can deal with their own death realistically, not as the enemy but as a part of life.
- Health professionals must recognize that the patient's continuing downward course may be a time of anxiety for the health professional, too, posing a challenge to the whole team.[2]
- Providing the best care possible means that as much imagination, competence, and energy must be directed to Mrs. Lykes's palliative interventions as would be devoted to someone's care when the patient does not have an incurable condition.

Throughout the patient's illness the goal of providing the best palliative care possible includes giving emotional support to people closest to the patient. This will help encourage the patient even though you might find yourself becoming frustrated with the patient's relatives and close friends because they are angry, confused, or feeling intense sorrow about what is happening to their loved one and may transfer their feelings to you. Their demands, worries, questions, and interference with treatment can be disconcerting, especially when their actions call into question your own best judgment or exacerbate your own anxieties about the patient's plight. It must be remembered that any time the patient's most intimate sources of support are alienated or harmed the patient also inevitably suffers deleterious consequences. At best, family and close friends are a great assistance to your efforts; at worst, they should not be unnecessarily excluded from your support and deprived of relevant information. Although their behaviors will differ according to culture and other family practices, they have a right to be included.[3]

In palliative care, stopping intense efforts to effect a cure must signal the beginning of an even more intense effort to engage in a regimen of clinical intervention aimed at reduction of discomfort. The words of a physician some years ago have always stuck with me:

> Even when we decide that our advanced technologies are no longer indicated, we can still agree that certain extreme measures are indicated—extreme responsibility, extraordinary sensitivity, heroic compassion.[4]

These words are especially valuable because often at the moment that you admit the person is indeed beyond medical intervention aimed at cure, you may momentarily feel at a loss as to how to continue to express your caring. We can imagine that Roy Moser had this feeling when he walked into Almena Lykes's room and noticed she had been crying, or when she confessed she does not "know what to do." Your own imagination may be thwarted by the knowledge that the patient's time is limited. This could deter you from setting attainable goals that may be of importance to the patient. Tonight is the future. Tomorrow is the future. Mrs. Lykes can be encouraged toward the goal of walking to the bathroom unassisted tonight or sitting up to write some business letters tomorrow. Sometimes, too, patients are hesitant to offer information about their desires because they fear the goal will seem irrelevant or even silly to someone else. For example, one young woman confided to the chaplain that she longed to go to the chapel for religious services but was afraid it was too much work for the nurses to get her there. Another woman who required large doses of pain-reducing medication told the medical technologist she was concerned that the "fuzziness" created by the medication would impair her judgment when her lawyer came to discuss her estate. The technologist relayed the information to the woman's physician, and the physician arranged to have the medication withheld during the lawyer's visit, with the grateful consent of the patient.

Another aspect of palliative care is to adjust your approach according to the probable time left before the patient's death. One has to be an artist of "good timing." The person who senses that the end is near often will ask to be left alone with only a few select people or, in some cases, with no one at all. To be cheerfully intrusive at such times denies a person her need to determine the use of her last moments. In contrast, to treat a person who may live for months or years with a slowly progressing illness as if she is about to die at any moment robs the person of her sense of belonging among the living. A 42-year-old woman dying of a slowly progressing leukemia went into her local hospital for her monthly blood tests. A laboratory technician who had not seen her for several months greeted her by saying, "You still around?" The woman told her husband later, "She was just teasing, but it made me feel funny—like maybe I was supposed to have died already or something."

Anyone who has experienced the ordeal of a loved one's prolonged dying knows that some of the tensest moments are those related to not knowing how long the person will be alive, of being afraid that one will prematurely "hang the crepe," and of not knowing how to make appropriate plans for the future. The art of palliative care includes being as sensitive as possible to the time frame the patient and family are living with and adjusting your own approach accordingly.

One highly successful alternative being explored for patients beyond medical cure is the hospice approach, which originated in England.[5] For the hospice patient the entire staff and institutional structure is directed toward maintaining the patient in as comfortable, pain-free, and humane an environment as possible.[6]

SUMMARY

Palliative care has many dimensions, among them your concerted effort to decrease physical, psychological, and emotional pain and attention to the patient's own timing and life situation and to the institutional option for the person such as hospice care.

Now that we have laid the general groundwork for what a caring response entails in this type of situation, I invite you to turn to the by now familiar process of ethical decision making to consider Almena Lykes's story in more detail.

The Six-Step Process in End-of-Life Situations

The art of caring requires that health professionals be keenly aware of when the moral aspects of the relationship hit a snag and an ethical problem appears.

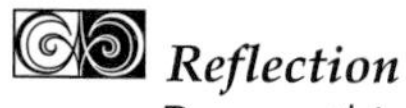

Reflection

Do you think Dr. Jarda Roubal and Roy Moser are faced with an ethical problem? If so, jot down why or why not and how their respective roles as physician and nurse are similar and different.

I believe they do have an ethical problem, given the seriousness of Almena Lykes's clinical condition. The life or death decision about life-prolonging measures must be negotiated to her satisfaction, and her present anxiety must be taken seriously into account. We begin here by reviewing the salient facts of her story to help highlight some details of the problems in her particular situation.

Step 1: Gather Relevant Information

The most important fact we have is that Mrs. Lykes has a noncurable condition, the pathology of which will continue to cause her muscles to grow weaker. She will have profound debility and, finally, failure of her heart and respiratory muscles. She will not be able to swallow. Eventually, she will die of her condition.

Dr. Jarda Roubal is monitoring this clinical course trying to maintain her respiratory functions. Roy Moser is a central, coordinating figure of the team of therapists, technologists, and others gauging how various interventions are helping to maintain the health she has remaining. They also are trying to stay in touch with her feelings, as well as keep her optimally functioning and comfortable. We know that all three of the key players in this story are at a crossroads. Should Mrs. Lykes's expressed wish to give up now be honored, or should the health professionals listen to her confusion in the lonely evening hours and again encourage her to hang on? Dr. Roubal will be the one to make the final call, medically speaking, about how to proceed. However, from an ethical viewpoint, that call must be made with as much certainty—and in as much accord with Mrs. Lykes's real wishes—as possible.

One key to her suffering is that she will be abandoned by her husband and will be (or already is) left alone by someone she deeply counted on. The fear and reality of such abandonment is common enough that it warrants your further consideration here.

Abandonment: A Patient's Reasonable Fear

Almena Lykes knows that things are not going to get better, clinically speaking. I have just mentioned how sometimes spouses, other loved ones, and friends fall away during the patient's process of dying. Some challenges facing family and other loved ones in regard to their role during a long-term course were mentioned in Chapter 12. Mrs. Lykes has a chronic, disabling, and incurable condition. For whatever reason, Mr. Lykes has disappeared and it is not possible to ascertain whether his absence is because of fear, weariness, or disgust and anger at her situation.

In addition to abandonment by loved ones, patients also sometimes detect that health professionals are distancing themselves, which exacerbates the patients' anxiety and suffering.

Health professionals seldom *physically abandon* patients who have an incurable medical condition. Sometimes, however, they are caught in policies that prevent them from giving a patient as much of or the type of treatment the professionals believe that person needs. For instance, in the United States, some managed care health plans have been accused of shortchanging patients, not paying for needed treatment for some groups.[7,8] Because health plans vary widely in their practices, you should check out the conditions of your employment site before signing a contract so as not to be forced into what seems to be abandonment by policy dictate.

Psychological abandonment is the greater danger that sometimes leads a health professional to physical neglect of the patient. Why? For one thing, their concepts of what health care interventions should accomplish may lead professionals to distance themselves, because the patient continues to "get worse." Others are repulsed by a patient's appearance, smells, and other disturbing manifestations of a patient's condition.[9] Psychological preparation for the pain of loss when a patient dies is advisable, and sometimes health professionals distance themselves to protect against the pain of that loss and feeling of failure. But psychological abandonment is distancing that far exceeds the use of necessary defense mechanisms. It follows that no matter what Mrs. Lykes's husband chooses to do, the responsibility for not abandoning her also falls on Dr. Roubal, Roy Moser, and the other health professionals working with her. Together they can support each other to overcome their tendency to abandon her physically or psychologically.

Reflection

Suppose you are Roy Moser that evening in Almena Lykes's room. What aspects of this situation might make you feel like fleeing? What steps can you take to help assure this type of harm does not befall her? What additional information from Mrs. Lykes might be helpful or necessary to provide appropriate care for her, thereby remaining faithful to your role?

Abiding: A Patient's Reasonable Hope

The idea of *abiding with* a patient may help you to think about what the opposite of abandonment looks like. To *abide* means "to endure without yielding," "to bear patiently," and "to remain stable."[10] Sometimes good care simply requires digging your heels in and standing firm.

The following are some general guidelines that can help you to maintain an attentive position toward Mrs. Lykes that she will experience as your abiding with her. You will recognize them as having themes similar to the ones you were introduced to as a part of personalized care and good palliative care in these situations. The guidelines include:

- Recognize your own feelings of fear, disgust, and repulsion. They are embarrassing, and the inclination is to pretend that they do not exist. Denial will not make them disappear.

- Encourage sessions in your workplace where everyone can share his or her feelings in a safe, constructive environment.
- Make efforts to talk to patients so that you will know them better and can focus on who they are personally. In many instances, the troubling feelings will become less important.

You deserve assurance that you have appropriate policies in place to help you show respect for her the way you are expected to do for all patients. You deserve assurance that the type and number of interventions you are offering do honor her considered wishes and her body's capacity for responding positively to them.

SUMMARY

Physical or psychological abandonment of a person who is dying can be countered by professionals who choose to abide with the patient. Professionals need support themselves in this situation.

Having touched some salient features of the patient's situation, please turn to the ethical decision-making process again.

Step 2: Identify the Type of Ethical Problem

At this stage of their decision making, both the physician, Dr. Jarda Roubal, and the nurse, Roy Moser, are faced with an ethical problem that comes from a high degree of uncertainty. This is a form of *ethical distress*. At the point we enter their picture, Dr. Roubal has made a clinical judgment that he believes is in Almena's best interest, but he certainly is shaken by Roy's report. Roy, too, must be in a situation where he cannot be sure what is going on. Both have additional work to do as moral agents. This juncture of their quandary is an apt place for you to consider a second related type of ethical problem that we have not often discussed as a separate focus of concern and which often accompanies situations of high uncertainty. This problem is termed a *locus of authority* issue (Fig. 13–1).

The locus of authority prototype of ethical problem requires two or more moral agents in the situation to decide which of them should be the final appropriate moral voice in the decision. To the extent that Almena Lykes is competent to make her own decisions, and the diagnosis of an incurable condition is confirmed, the ultimate answer is easy: *She* is. The physician has requested something that is potentially life saving so we want to be sure she is not making a decision to refuse it on partial knowledge or because she is depressed. She must not make a decision that she will not only regret, but that is irreversible.

Talking to her further is an obvious next step both the physician and nurse want to pursue. In Chapter 11 you were introduced to informed consent. The goal is to be sure that she is competent to

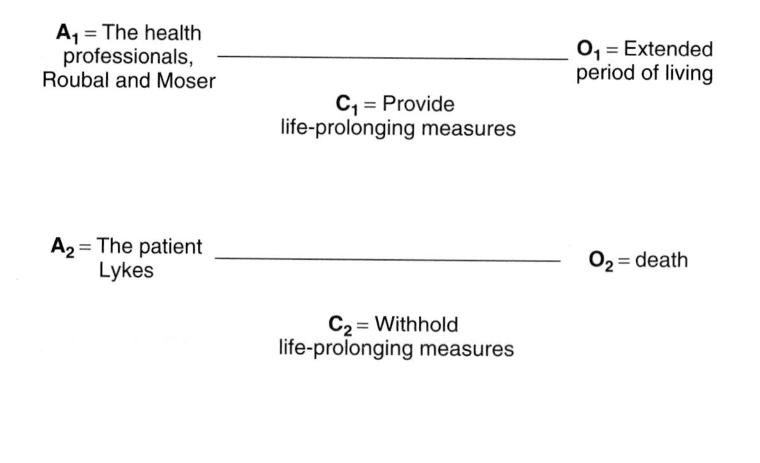

A = Moral Agent
C = Course of Action
O = Outcome

Figure 13–1. Locus of authority ethical problem.

make, and is making, an informed decision. There is virtually no basic moral difference between how this mechanism is used for showing respect to patients who will recover and how it is used for patients with irreversible conditions. The only psychological difference between the two types of patients is that a person such as Mrs. Lykes, with a seriously deteriorating incurable condition, is faced with a life and death urgency to make her informed wishes known.

Dr. Roubal believes she might be refusing the ventilator because she is depressed and that she will change her mind, suggesting that she will want to be put on the respirator when her depression lifts. This is not a judgment he should make lightly. A visit by the liaison psychiatrist can help ascertain whether she is depressed to the point of being unable to make this important decision. The position he apparently is holding—that of a paternalistic authority who will try to talk her into accepting the respirator—should not be maintained without the information about her mental status.

Step 3: Use Ethics Theories or Approaches to Analyze the Problem

What resources do each of these professionals need to arrive at a caring response in this type of situation? The ethics of care places virtues in a central place and provides a useful approach for assessing the ethical issues here. Much has been written about the virtue of compassion in health care and nowhere is it more important than when the patient has an incurable condition. The term *compassion* often is used in everyday language to indicate a warm or positive feeling toward the patient, which helps to convey sympathetic involvement with the patient's plight. Although that is not incorrect, it is more complicated than that, too. It is so important that we will pause here to examine it as a virtue, a duty, and as going beyond duty.

Compassion: Three Moral Faces of an Idea

There are three powerful components of *compassion*[11]:

1. The *character trait* or virtue of sympathetic understanding recognized as a virtue,
2. Willingness *to carry out your professional responsibilities* toward the patient, recognized as moral duty, and
3. Readiness *to go beyond the call of duty.*

We can observe these dispositions in others, but may not readily recognize them as compassion.

Compassion as a Virtue. The virtues of kindness and benevolence are recognizable as promoting a desire to treat people with gentleness and to "do good" when it is in your power to do so. Being able to do good depends first on the ability to imagine vividly how another feels, so that you become aware of the needs and wants of the other person. The word *compassion* comes from the Latin, *passio* ("suffering") and *con* ("with"). It entails the desire to treat others with sympathetic understanding. It is from this root meaning that compassion usually is understood solely as a disposition toward others, a virtue.

Reflection

Knowing as little as you do about Mrs. Lykes's situation, what do you believe are some of her needs that warrant your sympathetic understanding? To aid in your reflection, write them down.

The desire to be sympathetic is a resource in itself. You might find it expressed in something as simple as a reassuring arm across her shoulder, knowing she is discouraged, or a telephone call to assist Mrs. Lykes in making contact with a close friend or a person in religious life who has been a source of guidance or comfort to her in the past. To do so with understanding increases the likelihood that you will get it right in terms of the way you choose to express your sympathy.

Compassion as Willingly Doing Your Duty. A form of compassion sometimes overlooked is willingness *to carry out your duties* on behalf of the patient's best interests as you have discerned those interests through your sympathetic posture. As compassion compels you to do what is right, you can see how two aspects of ethical thought (character traits and duties) are brought together in an actual situation. Compassion, as a character trait in the type of person you want to be, aids you in the desire actually to *do* what you discern to be right. This helps you to keep to task, to pay attention to doing your work competently, and to not be careless about the well-being of the patient when you would rather be meeting a friend or golfing or even going about some other aspect of your daily work. In a word, it helps you to *abide with* the patient.

Compassion as Going Beyond Duty. Finally, the motivating force of compassion positions you to exercise *kindnesses that go beyond duty.* Acts that altruistically go beyond duty are called acts of supererogation. An example of such a person is the physician Dr. Bernard Rieux in Albert Camus's novel *The Plague,* who chooses to stay behind to minister to those dying of Bubonic plague rather than avail himself of the obvious life-preserving action of escape.[12]

The Principle of Nonmaleficence

Your general duty of fidelity or faithfulness to patients includes the stringent principle not to harm them. Do you remember the more philosophic term for this duty? If you said "nonmaleficence," you are right! The deliberate and diligent efforts of many before you to put in place procedures to assist you in providing compassionate care is one indicator that your moral obligation not to harm has been taken seriously by health professionals and society.

As you recall, when virtues and character traits guide your response you are acting within the context of what generally is called the ethics of care. That approach certainly is needed in Dr. Jarda Roubal's and Roy Moser's attempt to learn Mrs. Lyke's considered preferences. At the same time, their attention to the principle of nonmaleficence suggests that duty also plays an important function in your professional role. Therefore, an appeal to a deontologic approach will help guide each of them to do what is right. To learn more specifically the forms those right actions might take in the case of incurable conditions, we proceed to the next step of decision making.

Step 4: Explore the Practical Alternatives

You have already noted that if you were in the shoes of Jarda Roubal or Roy Moser you would have to find out what Mrs. Lykes really knows about the decision to be made, if she is too depressed to make an informed decision and, finally, what her considered choice is. You also can discuss your (and her) quandary with other members of the health care team who have been involved in her treatment. Once you have reached a point of greater certainty you will have to assume a function appropriate to your professional role on the team involved in Almena Lykes's care in regard to initiating, withholding, or withdrawing life-prolonging interventions. The issues of withholding or withdrawing are so important that you now have an opportunity to learn more about them. We will assume that Dr. Roubal's referral to psychiatry has deemed her to be competent. As a member of the team you are helping to determine the proper moral limits of clinical interventions designed to prolong her life. Therefore, one basic practical determination you have to make is whether life-prolonging interventions in this situation are "ordinary" or "*extra*ordinary" according to what Almena Lykes believes is the balance of benefits over burdens she will receive by initiating respirator assistance.

Employing Ordinary and Extraordinary Distinctions

Having introduced you, earlier in this chapter, to some problems that arise because health professionals stop treatment prematurely or psychologically withdraw, you now have an opportunity to consider the converse. Paradoxically, it is sometimes difficult for a health professional to withhold or stop a treatment. In recent years, the health professional's desire to "do all that is possible," coupled in some cases with the personal need not to "lose" a patient, have led to an overzealous approach. The ethical notion of heroic procedures or "extraordinary means" has been developed to help protect patients from such an assault.

From an ethical point of view, even treatments that are usual and customary or those considered ordinary treatment in medical parlance and practice can, under certain conditions, be judged extraordinary or heroic. The ethical criterion for considering a treatment heroic is that it may inflict undue physical, psychological, or spiritual harm on the person even though it serves to prolong the patient's life.[13] For instance, suppose that a relatively new treatment is being used successfully for amyotrophic lateral sclerosis. It could add several months to Mrs. Lykes's life. It has disturbing cognitive side effects, however. Mrs. Lykes rejects it out of hand. You must honor a competent patient's wishes. On that basis, this new treatment becomes extraordinary.

Summary

When a person makes a fully informed decision to refuse further treatment, that treatment is inappropriate, even though it may prolong life.

The "bottom line" in the ethical distinction between ordinary and extraordinary rests on the *patient's decision, not the health professional's judgment*. Any intervention, from the most simple and routine to the most technologically advanced, can be ordinary or extraordinary, depending on its fittingness for a particular patient. This is the most important thing you must bear in mind, not the fact of how "high tech" or, in your view, invasive or expensive or experimental the intervention will be. A relatively simple, safe, routine, or inexpensive intervention also could become extraordinary.

> **SUMMARY**
>
> Any treatment becomes extraordinary if the patient judges that the burdens decisively outweigh the benefits.

The same test can be applied to an incompetent patient, but the surrogate bears the weight of deciding what the patient would have found an unbearable burden and what would constitute a benefit.

Reflection

Suppose you are a member of the health care team who is treating Mrs. Lykes and it falls to you to talk with her about the possibility of starting experimental therapy for amyotrophic lateral sclerosis that may extend her life. It may also provide her with several more weeks without a respirator, but it has some disturbing side effects, such as a high likelihood of gastrointestinal and mucosal ulceration. Imagine a conversation with her to explore her willingness to try the new medication. What are key points you want to cover to be sure she is making a correct, informed decision?

____

____

____

____

Applying the Benefit–Burden Ratio Test. Why do patients refuse? Because they decide that treatments that may be promising from a medical point of view and which are administered routinely to others impose too great a burden on them to be worth it. In the story you read, that was what Almena Lykes said at one point. Patients may refuse for many reasons. Some may detest the idea of a treatment that will cause profound memory loss, or will require amputation or other disfigurement, or has side effects causing great discomfort, or is extremely costly to the family. At the same time, the reasons for refusal may be the benefit of gracefully "letting go." It is easy to imagine two patients who would receive similar physiologic benefit from a medical intervention, but who would assign different weight to the personal, human benefits accruing from the treatment. Mrs. Lykes might weigh the benefit of the experimental intervention or even permanent use of the ventilator quite differently than you or I because she believes she has accomplished what she hoped to in life and has a sense of being at peace with the nearness of death.

What happens when a competent patient refuses a treatment that the health professionals believe will be *highly* beneficial and effective?

They are not required to override the patient's decision even in this difficult situation. Sometimes patients choose to withdraw from clinical care altogether and go home, an option they have a right to choose.

Assessing Medically Futile Care. The notion of extraordinary care also applies when there is no reasonable hope that the patient will benefit from the care. It addresses the flip side of the coin of the above discussion of how patients have a prerogative, even right, to refuse a treatment that health professionals think are appropriate. Sometimes, however, patients demand interventions that health professionals judge are not designed to be of any benefit to the patient. In recent years, the idea of medical futility has become a point of lively debate, refining age-old ideas of what medical and other clinical interventions actually are designed (and able) to achieve.[14]

At first glance the idea of providing medically futile care seems ridiculous. Why does it even need to be discussed?

Sometimes interventions that did do some good initially are continued because to now withdraw them appears to be harming, even killing, the patient. The discussion of medical futility has created helpful guidelines for judging when health professionals justifiably may withdraw previously helpful interventions on the basis that the patient's condition has changed.

Futility always has meant that something would not help. But today, with so many interventions available, there is a need for a clear understanding by everyone of what "helping" and "not helping" means. The discussion of medical futility has led to a refined understanding of when an intervention may be withheld even though a patient wants it. In recent years there have been some legal challenges concerning how far to accede to a patient's, or surrogate's, demands in determining the degree or types of interventions that are warranted. The idea of futility has been useful in clarifying that medically useless treatments should be withheld or withdrawn, no matter how much a patient or surrogate wants them.

The ethically appropriate standard by which a procedure can be judged medically futile is the good of the whole patient, not that it can sustain a single organ or body system. The rationale for this should be clear because some medical interventions may allow an organ (e.g., the heart) to survive, but the patient's condition may otherwise be completely irreversible and devastating.

In today's exciting high-technology health care environment, the tendency to extend the arm of technical intervention can lead to a distortion of the art of clinical intervention.[15] From the earliest times our professional predecessors warned about this type of abuse, counseling always that our practice follow not only the science but also what we know about the effect on the patient's well-being. Elsewhere I have called the contemporary, technology-driven medical tendency to chase an organ or system at the cost of the whole patient's well-being a tendency to "spotwelding."[16] In many instances, health professionals are responding to urgent requests of patients or families who also place their trust more in the machine than in the professional and who subsequently fail to see the crumbling patient who is victim to the health professionals' frantic attempts to "spotweld" together the failing organs and organ systems.

The standard for declaring an intervention medically futile continues to be the subject of debate.[17] The most conservative approach is to hold to the traditional standard of physiologic futility, the judgment that an intervention will not, or no longer will, have any appreciable beneficial physiologic effect on the patient. One example would be the use of antibiotics for a viral infection. A second approach is to try to quantify the probability that an intervention will have an appreciable beneficial physiologic effect. Proponents of this position suggest that even though there may be times when the intervention works, it so seldom does that it should be dropped as a realistic intervention. A third position has been to try to develop either an individual or group standard of quality of life. In this position the benefit is framed in terms of a quality of life the patient would realize. Should, for example, an intervention that would bring a patient to the point of responding to light and sound but never to the point of responding to the environment in a more purposive fashion be judged futile? The risks of determining whole categories of persons who have qualities not worth supporting with interventions should be apparent in this approach.

Let us return now to the larger framework in which this discussion is placed, namely the criteria of ordinary and extraordinary care. Whether it will benefit this patient in this circumstance is the governing consideration.

> **SUMMARY**
>
> Any treatment also is extraordinary if it offers no appreciable hope of benefit to the patient (i.e., is medically futile).

You will be joining the ranks of the health professions at a time when this important topic undoubtedly will continue to be debated. Currently, all three standards of futility are being applied in different settings. Any time such a standard is set, certain interventions will be determined not to be of any benefit, in other words, to be "futile."

Keeping the Focus on the (Whole) Patient

The ethical reasoning about the limits of intervention that are morally appropriate (including consideration of ordinary and extraordinary distinctions) requires a focus on the individual patient's well-being as a point of reference. There are several helpful mechanisms for approaching the difficult question of ascertaining when enough is enough, their goal being to provide a more humane approach to patients who are critically ill or have irreversible conditions that will lead to their death.

The *health professions team,* headed by the physician who is the appropriate person to make the clinical judgment about the patient's medical status, should make the decisions, guided by the patient's informed wishes. However, as we have been discussing, the key considerations that arise are not solely about medical status.

Ethics committees are one mechanism to guide health professionals, patients, and their families in end-of-life care decisions. The committee's role is to make recommendations only, on the basis of ethical values, principles, and other considerations you have been using throughout the reading of this book and on the particularities of each patient's story.

There is one important difference between what you (as a current or future health professional) must do and what an ethics committee or ethics consultant does. You are in a position to carry out, or at least be on the team that carries out, the action. The committee or consultant stops with identifying the practical alternatives using the distinctions you have been reading about in this chapter. Often, the decision involves whether to withdraw or withhold measures that, under other circumstances, would be considered usual and customary to use, or, in other words, would be "ordinary treatment."

Withdrawing and Withholding Life Supports

When an illness is reversible, many technologies act as "bridges" between life-threatening symptoms and health, allowing the person to return to a healthy, or healthier, state. When an illness is not reversible, life supports* sometimes act as life-sustaining bridges between severe episodes within the dying process but ultimately are the literal bridge between life and death itself. Almena Lykes is faced with being put on life support in the form of a respirator. At this point she is refusing this treatment, and Jarda Roubal and Roy Moser are concerned about the enormity of her decision.

The proper moral limits of medical intervention described in the preceding discussion provide a general ethical framework for withdrawal and withholding of life supports. An intervention that the patient (or the patient's surrogate) finds much more burdensome

*This chapter uses the term *life supports* as it commonly is used in the medical, policy, and legal literature—namely, medical technologies that prolong life when a patient has an incurable condition. Sometimes they are called life-prolonging interventions.

than beneficial and from which there will be no escape may be withheld or removed ethically. An intervention that will not reverse the condition or symptom ("offers no appreciable hope of benefit") also may be withheld or withdrawn.

In such an act you, the health professional, are not killing the patient. It is an ethically justifiable act, the end of which may be the patient's death, but it does not meet the criterion of "killing." Killing is a direct act of commission, meaning that you—the agent—intend to bring about a patient's death and actively intervene to do so.

In other words, in withdrawing and withholding you are neither engaging in the activity with the intention of ending the patient's life nor are you the direct cause of her death. For example, in the case of Mrs. Lykes, she has a disease that will cause her death. Her death will probably come sooner without artificial, medically applied interventions to assist her breathing, heartbeat, kidney function, ingestion of nutrition and hydration, or other bodily functions, but eventually the medical condition directly will kill her. She does not have a respirator to assist her in her breathing. Dr. Roubal, her physician, determines that she will die shortly without this medical intervention, but she refuses it anyway. Her death will be brought about by the death-dealing force within her. At best her death can be delayed by your intervention.[18]

A decision to withhold or withdraw a treatment should be made openly and communicated with the team and documented in the medical record so that all health professionals involved in the patient's care will be aware of the decision. A physician may, in consultation with the patient or patient's family, decide that a patient will not receive a certain life support, but if there is no record of the decision, the nurses, residents, or others on duty will feel obligated to initiate it in the event of a life-threatening episode.

SUMMARY
Withdrawing or withholding treatment is not to be confused with acts of directly ending a patient's life.

This type of decision is psychologically difficult for health professionals. The process of withdrawing nutrition and hydration life supports is especially challenging. Although professionals may know rationally that they are not killing a patient, nevertheless it seems to be true when they disconnect the feeding tube. All the team support mechanisms discussed in Chapter 8 need to be brought into play to assist colleagues in these difficult moments.

Principle of Double Effect. The principle of double effect is a reasoning tool that can help you in situations in which you act with the intent of providing palliative care for a patient, but in so doing you have the unintended effect of hastening the patient's death. The most commonly cited example of this principle is the administration of a pain reliever that has a side effect of compromising respiration. Because the patient becomes more and more tolerant of the medication, doses high enough to relieve the pain will at some point stop the patient's breathing.

The principle of double effect acknowledges that one act can embrace two effects: an intended effect and an unintended, secondary effect. The intended effect governs the morality of the act. In this case the intended effect is the patient's comfort, acting on the presumption that the quality of life must be preserved. The inescapable but unintended secondary effect is that at some point in the continuum of this care the patient will succumb to the high dosage. Another aspect is that the increase in dosage must be the minimum necessary to achieve the patient's comfort. Finally, the unintended side effect cannot ever become the intended effect—that is, death cannot become the goal of the person providing the medication.

In summary, the most important thing for you to learn about this tool is that the intent is key. The intent to relieve the patient's pain or other serious discomfort governs the morality of the act, not the unfortunate and unintended secondary consequences (i.e., the patient dies). The second most important thing to learn is that the proportion of increase in the comfort-enhancing intervention must be only the minimum required to achieve the intended effect, namely the patient's relief of suffering from pain or other symptoms. Although only the physician has authority to prescribe such medication, nurses almost always must implement the procedures, and other team members also may be involved in assuring the patient's comfort.

Steps 5 and 6: Complete the Action and Evaluate the Process and Outcome

Going back to the story as written, Dr. Jarda Roubal and Roy Moser have several considerations to take into account before they decide whether to withhold the respirator and other life-prolonging measures. We noted that their first action is to get Almena Lykes wishes as crystal clear as possible through continued conversation with her and to take whatever steps necessary to learn whether she is so depressed that she is not in a reliable state to know her true wishes. Further action regarding intervention cannot justifiably be completed without knowing her informed preferences. Once they know this important information they will have an opportunity to work together with her and the team to continue each portion of her care motivated by the goal of a caring response. And at each decision point they also are well advised to use the tools of evaluation and reflection on the portion of the action they have just completed. These conditions will help assure that she does not become abandoned and that her care will remain competent and personalized.

Having assessed Mrs. Lykes's circumstances and the health professionals' considerations should provide you with a good general framework for a caring response in end-of-life care. However, before leaving the subject you will benefit from considering two additional facets of such care: the first being informed consent in situations where a patient clearly is not any longer competent to make decisions, and the second a brief discussion of clinically assisted suicide and medical euthanasia.

Advance Directives in End-of-Life Care

What should happen when a person is, or becomes, incompetent? Recall from Chapter 11 that their wishes then are "heard" through the voice of an appointed surrogate. One modern societal mechanism to assist surrogates and professionals alike in important decisions under such circumstances is the advance directive, and the process by which it is used, advance care planning.

Advance directives were developed to assure patients their end-of-life wishes would be honored as much as possible. They become effective only at the time the patient no longer is able to make her wishes known regarding the types and extent of medical intervention that she thinks appropriate.

Reflection

Because of their emphasis on the patient's wishes, what ethical principle are advance directives founded on?

If you responded "autonomy" or "self-determination," you are remembering well what you have learned so far. If you did not answer correctly, this is a good time to go back and review the discussion of autonomy in Chapter 3.

There are basically two major types of advance directives, although some documents bear slightly different names or combine the two:

- *Living wills* are designed to enable a patient to specify the types of treatment he or she would want to have and, more importantly, not have.
- *Durable power of attorney* documents are designed to enable a patient to specify who he or she wants to make the treatment decisions when he or she is no longer able to make them. This document often is used by someone who does not wish his or her "next of kin" to have to make such a decision.

Reflection

As you look at these two types of advance directives, what do you think are the major strengths of a living will? What are its major flaws or weaknesses? What are the major strengths of a durable power of attorney? What are its major drawbacks?

___

___

___

___

The living will and durable power of attorney are legally binding in all 50 U.S. states, but their wording may differ. You should familiarize yourself with those in the area where you live and work (and, by the way, where your loved ones live). Some limit the agent's decision-making power regarding any type of the life-sustaining treatment, and at the time of this writing, 13 U.S. states limit it regarding artificial nutrition and hydration.

In January 1990, a nationally mandated *United States Patient Self-Determination Act (PSDA)* made it necessary for every patient to be asked on admission to a health care institution whether he or she has an advance directive or wants to prepare one. For those who have one, it is placed in the patient's permanent health care record in that institution. If the person desires one but does not have one, the institution has forms for the person to fill out. Other countries do not have similar nationally mandated mechanisms such as the PSDA, although many share the task of trying to ascertain what is best for the patient in our current era where life can be prolonged almost indefinitely in some instances.

Although these forms are helpful in making an incapacitated patient's wishes known, far more important is that the patient talk to loved ones and professionals long before the moment of decision making arrives. There is no substitute for having had a long time in which to prepare loved ones for the challenge of having to make a life or death decision, as well as for having to make decisions that would honor the patient's understanding of the quality of life.

Clinically Assisted Suicide and Medical Euthanasia

No modern discussion of end-of-life care would be complete without a discussion of clinically assisted suicide and medical euthanasia.

Although assisted suicide often is called "physician-assisted suicide," I choose my words purposefully in calling it "clinically assisted suicide," because almost all health professionals who have interactions with patients could face patients who are contemplating this course of action and ask for assistance. Some health professionals, such as nurses and pharmacists, must join doctors in being directly involved in the chain of events leading to a patient's suicide when it is treated as a medical option in end-of-life care.[19,20] Many health profession organizations have issued position statements affirming their opposition to the practice on the basis that it is incompatible with professional ethics.

In the United States, the most decisive cases against this type of action occurred about a decade ago. In 1996, the Supreme Court ruled on two cases involving physician-assisted suicide and ruled against the rationale set forth for permitting assisted suicide in these instances.[21] What many people do not understand is that although the rulings are important in setting precedents against this practice, it does (and did) not preclude individual states from passing legislation permitting clinically assisted suicide. In fact, legislation permitting it currently exists in the state of Oregon.[22]

Most ethical debate identifies *intent* and *consequences* as key factors, distinguishing withdrawing and withholding life-prolonging measures from assisted suicide and direct euthanasia.[23] In all these, the patient dies after the act. As you now know from earlier discussions in this chapter, the intent is a morally relevant distinction between withdrawing or withholding life supports and those interventions designed to end a patient's life. In the former, the intent is not to cause the patient's death, rather to honor the patient's right to have certain invasive, life-prolonging interventions withheld or stopped. In assisted suicide, the health professional is the direct agent of administering the means by which a patient can effectively end her or his own life. The most commonly discussed form of clinically assisted suicide is the health professional who provides information about and a prescription for the lethal dose of a medication. In actual cases the health professional may or may not be physically present at the suicide. The question then is how involved the health professional must be to become an agent in the patient's death.

More fundamentally, the ethical debate steps back to a discussion of whether assisted suicide should be permitted at all. *Proponents* of clinically assisted suicide probably are in a minority among health professionals, although it is impossible to ascertain how strong the support really is. Proponents argue that respect for a patient is determined, first and foremost, by a respect for the patient's autonomy. They also argue that the professional promises to abide with a patient, show compassion, and be committed to providing comfort when cure is no longer possible and that these commitments extend to helping a patient gain access to the medical means to take her or his own life.

Reflection

Suppose Mrs. Lykes requests that Dr. Roubal give her the information and means necessary for her effectively to end her own life. What might her reasons be?

If you said things such as, "she cannot imagine going on in this condition—for her, life is no longer worth living," or "she knows it is going to get worse and she can't take it," you would be identifying themes that often are used in support of this procedure.

Opponents of clinically assisted suicide object to the idea that respect for persons is embraced fully by honoring their wishes, important as they are. Respect for persons must entail a respect for life, and the appropriate moral role of the health professional is to save life, not to assist in any way in taking it. Choosing to become an advocate of death is a distortion of the age-old ethical mandate of the health professions to save life. Neither faithfulness nor nonmaleficence can be honored once the line between being an advocate of life and being an advocate of death has been crossed. Opponents also assert that compassion never can be expressed by having a part in ending a patient's life to end her or his suffering.

Euthanasia within the medical context takes the direct moral agency of the physician (or other health professional) one step further. (See the following box.) The patient is truly a "passive bystander" while the health professional's intervention is carried out with the goal of ending the patient's life.

Assisted Suicide

1. The physician provides the medical means (instead of some other means such as a gun).
2. The physician is necessary but not sufficient for the act.
3. The patient needs to do the final act (take the lethal medication).

Medically Administered Euthanasia

1. Physician commits the act by medical means.
2. The physician is necessary and sufficient for the act.
3. The patient's illness simply provides the context.

Proponents and opponents in the ethical debate about medical euthanasia draw on arguments similar to the ones described earlier regarding assisted suicide. Proponents also often draw the line between voluntary medical euthanasia (where a patient requests euthanasia) and involuntary medical euthanasia (where requests cannot be made because the patient is incapacitated). In countries where medical euthanasia is permitted (i.e., the Netherlands, Belgium), most proponents do not accept advance directives as a legitimate mechanism for continuing such a request into a period when a patient no longer can speak for himself. Opponents add to their other objections that voluntary euthanasia inevitably will slip into involuntary euthanasia.

Concerns flowing from opponents to both types of procedures are that the trust health professionals accrue from their willingness to take the patient's life seriously when others devalue the patient will be fatally compromised and that health professionals themselves may become less diligent in seeking comfort measures for a dying patient if it is permissible, instead, to assist a patient in "ending it all." There also are serious concerns that minority patients and other socially marginalized members of society will be encouraged to end their lives (or have them terminated), whereas others will be offered alternatives. Alternatives in the form of diligent end-of-life care that stops short of assisted suicide then become the mandate guiding a professional's relationship.

Summary

Decisions about life and death in the health professions are among the most perplexing, from an ethical and a practical viewpoint. There is much we do not understand, so awesome is it to look at the death experience. You will do yourself a favor to take some time to be introspective about your feelings toward death. Just as the light and heat from the sun are useful and necessary in small doses, so it is true that health professionals must dare to look at death closely enough to gain insight into their roles as humble mediators between life and death, sickness and well-being. By so doing we all will better learn how the ethical tools of character traits, duties, and rights can help to build and sustain the moral foundations of the health professional–patient relationship in this challenging situation.

Questions for Thought and Discussion

1. When Nora Sugandi was a nursing student intern, part of her day consisted of making rounds with the medical and nursing staff and residents. Each day for several weeks one of the patients they saw was a withered wisp of a woman who was now semicomatose in the final stage of a long bout with cancer. The old woman had no known relatives and was never visited by anyone, but she lived on and on past the time the medical staff believed she would die. The group of physicians and other health professionals stood at the foot of her bed each day, glanced at her in bewilderment, read her medical record, said a few words to each other, and left.

Nora believed that the old woman would become tense during these discussions, and finally she mentioned it to some classmates. They scoffed at the idea, saying she was too weak and too far gone to know what they were saying or even that they were there. Nora became increasingly troubled in the presence of this tiny lady, who was lying in what seemed to be a gigantic hospital bed. Finally, one evening when Nora was walking down the patient's corridor, for some inexplicable reason she was drawn into the patient's room. The woman looked no different than ever—very small, very alone, and very still. Nora shut the door, gathered the woman into her arms, and held her.

Did the health professional respond appropriately to this woman's situation? Discuss with your classmates why or why not.

---

2. Is there a living will or durable power of attorney act in your state or province? What are its provisions? What are its limitations? What is the legal significance of such a document, and how does that differ from its psychological and ethical significance?

---

3. A patient with a rare, progressive liver disease that is invariably fatal after a long and arduous period of debility has stated several times that he wishes to end his life by his own hand "when the time comes." During his most recent visit to his physician he asks the physician to write him a prescription for "an assuredly lethal dose" of the medication he has been taking. The physician writes the prescription, then tears it up and says, "I can't do that." Then he tells the patient how many tablets would be needed for "an assuredly fatal dose." Did the physician do the right thing? Describe some of the legal and ethical ramifications of this conduct by the physician.

---

4. Currently, there is much discussion about assisted suicide and euthanasia in the medical context. Should health professionals ever have the power to administer euthanasia, even at the competent patient's request? Defend your position, drawing on the nature of a caring response including duties and character traits discussed in this book.

____

____

____

____

References

1. *Random House Webster's Unabridged Dictionary.* 2001. New York: Random House, p. 1398.
2. Field, M.J., Cassel, C.K. (Eds.). 1997. *Approaching Death: Improving Care at the End of Life.* Washington, DC: National Academy Press.
3. Crawley, L.V.M., Marshall, P., Koenig, B.A. 2001. Respecting cultural differences at the end of life. In Snyder, L., Quill, T. (Eds.), *Physician's Guide to End-of-Life Care.* Philadelphia: American College of Physicians, pp. 36–45.
4. Cassem, N. 1978. Treatment decisions in irreversible illness. In Cassem, N., Hackett, T. (Eds.), *Massachusetts General Hospital Handbook of General Hospital Psychiatry.* St. Louis: CV Mosby, pp. 573–574.
5. National Hospice and Palliative Care Organization (NHPCO). 2001. *Facts and Figures.* Alexandria, VA: NHPCO.
6. Lynn, J. 2001. Serving patients who may die soon and their families: the role of hospice and other services. *JAMA* 285(7):925–932.
7. McCulloch, D. 2002. *Valuing Health in Practice: Priorities, QALYS, and Choice.* Burlington, VT: Ashgate Press.
8. Furrow, B. 1995. Managed care and the evolution of quality. *Trends in Health Care, Law and Ethics* 10(1–2):37–44.
9. Toombs, K. 1997. Review essay: Taking the body seriously. *Hastings Center Report* 27(5):39–43.
10. *Random House Webster's Unabridged Dictionary.* 2001. New York: Random House, p. 4.
11. Dougherty, C., Purtilo, R. 1995. The duty of compassion in an era of health care reform. *Cambridge Quarterly* 4:426–433.
12. Camus, A. 1948. *The Plague.* (Gilbert, S., Trans., 1974). New York: Alfred A. Knopf.
13. Prendergast, T.J., Puntillo, K.A. 2002. Withdrawal of life support: intensive caring at the end of life. *JAMA* 288(21):2732–2740.
14. Stanley, K., Zoloth-Dorfman, L. 2001. Ethical considerations. In Ferrell, B., Coyle, N. (Eds.), *Textbook of Palliative Nursing.* New York: Oxford University Press, pp. 75–91.

15. Cassel, C., Purtilo, R., McFarland, E. 2003. Ethical and social issues in contemporary medicine. In Dale, D. (Ed.), *Scientific American Medicine* (vol. 1). New York: WebMD, Inc. pp. 3–7.
16. Purtilo, R., Donohue, W. 1992. Resources for medical decision making in situations of high uncertainty. *Nebraska Medical Journal* 70(10):277–280.
17. Helft, P., Siegler, M., Lantos, J. 2000. The rise and fall of the futility movement. *New England Journal of Medicine* 343(4):293–296.
18. Randall, F., Downe, R. 1999. The moral distinction between killing and letting die. In *Palliative Care Ethics: A Companion for all Specialties* (2nd ed.). New York: Oxford University Press, pp. 270–277.
19. Matzo, M., Emanuel, E. 1997. Oncology nurses' practices of assisted suicide and patient requested euthanasia. *Oncology Nurses Forum* 23(1):1725–1732.
20. Ganzini, L., Harvath, T., Jackson, A., Goy, E., Miller, L., Delorit, M. 2002. Experience of Oregon nurses and social workers with hospice patients who requested assistance with suicide. *New England Journal of Medicine* 347(8): 582–588.
21. *Quill v. Vacco,* 80 F3d 716 (2nd Cir., 1996) and *Compassion in Dying v State of Washington,* 79 F.3d 790 (9th Cir. 1996) (en banc).
22. Oregon Death with Dignity Act. 1997. Oregon Revised Statute 127800-127:897.
23. Sulmasy, D.P. 1998. Killing and allowing to die. *Journal of Law, Medicine and Ethics* 26:55–64.

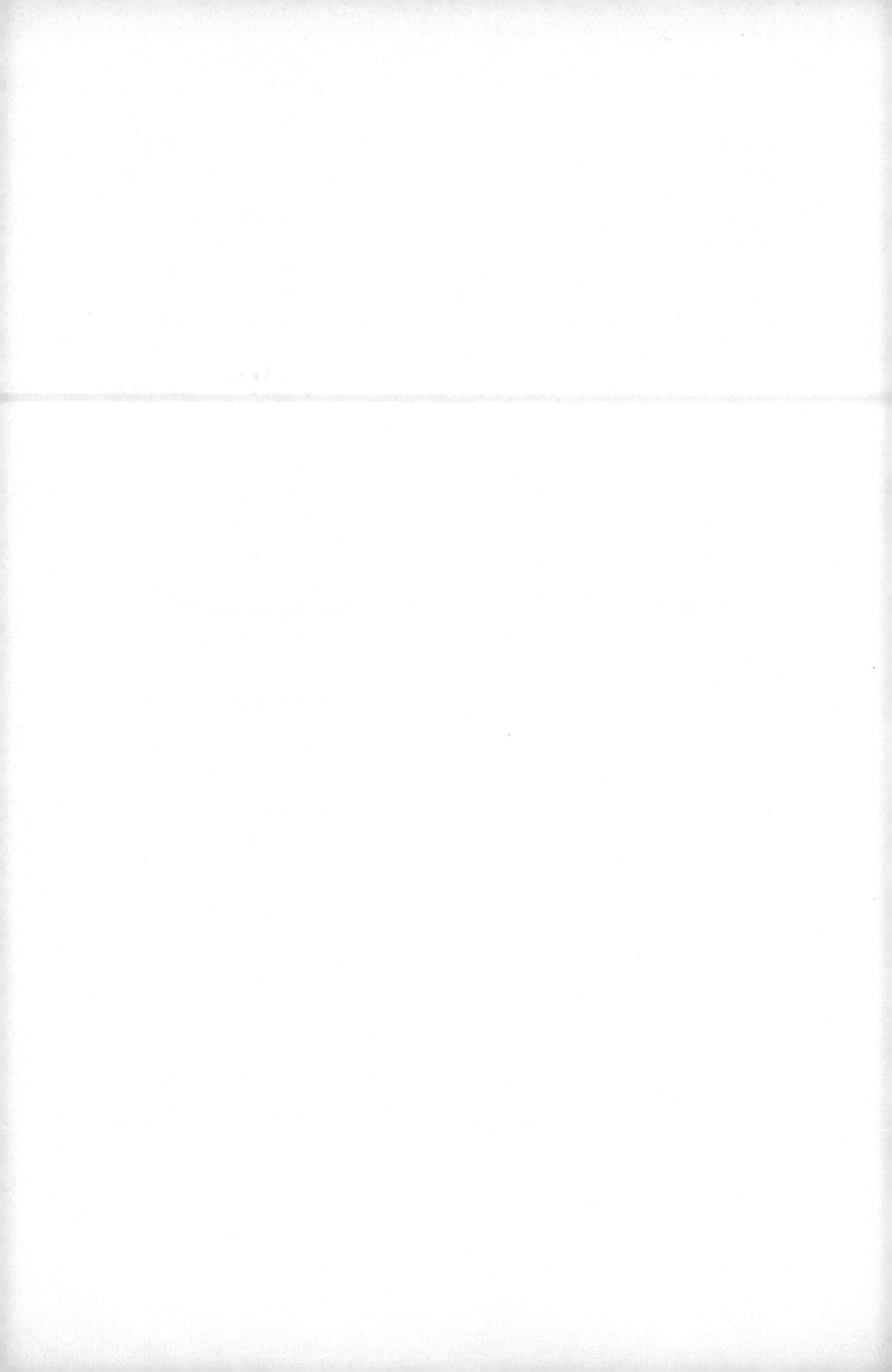

Section V

Ethical Dimensions of the Social Context of Health Care

14

Distributive Justice: Clinical Sources of Claims for Health Care

Objectives

The student should be able to:

- Describe what *a caring response* involves in situations requiring the allocation of scarce resources.
- Compare the concepts of *microallocation* and *macroallocation*.
- Distinguish the contexts in which fairness and equity considerations should be used.
- Describe two types of situations in health care in which fairness considerations are required for a just allocation of resources.
- Discuss the starting point of deliberation in distributive justice: treat similar cases similarly.
- Compare the ideas of allocation on the basis of a right to health care, on need, and on merit.
- Discuss the idea of *equity* in allocation decisions.
- Define the term *rationing*.
- List and critique five criteria for a morally acceptable approach to rationing of health care resources.

New terms and ideas you will encounter in this chapter

allocation of health care resources
universal access to health care benefits
a right/entitlement
microallocation
fairness
rationing
macroallocation
equity
random selection

Topics in this chapter introduced in earlier chapters

Topic	*Introduced in chapter*
Beneficence	3
Medical futility	13
Extraordinary (heroic) care	13
Principle of justice	3
Hippocratic Oath	1

Introduction

As this book is being published the United States has gone over the $1T (that's *trillion*) mark in annual expenditures for health care, the question of whether health care is a right continues to be debated, and as the number of possible interventions increases, managed care arrangements place caps on what a patient is eligible to receive. All nations face questions of limited health care resources and escalating costs. These issues worldwide create ethical challenges involving *the allocation of health care resources.* Such challenges fall within the category of dilemmas of distributive and compensatory justice discussed in this chapter and in Chapter 15.

Some of the important issues are best addressed by examining your direct caregiving role. For example, you may be faced with a personnel shortage in your workplace some day and will have to decide where to cut corners and why. You may work where there is not enough equipment or personnel to fully satisfy what your best effort requires. In deciding how to operate under that extenuating circumstance you are again making allocation decisions. These are termed *microallocation* decisions.

But some of the most critical issues regarding allocation of resources remove you from the arena of direct patient care to policy, where whole groups of similarly situated people are implicated. For instance, in the United States, a current lively policy debate surrounds organ transplantation. There is a serious shortage of available organs, therefore each year people waiting for a transplant die. Currently, more than 82,000 people are on the waiting list for organs, many of whom will die before a suitable organ becomes available.[1] Each group of potential recipients poses challenges regarding how this scarce resource should be allocated. Take the example of liver transplantation. One large population of patients needing lifesaving transplantation for survival are those suffering from alcohol-related end-stage liver disease. There have been many debates regarding the ethical responsibility to provide transplants to patients who are alcoholics.

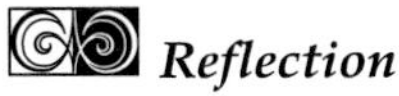

Reflection

Do you think a person whose liver has been damaged by alcohol or other substance abuse should have the same chance for a transplant as someone whose equally serious liver damage was caused by other reasons and not by self-destructive behaviors?

If yes, make a list of any conditions you would impose on the substance abuser and supports that should be in place to assure that he or she would not end up in the same situation again, knowing that the success rate depends in part on abstinence after the transplant. If you think he or she should be given exactly the same priority as anyone else with similar medical need, take a minute before reading further to think about why you feel this way.

Currently, in most countries where liver transplants are offered there is a waiting period for alcoholics to demonstrate that they are abstaining from alcohol, a criterion that appears to reduce the recidivism rate among those fortunate enough to be chosen for an organ.

SUMMARY

Debate about the priority list for scarce organs for transplantation often includes considerations of lifestyle and addiction.

Whatever the outcome, the decision about organ transplantation points out that in the allocation of health care resources conscious choices are made, and the choices do make a difference in the lives and well-being of whole groups of similarly situated people.[2]

Some policy decisions require that different types of societal goods be compared. For instance, an allocation decision may involve choices about whether during this year more roads will be built, or hospice beds increased, or existing national parks maintained. These decisions are called *macroallocation* decisions.

As previously, a case should assist you in your thinking about these complex practice and policy issues. The emphasis will be on microallocation decisions, although both will be addressed.

The Story of Christopher Lacey and Other Contenders for His Bed

One Monday morning as John Krescher, a critical care nurse specialist, is going into the intensive care unit (ICU), he is stopped by Mr. Christopher Lacey's sister, a nurse. John often has seen her and her husband there at her brother's bedside, although he has not had any lengthy discussions about Christopher with them. This morning Mr. Lacey's sister says angrily that Dr. Sidney McCally is planning to transfer her brother prematurely to the general medical unit. She believes it is because he is being urged to do so by the hospital utilization committee and the case manager for

Mr. Lacey's managed care plan. She and her husband are threatening a lawsuit against the hospital unless her brother is allowed to remain in the ICU and receive the fullest medical care there. John expresses his surprise and is about to ask her some further questions, but she rushes out of the unit, apparently on the verge of tears.

John goes over to Christopher Lacey's bedside and puts his hand on the man's shoulder. He studies the patient's face for some sign of response, but there is none. John's mind is flooded with thoughts. Mr. Lacey is a 28-year-old, divorced postal employee with no children. "He is only a year older than I am," John thinks. Initially, Christopher was admitted to the hospital complaining of severe, acute abdominal pain. After several days of tests that yielded no clues, the physicians did an exploratory laparotomy.* At that time an ischemic segment of bowel was resected. In the postoperative suite Christopher experienced respiratory arrest for reasons the doctors could not explain and was transferred to the ICU under Dr. McCally's care. Since that time, 3 weeks ago, he has been in a fluctuating level of coma and has never fully regained consciousness.

Christopher Lacey has had a stormy course characterized by multiple serious medical complications. A severe systemic infection developed immediately after surgery, at which time it was thought he would die. He was treated with massive doses of antibiotics and appeared to be recovered. But the antibiotics were severely toxic to his kidneys. He is now showing signs of renal failure, which may necessitate dialysis.

Some members of the health care team have become progressively more pessimistic about Christopher Lacey's prognosis. In the ICU rounds 2 days ago, Dr. McCally shared with the ICU nursing staff that he had had several discussions with the patient's sister and had tried to explain to her the likelihood that his condition would not improve. "But," Dr. McCally said, "she and her husband wish aggressive treatment as long as there is any hope of meaningful recovery or survival." Mr. Lacey had left no living will or durable power of attorney and had never expressed an opinion about long-term life support.

John goes back to the ICU desk where his colleague, Janet Cumming, is at the computer entering data in the patients' medical records. Janet says, "Mr. Lacey's sister is so upset because Dr. McCally has decided to discontinue intensive care therapy despite the family's objections. I guess we will be transferring him back to the regular medicine unit later today. I'm upset, too, John. My guess is that he will die there. Of course, we *are* 100% full, so I can see why there is a push to get him out, but he is being discharged from us before he is ready."

---

*A *laparotomy* is a procedure in which a surgeon enters the abdominal cavity to discover the source of a serious problem not detectable by other means.

The Goal: A Caring Response

This story raises a number of ethical questions. A seemingly healthy younger man becomes a victim of a series of events that leave him in a coma and dependent on medical life supports for his life and sustenance. What should be done for this man who shows no improvement and seems to be getting worse? In Chapter 13 you were introduced to some aspects of a caring response, namely, those characterized as palliative care. A widely recognized goal for health professionals is to do whatever is "best" or, in the language of ethics, *beneficent* for the patient. In this story the entire team has been working to make sure that Christopher Lacey is receiving the most caring response each is able to provide. It is what we expect of the health professional–patient relationship. We do not know if Mr. Lacey is dying, we only know that his condition is getting progressively worse. But in addition to his intensive and other clinical interventions, beneficence also requires any rehabilitation and other measures that may help maintain the patient's functioning.

Having examined the situation from the point of view of Mr. Lacey as an individual patient, this chapter provides you with an opportunity to think about him in relation to all other similarly situated patients and the professional's role in difficult allocation decisions. You might say you have to consider activities geared toward a caring response for *this* patient in the context of what it means for *all the other patients* from when you (and the team) are a moral agent. To do so, you can again use the six-step process as a decision-making tool.

The Six-Step Process in Allocation Decisions

Of the many issues involved in this situation, consider the following issues that are related to the broad questions of allocation of health care resources:

- Should care be continued in the ICU for patients who may get worse if they are transferred out but who do not seem to be getting any better?
- Should Mr. Lacey's care be continued in the ICU because the family has a right to require continued treatment of this sort?
- Should Mr. Lacey be transferred out because his health plan guidelines dictate that he has used up his fair share of the plan's resources, and, besides, this regimen for him is based on clinical information derived from many other people who were in circumstances similar to his?
- Should his financial situation be a factor in whether he is kept in the ICU?

In recent years the direct relationship between health professional and patient has become strained by institutional constraints, some of which were addressed in Chapter 7. Traditional health care ethics, with its emphasis only on the private transaction between you and the patient, often has not addressed the larger institutional questions. For instance, there is nothing in the Hippocratic Oath or even in most professional codes of ethics today that provides guidance for how to distribute health care resources fairly and equitably. The challenge is heightened when the allocation involves a scarce resource.

SUMMARY

Traditional professional ethics codes and oaths have not addressed the question of how to distribute scarce resources ethically.

Step 1: Gather Relevant Information

Patients such as Christopher Lacey bring the troubling aspects of resource allocation keenly into focus. Although, theoretically, it is possible to keep him alive indefinitely, the reality is that the technology required to keep him alive in the ICU is expensive. One problem is the uncertainty about whether Mr. Lacey will die if removed from the ICU, although it appears that he cannot go on for long without intensive care and dialysis. The treatment he requires is out of reach for his family financially and for anyone except extremely wealthy patients. Therefore, the majority of the benefits Mr. Lacey derives from treatment inevitably are at the expense of pooled financial resources (in the form of revenue from taxes, insurance premiums, and other common funds). Of course, Mr. Lacey has worked since he was 16 years old, so he also has contributed to these pooled funds over the years, with the knowledge that he himself might not need them. When viewed from the standpoint of one *person's* situation in relation to another (i.e., Mr. Lacey's need for the ICU compared with Patient B), the allocations considerations draw on ideas of fairness. When a whole group of patients (Group A with, e.g., AIDS) are compared with another group of patients (e.g., Group B has diabetes) the justice considerations draw on ideas of equity. We will examine each briefly.

Fairness Considerations

An understanding of the *principle of fairness* requires us to explore two issues raised by Mr. Lacey's situation.

First, resources he requires may keep someone else from receiving this valued, life-saving therapy in the ICU. Generally speaking, once a patient is in an ICU, he or she will not be removed for another similarly situated person. To intensify the problem, imagine that the ICU is full and that by keeping Mr. Lacey there a *number* of other similarly situated patients needing ICU care are prevented from receiving it. (One can imagine that Christopher Lacey himself would have died after his respiratory arrest had the ICU been full at the time with other patients as sick as he was.) Fairness considerations, therefore, often entail an assumption that if you happened to get there first you have a claim on the spot, knowing that sometimes this will assist the professional in otherwise impossible situations.

What kind of thinking supports the idea of a right to remain in your place as a consideration when an issue of space occurs? The reasoning begins with the acknowledgment that one major function of clinical intervention is to respond to clinical need when there is good reason to believe the intervention will help. As you learned in Chapter 13, interventions that are medically futile or overly burdensome from the patient's standpoint do not count on the basis that they are extraordinary or heroic. Thus, the principle of fairness guiding decisions within the medical context is "to each according to his or her need." If it appears that the medical need of one person is greater than another, fairness considerations would counsel that the person with the greater need be the one to receive the coveted place in the ICU. But fairness is not the only moral consideration in the final decision. The duties of beneficence and nonmaleficence to the patient already in the ICU (e.g., Mr. Lacey) may give that person the priority over others who have not yet been admitted.

Consider a second type of fairness issue. Theoretically, resources that Mr. Lacey is using to be sustained in his bodily functions could be channeled into other kinds of programs that could save the lives of hundreds or at least improve their level of well-being (e.g., in screening or vaccination programs).

Reflection

Should the idea that transferring a patient out of the ICU to save money that could be channeled into, for example, vaccinations for hundreds of children, enter the ICU personnel's decision about what to do in a particular case? Why or why not?

In everyday circumstances, this type of reasoning is a morally questionable guide for action at the level that decisions are made about a particular patient by his or her health care team. You have learned that a fundamental promise of professional ethics is that the individual patient's well-being is your appropriate focus as a professional serving in your clinical role. An identified patient cannot be placed in a faceless pool with risk for jeopardy. For one thing, the health care team cannot assure that funds and other resources "saved" by removing Mr. Lacey from the ICU will be channeled into saving more lives or increasing the level of health care overall because of the fragmentation that exists in the policies of health care financing. Even if we did have that assurance, the respect for a patient's dignity as a human being should preclude the health professional's willingness to compromise a single patient's well-being for the sake of others "out there." Later in this chapter we consider what happens to this general ethical rule of thumb in cases of crisis of great proportion or situations of dire scarcity. In those cases, priority must be given not to those in the most need necessarily, but must be decided on the basis of how to protect the good of the whole. Even though the usual thinking that governs in situations of relatively moderate scarcity is overridden in such crises, the goal is to bring the situation back to the usual norms on the basis of reasoning about fairness.

Equity Considerations

You will now have an opportunity to consider Christopher Lacey's story from the angle of similarly situated *groups* of individuals vying for a limited health care resource.

Social policy should be designed to protect the interests of everyone equitably. *Equitable* in this context means that policy decision makers have made every effort to treat each person in a similarly situated circumstance alike, basing differences among groups on criteria that are ethically acceptable. In Christopher Lacey's case, policies must be made and applied to everyone so that the health care ICU team does not have to take every case from scratch and try to figure out who is and who is not eligible. The policy may be in the form of federal or other government guidelines or an institution policy. It might be reflected in types of treatment that will not be covered by insurance, Medicare, or other third-party payers, or it might provide guidelines for types of patients who will not be treated because of excessive cost or unlikelihood of medical response to treatment. It is understandable that much thought should go into determining ethical allocation policies to help health professionals make good decisions. You are entering the health care environment in an era where "evidence-based" outcomes of treatment based on many similarly situated patients is being used as one criteria to guide equity. Critical analysis of such themes as the difference between policies based on insurance companies' assessments of what equity requires and those based on more traditional notions of professional ethics is helping everyone understand better what an "equitable" course of action requires.[3]

SUMMARY

Fairness deals with allocations among individuals; equity deals with allocations among groups.

We turn now to the type of ethical problem that includes the notions of fairness and equity within it, namely, *distributive justice.*

Step 2: Identify the Type of Ethical Problem

In Chapter 3 you were introduced briefly to the idea of justice. In review, justice can be thought of as an arbiter, useful for analyzing and resolving ethical problems regarding what is rightfully due each individual or group who presents a claim on resources. In Chapter 2, you were introduced to the schematic representation of this basic type of ethical problem accordingly:

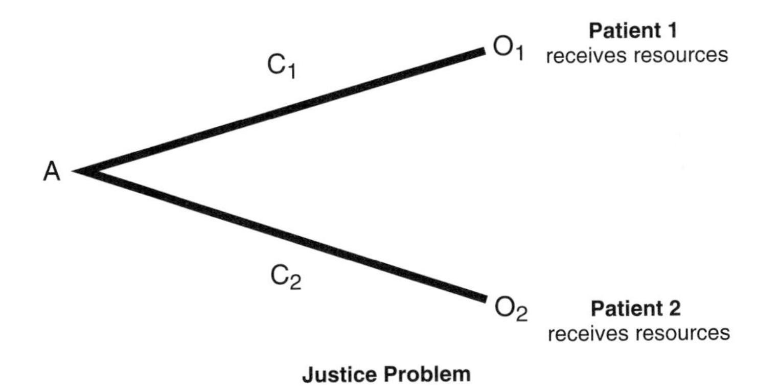

Justice Problem

In society, claims are taken into account according to individuals or groups of people who are judged to be similarly situated according to need, merit, or other considerations. On one hand, Mr. Lacey is a focus as an individual, but also as one who belongs to a group of people requiring ICU care. In fact, a general rule of justice when there are goods and burdens to be allocated is to "treat similar cases similarly." You will recognize this stance as the conceptual basis from which the notions of fairness and equity, discussed earlier, are derived. Obviously, the idea of simply treating similar cases similarly presents some difficulties because you can treat whole groups of people poorly (e.g., slaves in the United States and elsewhere).

Justice as a Principle

The idea of justice is to show respect for people by not making arbitrary or capricious distinctions and by not discriminating against some groups on that basis. Justice requires that morally defensible differences among people be used to decide who gets what.

To apply justice as an ethical principle, you must be dealing with a resource that is prized but is in short enough supply that not every group who wants or needs it can have it. The resource in this case may be hospital beds or hospitals, health professionals, medications or other types of treatment, or diagnostic modalities. Because of the way our health care financing and delivery system are tied together, sometimes resources are available, but groups of people cannot avail themselves of the benefits because they cannot pay for them.[4] Currently, approximately 50 million people in the United States are uninsured or seriously underinsured for health care needs. These figures raise serious ethical questions about how our society views the cherished resource of health care and who should have priority when access to it is being granted. What ethical tools do we have to deal with such challenges?

SUMMARY

Justice requires that decisions about the distribution of goods and imposition of burdens among individuals or groups be based on consideration that can be agreed on as being morally justifiable.

Step 3: Use Ethics Theories or Approaches to Analyze the Problem

At least three approaches can help the moral agent to participate confidently in the allocation decisions even though the professional's clinical role of doing what is optimal for each individual patient necessarily may be compromised if the resources are *very* scarce.

Health Care as a Right

One fundamental approach to the issue is to treat health care as a *right,* and if so to decide how much and what kind of health care an individual or group is entitled to receive. A right is a stringent claim. The stronger the claim, the more likely a society will accept responsibility for developing policy designed to meet the claim on behalf of all its citizens.

Reflection

From what you know about the current policies regarding health care in your country, do you think it views health care as a right?

Your answer depends in part on your understanding of the idea of rights. The concept sometimes used in discussing a rights approach is that of *entitlement.* This is called a positive right. This approach, adopted by many countries in the world, supports policies that enable everyone to receive health care benefits. At minimum, access has to be *universally available.* People such as Mr. Lacey and the other patients who need ICU beds should be able to have them. The societal challenge is to find money to support an adequate supply of ICU beds so that such a basic resource is available for those who will benefit from this type of care. A rights approach does not mean that everyone could decide they wanted the most expensive modality or could choose where they wanted treatment. Considerations of equity in the face of limited resources must guide such decisions.

Health Care as a Response to Basic Need

A second approach is to base allocations on *justice according to need.* Health care addresses a basic human need: healthfulness. Therefore, everyone ought to receive a response to this need. In this approach you could still think of health care as a right, but only because of its power to help maintain health, attend to suffering, and alleviate the dysfunction and discomfort that comes from an illness, injury, or other affliction. As you can imagine, one of the greatest challenges in this type of approach is to define the severity and nature of need and likelihood of benefit among different groups. It is the approach that most fully characterizes the ideals in traditional health care codes of ethics and oaths. People with similar needs should be treated similarly. All things being equal, those with more need should have greater priority unless there is evidence that the expenditure of resources on this group would not yield positive results.

Health Care as a Commodity

A third approach is to base allocations on *justice according to ability to purchase it.* Health care is treated the same as any other type of product in a free market society. Many policies and practices in the U.S. health care arena currently are based on this type of reasoning. A treatment is a commodity to be bought like a summer vacation package, or trash masher, or DVD. The informed consumer decides and makes choices. Money is the key resource that governs such an approach. In this approach it is not the responsibility of society to provide money (or vouchers or employee-based health insurance plans) so that people will be able to pay for health care when they wish to purchase it, although some societies may choose to provide the means. Everyone buys what he or she wants and, in addition, can afford. People situated like Christopher Lacey are free to buy more time in the ICU if they are able to pay for it.

Sometimes this approach includes a component that places a claim on government and other pooled societal resources. It is recognized that even in a free market society some interventions will be well beyond the personal means of the majority of individuals. Societal resources will best be spent on individuals or groups viewed as a "good investment." This becomes a tricky decision to make because the justifiable emphasis on a group being able to benefit from intervention can cross the line to become discrimination—for example, giving priority to conditions affecting people who are younger, have higher basic intelligence, or are better situated to go back to being income producers.

For example, suppose two men are brought into the emergency department after an auto accident. Both need ICU care and are expected to benefit from this care, but there is only one bed available. Mr. A., a brilliant, 26-year-old PhD student, is on the brink of making a major breakthrough in Alzheimer's disease research. His ability to pay for care is limited because of his need to pay off large student loans. Mr. B., who is 75 years old, is a wealthy, world-renowned, retired concert pianist.

Reflection

What qualifications does each have that might influence the type of thinking that an "investment" approach would take? Do you agree with this approach? Why or why not?

These three basic approaches—rights, needs, and merit—are presented here in somewhat "pure" form, as if they are completely distinct from each other. In fact, policies usually are based on many factors and may include components of each of these approaches. For instance, a health care benefits package that takes shape from the basic premise that health care is a right may be founded primarily on assessments of relative need. The decision, however, should be tempered by an assessment of the amount of benefit individuals with type A need will realize versus the amount enjoyed by type B. Additional types of health care interventions may be judged as being so far removed from a social consensus about their necessity for health that they are made available only as out-of-pocket purchases.

SUMMARY

In situations of moderate scarcity justice decisions about the distribution of goods depend on assessments of rights, relative need, or relative merit.

Because you are considering groups of people, name some characteristics of individuals/groups to whom you might give high priority if you were setting policy to address these difficult decisions.

Steps 4 and 5: Explore the Practical Alternatives and Complete the Action

In previous chapters the application of Step 4 almost always placed you (or the clinicians in the story) solely in the moral role of advocate for an individual patient. That is the role John Krescher has to maintain throughout his relationship with Mr. Lacey and Mr. Lacey's family. At the same time, this chapter is focusing on a piece of the larger social context of which health professionals also are a part, and in these instances moral agency shifts to focus on participation in policy. The exercise of one's professional influence here takes the form of policy making and review activities. The practical alternatives simply are either to let others make policy decisions or to offer one's services to help shape allocation policy. This avenue of moral action was discussed in relation to general policies of one's institution in Chapter 7, and there are no appreciable differences when the specific content focus is on allocation issues. However, allocation policy often is set by private insurers, government bodies, and other extrainstitutional bodies so that to have a positive effect means being willing to participate in commissions, review committees, and other public forums. There you will have an opportunity to contribute your considered opinions regarding the questions posed at that the end of Mr. Lacey's story regarding such important issues as the following:

- Once in the ICU, what criteria should be used to move a person out when the beds are full and new patients need ICU care?
- Should a patient's ability to pay influence the length of time he or she stays in the ICU?

Your reasoning about how fairness and equity concerns should guide the situation may convince others. You will be able to add your insights into current debates about whether health care is a right, should be a resource to respond to basic need despite ability to pay, or is a commodity. In other words, in allocation decisions your moral agency can be effective at the policy level.

Step 6: Evaluate the Process and Outcome

My grandmother liked to say, "The proof is in the pudding," meaning that only if the pudding tasted as good as it looked or smelled should one conclude that the chef has succeeded. The proof of a just policy process and outcome includes that all of the basic fairness and equity considerations have been taken into account and that the amount of compromise of resources for an individual patient such as Mr. Lacey is strictly proportionate to the actual scarcity. This factor is so crucial in allocation decisions that I turn now to a more focused discussion on rationing to complete your study of distributive justice considerations.

Rationing: Allocation and Dire Scarcity

Having given careful attention to the way the general principle of distributive justice works, consider the notion of rationing. Some use the term *rationing* to denote any intentional method of distributing a desired good when there are too many qualified claimants for a good, or the good is too costly for all to have it. As you can easily discern, this is the way we have been describing distributive justice as a general principle of allocation. Traditionally, rationing decisions were made when there was a dire or severe shortage of the good, and it is from this traditional stance that it is addressed in this chapter. Currently, an active discussion about this type of rationing focuses on the sobering prospect of an inadequate supply of antidotes or vaccine against agents used for the purposes of bio-warfare on large civilian or armed forces populations.[5]

Almost everyone would agree that giving priority to guidelines geared to the survival of the whole society is appropriate in situations of dire (but only dire) scarcity. In situations of moderate scarcity, individual or group rights, need, or merit should govern, tempered by the considerations discussed throughout this chapter. Currently, another impetus to create rational approaches to the limits placed on access to health care resources is being occasioned by new technologies. Fleck[6] proposes that the need for rationing "will become more painfully acute during this decade, especially because we are likely to see the rapid proliferation of costly 'last chance' therapies." He names the totally implantable artificial heart and the left ventricular assist device as just two examples currently available in the United States. The artificial heart would generate an annual need for 350,000 such life-saving interventions at an aggregate cost currently of $52 billion. Everyone lucky enough to receive one will enter a group where the average extra years of life expectancy is 5 years.[6]

Criteria for a Morally Acceptable Approach to Rationing of Health Care Resources

Several criteria have been developed to assist in the difficult, sometimes tragic, situation occasioned by the severe shortage of an important good or service.

There Must Be a Demonstrated Need That Rationing Is Necessary

Rationing means that some groups who would benefit will not receive any of the desperately needed services or goods. The idea that health care responds to a basic human need requires that the burden of proof be placed on anyone declaring that it is time to ration the good.

It Must Be a Last Resort Move

It follows from the preceding criterion that every other approach must be exhausted before individuals who would benefit will be totally excluded from care. For example, one necessary exercise is to place priority on research to find less expensive but equally effective modes of treatment that would be offered to everyone for a given type of problem. (Managed care arrangements, such as the one in which Mr. Lacey is enrolled, attempt to keep costs in check by limiting the number of treatment days or costs a patient may incur on the basis of pooled data from many similar patients before him.)

A Standard of Care Must Be Established and Honored

Many groups have attempted to establish a baseline level to help assure equity for everyone. For example, the Ethical and Religious Directives for Catholic Health Care Services require that poor people be a focal point of consideration. If their needs are met, it is likely that others' needs will be, too.[7] Philosopher John Rawls's proposal is that an unequal distribution of basic goods in a society must be acceptable from the standpoint of the least well off.[8] Many nations have used a basic set of benefits that *everyone* must receive as a bottom line standard, no matter how minimal.

The Process Must Be Inclusive

Representatives and advocates for all groups that will be affected should participate in the policy-making process. An interesting experiment in rationing was conducted by the state of Oregon in regard to its Medicaid recipients. A random group of taxpayers was asked to rank many treatment interventions according to priority, the idea being that when the results were tabulated, the state dollars allocated annually to health services would be directed only to people needing those treatment interventions. When the money ran out, no more payment would be made that year, which translates to patients not recovering that particular intervention that year no matter their need.

Reflection

What is your reaction to Oregon's rationing approach to the allocation of health care resources? Would a strictly random chance distribution have been more ethically acceptable? Why or why not?

Proportionality and Reversibility Are Required

The beneficial services that are withheld must be proportional to the actual scarcity. Cuts or cutbacks are justifiable only as long as true and serious scarcity exists. (See Box 14–1 for a summary of all five criteria for rationing.)

Tragic Choices

In the awesome possibility of eliminating some people from receiving resources altogether, a *lottery* approach, or process of *random selection,* has been suggested by some as a procedure that can help to make a decision more just when the claim is for a particular medical treatment simply not available to everyone who needs it.

BOX 14-1 CRITERIA FOR A MORALLY ACCEPTABLE APPROACH TO RATIONING OF HEALTH CARE RESOURCES

1. Rationing is necessary.
2. Rationing is a last resort move.
3. A high standard is the goal.
4. The process is inclusive.
5. The cuts are proportionate and reversible.

In random selection a prior medical judgment of medical need and suitability has been made, and the patient's freedom to refuse possible treatment has been ascertained. In an attempt to be as impersonal as possible in selecting who is to receive treatment among those still found eligible, "rolling the dice" has been suggested as a model. In extreme circumstances such as this the method has been upheld in the courts of the United States as a procedure that fully expresses an equal consideration of the equal right of each person to his or her life (*United States v. Holmes*).[9]

It affirms that there is no way of justly determining a person's social worth to others, and therefore removes the necessity of an arbitrary decision among those who are equally medically needy but otherwise differ.

It also has been argued by proponents of this position that those unfortunate people who are excluded from treatment may find it easier to accept because they have not been excluded on the basis of individual traits they have or do not have.

Nonetheless, not everyone agrees that random selection always is the most humane way of proceeding. Some maintain that once patients have been selected as being similarly situated in terms of medical need it makes sense to give weight to such merit-related social factors as the likelihood of future service to society, the extent of past services, or family responsibilities. These positions take seriously into account that people are seldom viewed in isolation but rather as members of their larger communities.

SUMMARY

Random selection attempts to remove the opportunity for discrimination, but some criticize its deeply impersonal nature.

Summary

In conclusion, discussion of the proper moral response to Christopher Lacey's situation, viewed from the lens of what justice would require, raises many questions regarding the most morally defensible way to proceed in his case. Inherent in the judgment are considerations of fairness and equity and the appropriate criteria for a rationing approach if one is needed.

What Sidney McCally, John Krescher, and the other members of the health care team decide to do will be based on clinical and policy considerations. In the ethical dimensions of the decision, they will be faced with the issues of fairness and their duty to be faithful to the patient and to do no harm. They will need courage to act on their decision in addition to wisdom to decide well. Although questions of distributive justice are at the heart of the case, much more is at stake in the actual decision-making situation for this man, his family, and their relationship with the health professionals. The policy makers who take seriously what equity means in this type of situation will help the health professionals do the morally correct thing.

Questions for Thought and Discussion

1. Imagine that a friend of yours has AIDS and a highly experimental but potentially lifesaving medication has been found. Currently, the supply is too scarce to distribute to everyone who needs it. What type of decision-making procedure for deciding who should receive the drug is the most fair?

2. Discuss some difficulties in using the criterion of medical need as the basis for distribution of health care resources among various groups and individuals.

3. (This exercise can be performed as an individual or group exercise.) You have an opportunity to argue for which services should be included and excluded in your state's health care rationing plan for Medicaid recipients. You have taken this task seriously for many reasons, but one is that the federal government has given your state the opportunity to develop a rationing plan for Medicaid recipients nationally.

On the basis of the Oregon plan, the first step was to poll a random group of citizens to set priorities among services. Your task force has gone one step further than the Oregon plan. Oregon polled only voting citizens. You set a mechanism in place that assured input from a large contingency of Medicare recipients from across your state. (One criticism leveled at Oregon policy makers was that their pool of voters did not include a proportionate number of Oregon Medicaid recipients.) Now the real crisis has come because several important services that the members of the task force thought would be included are not. You will now decide among yourselves how to make the final cuts but will not alter with the list created by the first part of the process (as described earlier). The task force has before it six possible services that could be included for the state's 20,000 Medicaid recipients (all estimated costs are annual, and the task force has $26,136,000 to allocate):

a. Preventive dental care for children ages 2 to 6 years (includes a yearly check-up, teeth cleaning). Does not include fillings, orthodontics, or other acute dental or surgical services. **Estimated cost: $2,760,000.**
b. Outpatient mental health services (initial evaluation and up to 12 visits) for children and adolescents (ages 4 to 19 years). Does not include medications or hospitalization. **Estimated cost: $6,000,000.**
c. Smoking-related asthma treatments. **Estimated cost: $4,960,000.**
d. Liver transplantation and follow-up. **Estimated cost: $9,900,000.**
e. Mammograms for women younger than 50 years. **Estimated cost: $4,900,000.**
f. Coverage for pain management for patients with chronic back pain, including medications, rehabilitation, and pain centers, but not including surgery, which could be covered in another surgical category that ranked higher on the list of services. **Estimated cost: $10,040,000.**

Rank order, with highest priority number 1 and lowest 6, and write your rationale below each one.

1. ______________________________

2. ______________________________

3. ______________________________

4. ______________________________

5. ______________________________

6. ______________________________

References

1. Sheehy, E., Conrad, S.L., Brigham, L.E., Luskin, R., Weber, P., Eakin, M., Schkade, L., Hunsicker, L. 2003. Estimating the number of potential organ donors in the United States. *New England Journal of Medicine* 349(7):667–674.
2. Surman, O., Purtilo, R. 1995. Re-evaluation of organ transplantation criteria: Allocation of scarce resources to borderline candidates. In Thomasma, D., Marshall, P. (Eds.), *Clinical Medical Ethics Cases and Readings*. New York: University Press of America, pp. 356–366.
3. Hoffman, S., 2002. Actuarial fairness vs. moral fairness in health insurance. *Law and Bioethics Report* 1(4):2–4.
4. Cunningham, R., Sherlock, D.B. 2002. Bounce back: Blues thrive as markets cool towards HMO's. *Health Affairs* 21(1):11–23.
5. Ruben, E.R., Osterweis, M., Lindeman, L.M. (Eds.). 2002. *Emergency Preparedness: Bioterrorism and Beyond*. Washington, DC: Association of Academic Health Centers.
6. Fleck, L.M., 2002. Rationing: don't give up. *Hastings Center Report* 32(2):35–36.
7. Committee on Doctrine of the National Conference of Catholic Bishops. 2001. *Ethical and Religious Directives for Catholic Health Care Services*. Washington, DC: United States Catholic Conference.
8. Rawls, J. 1971. *A Theory of Justice*. Cambridge, MA: Harvard University Press, pp. 54–114.
9. *United States v. Holmes*. 1842. 26F Case 36 (No 15, 383) C.C.E.D. Pa.

15

Compensatory Justice: Social Sources of Claims for Health Care

Objectives

The student should be able to:

- Distinguish some key differences in approach to distributive justice and compensatory justice.
- Identify a range of policy options that could be adopted in situations in which compensatory justice is being considered as an appropriate response to a group that has been harmed.
- Describe some cautions that should be taken into account when compensatory justice approaches are being applied toward the goal of a more equitable society.
- Evaluate why stigma and social marginalization are societal factors influencing attempts to create just health care policies.
- Identify and evaluate the role of personal responsibility for health maintenance from the standpoints of distributive justice and compensatory justice considerations.

New terms and ideas you will encounter in this chapter

compensatory justice
collective responsibility
social marginalization
personal responsibility for health maintenance
vulnerability
communitarianism
social justice
labeling
altruism
solidarity

Topics in this chapter introduced in earlier chapters

Topic	*Introduced in chapter*
Beneficence	3
Nonmaleficence	3
Distributive justice	3, 14
Equity	14
Disability	12

Introduction

Justice issues often are difficult to grasp because they require us to move beyond the usual one-on-one situation of health care interaction and consider whole groups of people. In Chapter 14 you began your inquiry into the questions of justice, so you are already familiar with this concept.

This chapter introduces another dimension of justice that is pertinent in some of the situations you will face as a health professional. The issue of compensatory justice arises when groups of people have health problems related to their position in the larger society. The story of the Maki brothers will help you focus on how compensatory justice is relevant in the context of patients' work, and it also will help you think about other contexts in which compensatory justice considerations arise.

The Story of the Maki Brothers

Mr. Eino Maki is an asbestos miner who emigrated from Finland to the United States in 1965. He was born into a poor rural family who lived in a small remote village near the Russian border. Eino did not attend school in Finland after the first grade because he was a "slow learner" and could not keep up with the other students. Although most students in this country received excellent educations, his family refused to send him to a special school in Tampere, some 300 miles away, saying they needed his help on the farm.

One dreadful morning in 1963 a fire destroyed the family's home and Eino's parents perished in the fire. Eino and his sister were sent to live with an aunt and uncle in Helsinki. At the age of 18, he could not find work in Helsinki, so he emigrated to the United States to live with his unmarried older brother in an area where there are many asbestos mines. The community where his brother lives is about 90% Finnish.

When Eino arrived in the United States, his brother, John, attempted unsuccessfully to find him a job in the railroad construction company where he was employed as a section worker. After several months Eino did secure a job in a nearby asbestos mine.

He has been employed by this same mining company and has held essentially the same position for the last 37 years. Although at work he still suffers the stigma associated with his being "slow" at grasping ideas, he is an excellent worker and participates in the social life of the community. Many evenings are spent reminiscing about the "good old days" in Finland, and everyone talks about going back. Privately, however, John and Eino agree that it is unlikely they ever will return.

In the last 2 or 3 months Eino has had increasing difficulty breathing. Occasionally he has coughed up blood-tinged sputum and often has pains in his chest when he awakens, but they disappear after he has been up and around for a couple of hours. At first he does not say anything to John, but one November morning he realizes that he cannot make it to work. He asks John to take him to the company physician.

Eino has never liked doctors. In all of his years of employment he has visited the company physician only for the required routine annual physical examinations and once when he suffered a dislocated shoulder in a fall from a mine platform. He has always passed the physical examinations with a "clean bill of health."

After the examination the physician assistant who has conducted the initial tests tells Eino that some further tests are needed and that he will have to be admitted to a hospital, which is about 120 miles away. Eino is angered at this news but realizes that he cannot go back to work feeling the way he does. He tells John he wants to rest at home until he feels better, but John, seeing the trouble his brother is having, urges him to go to the hospital and drives him there.

Five days later in the hospital Eino takes a sudden turn for the worse. John is called and drives back to the hospital. When he arrives he is met by Dr. Kai Nielson, a young physician who looks to John as if he cannot be a day older than 16 years. Dr. Nielson asks John to come with him to a little room next to the nurse's desk and closes the door. "Mr. Maki, I'm afraid I have some bad news," he says. "Your brother has cancer and has had it for quite a long time. Ideally, we should start a type of treatment immediately that his company's health plan does not totally cover."

So far John has barely been hearing what the young doctor is saying. His mind is racing wildly. He vaguely recalls Eino's report of a discussion at a union meeting a year or so ago regarding a rumor that work in the asbestos mines causes cancer and that their union was looking into it. This concerned John greatly, but Eino brushed it aside, said it was "a bunch of hogwash," and he was "healthy as a horse," refusing to discuss it further. Knowing that Eino was not only "healthy as a horse" but "stubborn as a mule," as he told a friend later, "What could I do? I let the matter drop."

Finally, John realizes that Dr. Nielson has been talking to him. "We could do the treatment, but unless Eino has additional insurance coverage, the treatment is going to cost him a lot of money."

John tells the physician that they own a small cottage together, with about two acres of unfarmed land around it. They have no savings, only the pension that their respective companies will provide, but that benefit cannot be realized until Eino is 65 years old. Dr. Nielson replies sympathetically, "Well, there is a chance your brother will be eligible for federal assistance, but unfortunately it may mean you will have to sell your house to become eligible for it once you've expended the earnings you'd realize from that. I don't know exactly how it works, but I'll have the social worker talk to you. Of course, we can't guarantee that the treatment will beat the disease, but we feel reasonably sure that it would at least slow down the rate of growth of the cells."

There is a pause. Then he adds, "It is, of course, a big decision. It is entirely up to you and your brother what you decide to do. We haven't talked to him or rather been able to talk to him. He doesn't like doctors much! Why don't you two talk it over with the social worker? Remember, it's your decision and your brother's. But don't take too long in deciding. . . . I think every day counts. Do you have any questions?" John shakes his head "no." "Well," Dr. Nielson concludes, "if you do after talking with the social service department, have them set up an appointment for you to see me again."

As John stands, Dr. Nielson extends his hand and John shakes it warmly. John glances up into the doctor's face and sees an expression of genuine pity in the young man's eyes. John blurts out, "Was the cancer caused by the mines?" The young doctor drops John's hand and studies his own hands as he answers, "Mr. Maki, the cause of cancer is often complex. It can be the result of a combination of factors. But the type of cancer that your brother has is the same type that asbestos miners get at a higher rate than the general population. Primarily it affects the lungs."

John thanks Dr. Nielson. Outside the doctor's office he wanders over to a window and stares outside into the snowy darkness for a long time, his hands in the pockets of his overalls. He has not cried since their brother Matt was killed in a tractor accident many years before, but he feels a lump rising in his throat now. He feels totally unable to move, as if he is glued to the floor. He struggles to think clearly, but his mind remains a blank.

The story of John and Eino Maki raises numerous ethical issues. For instance, some people reading this story have questions about why Dr. Kai Nielson was sharing all of this potent information with John when it was Eino, a competent adult, who is the patient. Is it a good enough reason for the physician to put the burden of sharing the bad news with Eino on John's shoulders? What more might you want to know about that part of the story before making a judgment about Kai Nielson's behavior in this situation?

The lens through which we focus our attention (care) in this chapter is the issue of justice that patients similarly situated to Eino raise. This, too, is of moral relevance to your role as a health professional.

The Goal: A Caring Response

This story, like the one in Chapter 14, raises a number of ethical questions. A seemingly healthy, hard-working man becomes a victim of circumstances that leave his health compromised. A caring response by health professionals requires that they do whatever is "best" or, in the language of ethics, is *beneficent* for the patient. In our story, Dr. Kai Nielson has been doing just that while he has been engaged in the process of diagnosis and communication. However, this professional also knows that in some regards matters are now slipping out of his hands. Although he may have some agency in securing the necessary services for Eino Maki, he also knows that other forces also will have to come into play. Mr. Maki's situation reminds us that a caring response requires the foundation and infrastructure of a larger society willing to support individuals in his predicament. Society will tend to place Eino within a whole category of similarly situated persons to assess whether and how much of societal resources will be allocated for them.

The Six-Step Process in Compensation Decisions

Mr. Maki's story raises several ethical issues, but none is more important than the idea of compensation for illness or injuries. In Chapter 14 you had an opportunity to think about allocation dilemmas when whole groups of individuals were making claims for the share of scarce resources on the basis of medical need.

Does it make any difference when the medical need is caused by "injury" to the patient's body occurring on his or her job, a type of work injurious to his or her health but taken in part because of low social and economic status in society?

Thoughtful individuals have pondered the role that such differences among patients should play. To help elucidate some of the thinking, let us consider the relevant "facts" in the story of the Maki brothers.

Step 1: Gather Relevant Information

Eino, and people like him, carry out labor tasks and other societal functions that are needed for the society to function well but are not valued in other ways and often carry high risks to the workers. Of course, some "high-risk" situations are respected, and individuals who carry out the tasks are given extra financial benefits, as well as a high status. Examples are fire fighters, members of a police force, or Navy Seals. Others, like Eino, are relegated to the greater risk and "less desirable" jobs because of their lower social status, often accompanied by poverty or other characteristics that carry a stigma with them. It can be argued that Eino did not have the full capacity to comprehend the danger he was in, and if he had, he would have been able to do little to change his situation.

The idea of "compensation" arises out of society's consciousness that there is something unfair about this situation. Not everyone has the same chance at the benefits from the get go. Some people are born into situations that, through no fault of their own, force them into disadvantageous situation. They are "handicapped" in the sense that a sports participant may be handicapped and therefore given additional "points" on that basis alone. It is not surprising that the problem it raises in society is characterized as a problem of justice.

Step 2: Identify the Type of Ethical Problem

People in situations such as Eino finds himself experience medical need, and from the way the physician, Dr. Nielson talks, there is some hope of "beating the disease" if the "most appropriate treatment" is made available. Chapter 14 explains that if treatment is justly distributed to each according to his or her medical need, there should be a way for patients such as Eino Maki to receive optimum treatment, and in so doing the demands of distributive justice would be met.

From a justice standpoint, however, Eino's situation raises serious questions of justice not solely as a distributive justice challenge but also requires consideration from the perspective of compensatory justice.

Compensatory justice acknowledges due regard for groups of individuals by offering them compensations for wrongs they have suffered. The compensation is not necessarily for a consciously perpetrated wrong.[1] The underlying idea is that because of the socially vulnerable position these individuals are in through no fault of their own, their positions becomes a morally relevant consideration.[2] As for Eino, we have reason to believe that his work in the mines led to a life-threatening, industry-related condition. If the company knowingly placed workers at risk, the moral responsibility squarely can be placed on management. If they, too, are surprised by this bad news, society's understanding of the wisdom of compensating individuals in such a situation has led to certain mechanisms for spreading the cost of the compensation across the larger society by using taxes and other common resources. ("Workmen's compensation" grew out of this idea originally, but since has come to be considered a protection for anyone injured on any job, no matter their social status, economically secure position, or other variables.) Sometimes the "wisdom" of providing compensation has come from pressure by interest groups such as unions or other organizations who try to provide a voice for those who are not in a position to speak effectively for themselves.[3]

In any case, the idea that a moral claim for compensation may require that medical (or other) resources that could be used for something else should be used for this purpose makes this problem a justice dilemma.

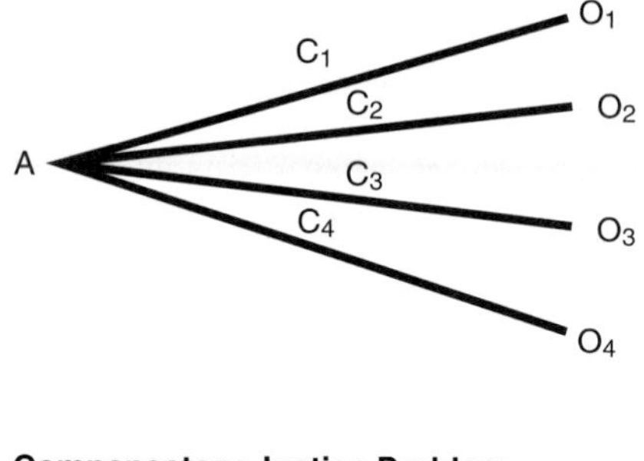

Compensatory Justice Problem

A = Moral Agent
C_1 = Action taken on behalf of claimants whose social "handicaps" are added to their medical need
O_1 = Outcome is priority on allocation of resources to those whose social "handicaps" are added to medical need
C_{2-4} = Action taken on behalf of other claimants
O_{2-4} = Outcome determined by priorities on basis of claimants in 2–4

Similar reasoning has been applied to priority setting for shelter, food, or other basic goods of society, the underlying assumption being that not everyone comes equally equipped to enjoy life's basic benefits.

SUMMARY

Compensatory justice assumes that allocations of scarce resources should be made to address health care problems of an individual or group on the basis of more than medical need alone.

Step 3: Use Ethics Theories or Approaches to Analyze the Problem

In Chapter 14 you were introduced to several aspects of theories of justice that are relevant to the current discussion.

Equity Considerations

For instance, there is the idea of equity. To review, equity means that every effort must be made to treat each person in a similarly situated circumstance alike, basing differences among people on criteria that are ethically acceptable. This idea is relevant to the discussion about Eino Maki. One could say that *anyone* working in such a dangerous situation, and doing so because of his social and economic situation, would be "similarly situated," and therefore would fall within the same general category of claimants. You also were introduced to the ideas of health care as a right, and of allocations according to medical need or merit. It certainly helps support the idea of compensation if health care is viewed as a right in contrast to the opposite extreme that health care is a commodity like all other products to be bought by those who can afford to do so. And as for the criterion of medical need as a basis for making a claim on resources, in thinking regarding compensatory justice, the basis of the claim *includes but goes beyond* the idea of medical need alone. One has to go to the larger base of social need.

The Principle of Nonmaleficence

How is "social need" established, and on what ethical principle might it become a moral claim on others?

In Mr. Maki's case, the compelling argument in favor of supporting his medical treatments financially is not only that he has a terrible medical condition (which, indeed, he has) but that he has the condition *because* he was in a job that carried with it the albatross of a carcinogenic agent that is well established scientifically and can be tested for before the damage he has incurred to his health. For many people examining Eino Maki's plight there is an intuitively sympathetic response in favor of compensating him for his job-related cancer. It seems basically wrong, from a moral point of view, that he should have to suffer the ravages of a debilitating, painful, and fatal disease because he has been working in a setting that economically disadvantaged individuals are forced to endure and that carries a life-threatening hazard with it. The principle of nonmaleficence, "do no harm," includes the idea that there should be a disposition to *prevent* harm and *remove* harm when possible. Compensation is a response to harm. For many, this case for compensation is strengthened by the fact that the company might have known about the problem and failed to take humane measures and precautions on behalf of its workers.

SUMMARY

Compensatory justice reasoning acknowledges that some persons are socially disadvantaged in ways that put a moral claim on the larger community to respond to the harm that accompanies this situation.

It follows that in the reasoning about compensatory justice, for groups with conditions generally judged to present similar medical need but one is at a greater social disadvantage, the latter will have the relativity greater claim on medical resources. Of course, in many instances, the distinction is moot because a position of social disadvantage often creates disparities in health status, so that the resulting situation looks the same viewed from either perspective.[4]

Step 4: Explore the Practical Alternatives

The compensatory justice issue can be highlighted by comparing several policies that might be adopted by companies, governments, or other policy-making bodies. All of them suggest that there may be a collective responsibility to respond to harm. You have an opportunity to explore these alternatives in some detail. As you do, try to think about which one(s) you could support from an ethical standpoint and why. In each case, you can choose whether you support or do not support the policy and some considerations to help you defend your decision.

1. The company should offer Eino (and all similarly situated employees) a sum of money equal to that which would pay for their treatment and provide early retirement with all retirement privileges if the person is unable to return to work. It is up to the affected employee to decide whether to spend the money on treatment or something else.
   Support _____ Do not support _____
   Consider:
   the most caring response overall to all similarly situated employees;
   Eino's rights, autonomy, and moral responsibility;
   the company's moral responsibility and rights and needs; and
   the larger society's involvement.
2. The company should pay for the employee's treatment with the understanding that he or she will return to work if medically able and, if unable, will be retired with full privileges of retirement that would have accrued if he had worked until regular retirement age.
   Support _____ Do not support _____
   Consider:
   the most caring response;
   Eino's autonomy and moral responsibility;
   the company's moral responsibility and rights and needs; and
   the larger society's involvement.
3. The company should pay for the employee's treatment with the understanding that he or she will return to work if medically able. If unable, the person will be terminated with whatever retirement has accumulated up to the time of termination.
   Support _____ Do not support _____

Consider:
the most caring response;
Eino's rights, autonomy, and moral responsibility;
the company's rights and moral responsibility; and
the larger society's possible involvement of supplementing Eino's income if he has little or no retirement income (society as a "safety net").

4. Federal or state funds from tax dollars or other public sources should provide Eino (and all similarly situated people) a sum of money equal to that which would pay for treatment and arrange to supplement his current retirement earnings up to his company's full retirement level if he is unable to return to work. It is up to the affected person to decide whether to spend the money on treatment or on something else.
   Support _____ Do not support _____
   Consider:
   the most caring response;
   Eino's rights, autonomy, and moral responsibility;
   the company's lack of involvement for compensation beyond what Eino has already earned; and
   the larger public's collective contributions and assurance of being able to be supported in Eino's situation.
5. Federal or state funds from tax dollars or other public sources should pay for full medical coverage for people like Eino but not offer them a cash equivalent. That is, the compensatory considerations are limited to medical treatment directly related to the "injury." The understanding is that the person will return to the former employment if medically able. If unable, he or she will be retired by the company with full privileges, and the company will receive a subsidy from the government.
   Support _____ Do not support _____
   Consider:
   the most caring response;
   Eino's rights, autonomy, and moral responsibility; and
   the shared moral responsibility of company and the larger public and how it is divided (society as provider of medical compensation, "safety net" of the company).
6. No company or public compensation should be provided for Eino or similarly situated people.
   Support _____ Do not support _____
   Consider:
   the most caring response;
   Eino's rights, autonomy, and moral responsibility;
   the company's rights, autonomy, and moral responsibility; and
   the public's rights, autonomy, and moral responsibility.

As you can see, each of these options provides a variety of possible conflicts of interest or opportunities for community-wide solidarity efforts. The conflicts may be seen as competing interests of similarly situated harmed individuals, the private sector of society, and the larger public sector of society. Questions of the most caring approach (all things considered), rights, autonomy, and the sphere of moral responsibility of each should be taken into account in the analysis of any of these options. Options 1 through 5 support the compensatory justice position that compensation should be provided for the harm suffered by people such as Eino Maki, although the form, amount, and source of compensatory funds will differ according to the political and social context in which the compensatory mechanisms are situated. Many ethicists viewing the situation from the standpoint of health care as the good being distributed support the position that at least a basic safety net of health care benefits should be provided by federal, state, or local governments (the public sector). The position that the whole community of society should work together to find common solutions because it will, in fact, more likely benefit all is called a "communitarian" approach.[5] Although there are several varieties of communitarian thinking, they reflect a basic theme of interdependence. The first five options all have elements of such thinking. Each would provide some compensation for Eino and other people made vulnerable by circumstance. The tradition of the United States has carried some communitarian themes in it but is largely based on the individual autonomy of individuals living within structures and institutions where markets will drive what each individual or group will rightly enjoy.[6] Canada and almost all European countries take a more communitarian approach. Eino and John Maki are good examples of people who want to "earn their own way," the hallmark of this type of thinking. There also are several varieties of this liberal approach within modern society. The sixth option most fully conveys the extreme of the liberal society free market approach, which leaves no room for the idea of compensatory justice, except in criminal justice where the victim should be compensated.

SUMMARY

Compensatory justice requires an assumption of deep interdependence of people in society.

The above discussion illustrates that compensatory justice cannot be discussed apart from also determining who in the population should bear the burden of costs incurred as a result of policies based on compensatory reasoning. For example, the first three options suggest that the cost should be borne privately, in this case, by the company. Options 4 and 5 remove the responsibility from the private sector. Taxes to pay for compensation plans come from those people who, under the U.S. doctrine of personal liberty, have been able to become and remain self-sufficient. As taxes increase for the purpose of supporting groups or individuals with situations such as that of Eino Maki, compensatory justice may be viewed as impinging on the personal liberty of people who currently are not ill or in need of medical services. They argue that they may not be able to send their children to colleges they otherwise would choose, put additions on their homes, buy sports and exercise equipment to keep fit, or, for some, even heat their homes properly.

Step 5: Complete the Action

To arrive at a policy, the question is how much personal liberty members of society are willing to contribute towards mechanisms allowing justice to be upheld. The concern that self-interest will prevent collectively agreed on approaches has promoted more community-spirited ways of thinking about this act as a "contribution" instead of a "sacrifice" or loss. One example is that such a contribution yields the rewards of altruism. Another is the idea of a reciprocity ethic. In the latter, a contribution to someone else's well-being creates a societal environment in which others will be willing to contribute to one's own well-being when the need arises.[7]

Reflection

Having considered all the ramifications, suppose that you are a member of a policy-making body that must vote on the six policy options discussed earlier. On the basis of what you have learned so far about the various approaches and possibilities for private versus public sources of support, who do you think should be responsible? Why?

Even though you have been a responsible committee member, what (if any) lingering reservations do you have regarding your choice?

In making this policy decision you have exercised your moral reasoning in a manner similar to that which you will be asked to use in the policy-related aspects of the practice of your profession: in your process of coming to a decision you have had an opportunity to engage in the step-by-step process of decision making. You have brought to consciousness the expressions of caring, considered the relevant facts, dealt with the ethical dilemma of justice in the situation with which you are faced, and, through that, arrived at the above selection of your option.

Step 6: Evaluate the Process and Outcome

Although much can be said in support of compensatory justice, the determination of groups in society to be singled out for preferential treatment requires that they be designated as a special class.

This raises at least two important caveats: one is about the double edge of labeling, and the other is about the specific label of "vulnerability," the latter being a term often applied to establish disadvantageous circumstances of the kind that Mr. Maki illustrates.

Labeling: A Double Edge

Labeling assures that already vulnerable groups become readily identifiable as different. However, Martha Minow[8,9] points out that "Difference . . . is a comparative term . . . different from whom? I am no more different from you than you are from me . . . But the point of comparison is often unstated . . ." She says that at the root of this issue is "the dilemma of difference."[8]

> "When does treating people differently emphasize their differences and stigmatize or hinder them on that basis? And when does treating people the same become insensitive to their difference and likely to stigmatize them or hinder them on that basis?"[9]

The problem, she concludes, is that when societal arrangements are designed only with the included in mind, the excluded cannot meet the standard because of something in their makeup. Such groups are not always given the positive treatment promised them and may be even further discriminated against.

A case in point is an extensive screening program for sickle cell disease that was initiated in the United States in the latter quarter of the 20th century. Sickle cell disease affects primarily African Americans. It is a painful condition manifesting itself in infancy and continuing throughout a shortened life span. Symptoms associated with it include infarction of the soft tissue and bone, causing acute pain. It also affects the spleen, liver, and kidneys.[10] The screening designed to identify affected individuals and therefore *identify them as a group deserving of special attention* was not accompanied on a large scale by treatment programs. Instead, in many instances, African Americans identified through the screening process have found that insurance, employment, and other records carry stigmatizing information regarding their status as carriers of the sickle cell trait.[11] In summary, people in a labeled group who have experienced previous social wrongs do not necessarily find redress or medical need are sufficient conditions to place them in a position of receiving appropriate attention and treatment.

The "Vulnerability" Criterion Considered

Chapters 3 and 14 introduce the basic justice presumptions on which all resources are allocated in the United States. At the root is a notion of equality, an egalitarian concern arising from this nation's very founding documents. This, in turn, gives rise to various understandings of the role that justice plays in making a good community for all. Chapter 14 shows that in the overall approach to health care allocations there are compelling reasons why a concern for equality cannot be met through providing equal amounts of resources to everyone. So far in this chapter you have learned that, in Western societies' understanding of justice, distributive justice reasoning alone has shortcomings in situations where socially stigmatized groups are not viewed as meriting equal concern when compared with more powerful, mainstream groups. Therefore, the stigmatized groups are at risk for (i.e., vulnerable to) being left out of the benefits realized by that mainstream. Some at-risk groups include women, the elderly, people with disabilities, poor people, groups of people in racial and ethnic minorities, and other people who realize low social status within the mainstream society. Collectively, they are socially marginalized from the goods of society.[12]

Our acknowledgment of sexism, ageism, and other discriminatory attitudes have helped to shift the cause to the larger society. It is out of such a current social environment that the idea of what compensatory justice entails has continued to develop to include an onus on society to make it more inclusive.[13]

SUMMARY

We have come a long way in acknowledging the major role that mainstream society plays in social marginalization and that the appropriate moral response must be found in more equitable societal arrangements. Traditionally, socially stigmatized groups were viewed as the cause of the "unfortunate" situation they were in because of some personal, genetic, or cultural "defect" or sin.

Anderson[14] summarizes this shift well in her article, "What Is the Point of Equality?" She points out correctly that the dominant philosophic view (translated into public policies) currently is that "the fundamental aim of equality is to compensate people for undeserved bad luck—being born with poor native endowments, bad parents, and disagreeable personalities, suffering from accidents and illness, and so forth."[14] The compensatory justice goal for such individuals having drawn a so-called short straw in the natural lottery of life is to mitigate or eliminate the negative impact of their predicament. But ultimately, Anderson rejects this concept of the goal of compensatory justice because, she argues, in it the source of claims by the disadvantaged group is that they are inferior to others in the worth of their lives, talents, and personal qualities, "thus its principles express contemptuous pity for those the state stamps as sadly inferior." Furthermore, it creates a situation characterized by "demeaning and intrusive judgments of impaired people's capacities to exercise responsibility and effectively dictates to them the appropriate uses of their freedom."[15]

In contrast, she proposes (with many other thinkers today) that a more considered understanding of justice would work toward the aim of creating "a community in which people stand in relations of equality to others" based on true and deep respect. She joins Silvers[16] in emphasizing that for equity to be realized, compensation reasoning must be replaced by prior distributions to assure social conditions for everybody to optimize their freedom at all times. In this approach, groups who make claims on another can do so through virtue of their equality with, not inferiority to, mainstream groups.

In the situation of Eino Maki, if his company met all requirements for safety within the work environment—and was responsive to data regarding types of changes that would protect employees who have mental or physical susceptibility to harms in that workplace—the company not only would meet the demands of justice as Anderson understands it, but also would meet the company goals of employee retention and the opportunity for greater productivity. In summary, it would be consistent with a correct conception of what equality requires. With this perspective beginning to emerge, one can imagine a time when current conceptions of compensatory justice will be replaced in our social–political structure. The construction of an inclusive social environment may be viewed by some as utopian, but substantive changes that already have been made show it to be a practical alternative. From a cost-sensitive approach alone, the costs to society of lost productivity and need for caregivers (professional and otherwise) makes the neglect and exclusion of whole groups of people a bad idea. Health professionals are in a good position to be one important voice advocating for such changes.

In the meanwhile, the idea of compensations for harms continues to have a large social function (and at times be tested in the court and other environments). It would seem unjust to withhold considerations about whom and under what conditions compensations should be made for harms imposed by current unjust environments.

The Patient's Responsibility for Health Maintenance

The story of Eino Maki raises important questions about how to allocate health care and other resources when some people in society are more disadvantaged than others because of their social situation. But we never fully addressed the question of what Eino's role should be in preventing his current ill health. Eino was a hard-working miner in a dangerous environment, and at least some people who read his story probably are sympathetic toward him. Today, there is a lively discussion about how the social responsibility to allocate resources justly can be balanced against each individual's personal responsibility to try to stay as healthy as possible. The story of Jane Tyler and Sam Puryo illustrates some of the complexities that arise in the process of trying to exercise justice for everyone in a society. Jane also has a life-threatening situation (emphysema), but her situation is different from Eino Maki's in some striking ways.

The Story of Jane Tyler and Sam Puryo

Jane Tyler, a 32-year-old single woman and mother of three children (5, 8, and 12 years old), has been living on public assistance since her first child was born. Jane lives with her mother, who helps with light housekeeping and child care. Now that the children will be in school she has successfully applied for a grant that will allow her to train to become a business information technology assistant so that she can make a living for herself and her family. Receiving this award was a tremendous boost to her self-esteem, and she sees it as a bright doorway out of her "no exit" life situation.

Therefore, it comes as a devastating blow to her to learn that she has emphysema. She has been threatening to stop smoking for a long time, but her two-pack-a-day habit has had a strong grip on her. It is an even greater shock to learn that although the emphysema is only in the beginning stages, she may not be eligible for state-of-the-art curative treatment because she is on public assistance. It seems that the state legislature presented to the voting public the opportunity to decide priorities for high-cost interventions provided through public funds by sending a questionnaire to a sample group. Some readers will recognize this general approach as the innovative tactic passed by the Oregon state government in 1989 (Senate Bills 27, 534, and 935, 65th Oregon Legislative Assembly). It has now become known as "The Oregon Experiment." There have been numerous critiques in the medical, social policy, government, and lay literature. The public sample of taxpayers eliminated "debilitating or life-threatening disease clearly caused by smoking" from the list of priorities (as well as many other conditions). Three physicians have concurred conclusively that Jane's emphysema is caused by her smoking. One of them believes there may be cofactors that lead some people to actually manifest the symptoms of emphysema, whereas others do not. The other two are completely convinced her smoking directly has created her serious health problem. As only two concurring physicians are needed for this policy to take effect, she is able to receive only cursory treatment. Her only opportunity for an adequate treatment regimen is for her to find some way to pay for it.

Sam Puryo is a caseworker in the public assistance office. Jane has been one of his clients for several years. He is upset at what he judges to be the apparent injustice of the laws that have put her in her current dilemma. He tries to call his state senator to see if there are any loopholes in the law that could help her or if an exception can be made for this woman who Sam sees as exceptional. The senator is not encouraging; she is sympathetic but knows of no loopholes and is pessimistic about an exception being made.

During a coffee break, Sam gets into a discussion of the new rulings with his colleagues at the welfare office. His fellow social worker is strongly in favor of the approach taken by the legislature. All the people at lunch agree that it is important to be willing to consider the arguments.

As you have already learned, justice has been defined in various ways, each of them based on the presumption of equality but adding the fundamental idea of giving to each his or her due when their situations call for it.

Reflection

Consider the following questions. What *is* due Jane Tyler and other people in similar situations? More importantly, how should her situation be approached to ascertain what is due her ethically?

There are at least three variables that might be relevant in trying to sort out what is due to Jane Tyler. One is her medical need, a second is her low economic status, and the third is her apparently self-inflicted condition.

The first variable, her medical need, was introduced in Chapter 14 as being relevant from the point of view of distributive justice. If I were looking at Jane's situation solely from a distributive justice stance, I would conclude that the medical care is due her on the basis of her medical need. However, her second variable is low socioeconomic status with its tendency to socially marginalize her and exclude her from services. This chapter introduced the idea of compensatory justice. From a compensatory justice standpoint, we also would have to consider Jane Tyler's poverty. Her economic status may become another decisive variable according to the following lines of observation: poor people often are at a disadvantage in their opportunities to acquire an education, and therefore obtain employment that requires special skills or contacts. Women born into poverty are more economically disadvantaged than men. Finding an avenue to a skilled job could be an important turning point in her life and in her children's welfare. She has found funds but now her health needs may be the barrier. From the standpoint of compensatory justice, she deserves a high priority position for allocation of health care resources rather than the low one she faces.

Now comes the further complication of her smoking-induced condition. You can see compensatory justice reasoning being applied again, but this time it is working against Jane Tyler. Most of us believe—in theory, if not in practice—that responsible citizens should attempt to refrain from self-destructive behaviors. Now she is viewed tacitly, if not explicitly, as *creating* a harm through her carelessness and abuse, the harm being not only the destruction of her lungs but also the drain on tax money that might be required for her care and that of her small children as her condition deteriorates. Do you think that she *is* voluntarily harming herself and others, or is this an example of blaming the victim, a person who is a victim of society's unjust social arrangements?

One defining factor is whether in fact Jane is in a social position to be held accountable for her smoking and the ensuing difficulties it has brought on her. Distinguishing between disadvantages that a person brings on himself or herself and those resulting from external forces over which he or she has no or little control is not easy to do. Although most readers know that a person's conduct is determined in early childhood and is reinforced by one's cultural, ethnic, and socioeconomic group (to name some influences on behavior), many join society's judgment that all she has to do in liberal free societies is "just say no" to change her behavior.

This discussion and your responses are germane because you are entering the health professions at a time when there is much debate about how much responsibility individuals must take for their own health.[17] According to one position in this debate, someone who has liver failure caused by heavy alcohol intake should not be eligible for public aid for health care services because the disease resulted from his or her chosen lifestyle. However, those taking the other position point out the great risk for injustice in such a strict accounting for our knowledge about the determinants of alcoholism is still quite limited. In addition, one could argue that the alcohol-dependent person is a victim of an unfavorable social situation, unhappy childhood, or psychiatric disorder.

Although you cannot help but have opinions and personal feelings about issues related to others' self-destructive habits, it is important to remember that the relevant arguments are usually general, not specific. Therefore, a caring response to a group in deciding what role their self-destructive behaviors should play in the allocation of publicly generated resources for health care (or other basic goods) must begin with humility toward the complexity of "what makes people tick." Although it cannot be reasonably expected that the larger society will support any and all types of self-abuse and self-neglect, the prior moral responsibility is to get to the root causes of a group's behavior. Each and every one of us belongs to more than one group. Therefore, this cannot be accomplished without skills that allow for culturally competent approaches to the variety of situations we and others like us in terms of the societal place—economic, sex, or other life situations—we find ourselves in at anytime allocation decisions are being made.

SUMMARY

Currently, there is much debate about the role each individual must play in assuming responsibility for his or her own health. Such assessments must be made within the larger societal context in which individuals reside to assure that inequities are not placed on them.

Summary

The justice-related issues raised in this chapter (and in Chapter 14) admit of no easy answers, theoretically or in their practical application. You will have opportunities to reflect further on the implications of how distributive justice and compensatory justice approaches foster the larger societal goals of a caring response in the face of limited resources. The underlying concerns presented by social marginalization and the complementary roles that individuals, their institutions, and the larger public should play in upholding the tenets of a flourishing society all are relevant considerations in implementing just policies. Only when just policies are in place can individual health professionals and others be confident that just practices will be possible.

Questions for Thought and Discussion

1. Some have argued that because the extent to which people value health in relation to other goods (such as food, shelter, clothing, a car, living where there is fresh air, and so on) varies from person to person, the most just health care resource distribution would be to give the same amount of money to each citizen (a "voucher" or "savings account") and let him or her spend it however he or she chooses over a lifetime. Discuss the strengths and weaknesses of this arrangement.

   At what age should this allocation be made? Why?

2. Discuss the pros and cons of the following proposed legislative bills from the point of view of compensatory justice considerations:

____

____

____

____

Condition A is a progressive disease of the central nervous system. It first affects the spinal cord and in its later stages infiltrates the brain, resulting in progressive spasticity and later in multiple movement and thought disorders. It occurs primarily in white, middle-class men 40 to 55 years of age and leads to certain death within 15 to 20 years. The cause and course of the disease is well understood. It is an autoimmune condition. Recently, a medication has been discovered that can help to slow the progress of Condition A dramatically. Currently, however, the cost of the medication required for treatment is estimated to be about $10,000 per year for each patient. About 7500 people in the United States have been diagnosed with the disease, and the incidence seems to be increasing. It is believed that many more cases will surface if the medication becomes available for any who need it.

Legislation has been introduced into the U.S. Congress to make possible the processing and administration of the drug to all patients "in the name of humanity." A conservative estimate is that the cost to U.S. taxpayers will be about $17.5 million per year.

When the bill is being debated, a counterproposal is introduced. Proponents propose that the funds be allocated to provide full dental care, free of charge, to any Hispanic or Latino child in the United States up to 8 years of age whose parents fall under the poverty line economically. This free dental insurance will be compartmentalized from other federal or state funding for medical care, because some of those plans do not cover dental care and some do not cover the children of undocumented (i.e., illegal) immigrants. The estimated total cost is close to that in the competing bill, but "will serve ten times as many, each of whom is equally deserving of services as the people in the competing bill." The core of their argument is that in general the latter individuals have been discriminated against in the United States, that only the poorest among even that group has been targeted, and that legislators and policy makers must take this factor into account in determining health care priorities.

REFERENCES

1. Beauchamp, T., Childress, J.F. 2001. *Principles of Biomedical Ethics* (5th ed.). New York: Oxford University Press, pp. 259–260.
2. Rawls, J. 2001. In Kelly, E. (Ed.), *Justice a Fairness: A Restatement*. Cambridge, MA: Belknap Press of Harvard University.
3. Tweedale, G. 2001. *Magic Mineral to Killer Dust: Turner and Newell and the Asbestos Hazard*. New York: Oxford University Press.
4. Adler, N.E., Newman, K. 2002. Social-economic disparities in health: Pathways and policies. *Health Affairs. The Determinants of Health* 21(2):60–76.
5. Habermas, J. 1999. Three normative models of democracy. Liberal, republican, procedural. In Kearney, R., Dooley, M. (Eds.), *Questioning Ethics. Contemporary Debates in Philosophy*. New York: Routledge, pp. 135–144.
6. Appiah, A. 2001. Liberalism, individualism and identity. *Critical Inquiry* 27:305–332.
7. Kittay, E.F. 1999. *Love's Labor: Essays on Women, Equality and Dependencies*. New York: Routledge, pp. 67–68.
8. Minow, M. 1990. *Making All the Difference: Inclusion, Exclusion and the American Law*. New York: Cornell University Press, p. 21.
9. *Ibid.* p. 20.
10. Purtilo, D.T., Purtilo, R.B. 1989. *A Survey of Human Diseases* (2nd ed.). Boston: Little, Brown, pp. 295–297.
11. Anionwu, E., Atkin, K. 2001. *The Politics of Sickle Cell and Thalassaemia*. Philadelphia: Open University Press.
12. Danis, M., Patrick, D.L. 2002. Health policy, vulnerability and vulnerable populations. *Ethical Dimensions of Health Policy*. New York: Oxford University Press, pp. 311–334.
13. Carlson, E.A. 2001. *The Unfit. A History of a Bad Idea*. Cold Spring Harbor, NY: Cold Spring Harbor Press.
14. Anderson, E.S. 1999. What is the point of equality? *Ethics* 109:287–337.
15. *Ibid.* p. 289.
16. Silvers, A. 2000. The unprotected: Constructing disability in the context of antidiscrimination law for individuals and institutions. In Francis, L.P., Silvers, A. (Eds.), *Americans with Disabilities: Exploring Implications of the Law for Individuals and Institutions*. New York: Routledge, pp. 126–145.
17. Callahan, D., Koenig, B., Minkler, M. 2000. Promoting health and preventing disease: Ethical demands and social challenges. In Callahan, D. (Ed.), *Promoting Healthy Behavior: How Much Freedom? Whose Responsibility?* Washington, DC: Georgetown University Press, pp. 153–170.

16

Good Citizenship and Your Professional Role:

Life as Opportunity

Objectives

The student should be able to:

- Describe two key characteristics associated with having a career as a professional person.
- Compare the focus of *shared fate* and *self-realization* careers.
- Discuss what a caring response entails when the "patient" is the public at large.
- Identify two ethical principles that apply to a health professional's obligations to society.
- Describe the role of moral courage in pursuing possible wrongdoing and some common themes expressed by people who act courageously.
- Recognize the difference between a professional's moral responsibility to promote service focused on the public interest versus the common good.
- Discuss three criteria of suitability that will help professionals set priorities that are appropriate when faced with opportunities for service to the community.
- Describe how the idea of a *civic self* becomes an orienting notion when acting on behalf of the common good.
- Reflect on how a basic respect for people may mean that the health professional will become involved in pressing social issues outside of health care.

New terms and ideas you will encounter in this chapter

good citizenship	"shared fate" orientation of the professions
right to work	public interest versus common good considerations
social responsibility	civic self

Topics in this chapter introduced in earlier chapters

Topic	*Introduced in chapter*
Professional role	2, 4, 6, 7, 14, 15
Responsibilities to self	7
The caring response	2
Ethical distress type A	2
Nonmaleficence	3
Beneficence	3
Common good	3

Introduction

Sometimes the health professional is involved in taking risks with dangers that are little understood. The little prince in Antoine de Saint-Exuperéy's famous children's story of that same name identified these dangers as "baobabs." This final chapter addresses the risks you may choose to take as a professional person and a citizen with baobab issues that endanger basic moral values of a society.

Good citizenship is everyone's responsibility. In fact, the demands of good citizenship and of being a good professional have much in common. Each requires a measure of personal and social confidence, communication skills, and a willingness and ability to work with others. The basic question, and an interesting one, is whether you have any *special* rights, duties, and responsibilities as a citizen because you are a professional.

Reflection

Are professionals required to have any special virtues? Are there special rights and responsibilities? What do you think?

To help focus your thinking, consider the following story.

The Story of Michael Merrick and ExRad Corporation

Two years ago the residents of Peetstown, a small town in the northeastern United States, welcomed the arrival of ExRad Corporation. The town had suffered terribly when Cal Mode Textiles Corporation had left, leaving in its wake more than 400 unemployed individuals, and a major recruitment by the residents had resulted in ExRad's choice of their town for its new location.

Michael Merrick is a pharmacist working in Peetstown. He grew up in the beautiful hills 10 miles from where he now works, although for several years he went to school and worked in New York City. He, his wife, and their three children moved back to Peetstown 2 years ago.

Recently, Michael and his family went on a walk along a path by the stream that flows through the small town of Peetstown. The stream provides recreation for children and adults alike along its banks, as well as fishing and swimming. All of them simultaneously smelled a strong, sweet odor. Michael's 10-year-old son, John, ran upstream and discovered a small pipe just under the surface of the water. The odor was distinctly stronger in the pool that had formed there and the water was purplish.

Michael suggested that they not go too near the water. They continued their walk. But that night he took a small jar and went back to collect a sample of the water. The next day he drove 40 miles to visit a chemist friend who works in the chemistry department at the community college. The friend agreed to analyze the water and a week later called to say it contained large amounts of trichloroethylene, a toxic chemical that Michael remembered had poisoned the water supplying a town in Pennsylvania not long ago. Alarmed, Michael told a physician colleague who makes biweekly visits to the local clinic in Peetstown about his findings. The two decided to go to a county health official, who then promised to take care of the problem. But a month went by and Michael heard nothing. He tried calling the county official with no success. Finally, he saw the man at the monthly Rotary Club meeting and asked him what was happening. The man took him aside and said, "Don't worry about it. It was nothing. The injection well belongs to ExRad Corporation, and they are looking into it." Then he added, "You know we need that corporation."

The next day Michael returned to the stream again. The odor was stronger than ever. When he got back to the clinic, he called the physician and related his story. She said, "I guess we had better pursue this ourselves, Mike." That night after dinner Mike discussed the matter with his wife. Both of them were worried about what lay ahead. Michael called the physician and told her he felt he had to pursue the matter as best he could on his own because he was concerned about the effect of this toxin. She said, "It's the right thing to do. Count me in. We'll talk next week when I'm there."

Reflection

The threat of an environmental health hazard has come to their attention, and they must now decide what to do. What, if anything, do you think they should do? Why?

____

____

____

____

Now that you have made an initial judgment, let us go through the story to highlight some basic ethical considerations. Then when the chapter is completed, you can see if you change your mind regarding the course of action they should take.

The Goal: A Caring Response

Michael and his physician colleague are not faced with a clinical or even health policy situation. Yet, they feel as if they should do something as citizens. They may have no thoughts at this point about whether their decision to try to get at the root of a problem they believe is potentially causing harm to their community is related to their professional roles. Their lack of imagination or understanding about this issue is understandable because, as has been highlighted in the Chapters 14 and 15, the health professional's idea of "care," in common parlance, usually is thought of as being contained to situations between individuals. But you also have now had a chance (in Chapters 14 and 15) to begin to expand your horizon regarding the focus of your caring. So you have at least a small foundation on which to build your thinking about care with the public in general as the goal of your caring response. That is something you have a chance to think about as we walk with Michael and his colleague through the six-step process of decision making.

The Six-Step Process in Public Life

What information can help us (and them) discern whether their role as a health professional puts any special claim on them to pursue this potential environmental and health hazard? Well, one thing we do know is that professionals are a privileged group in society. In the first place they have had an opportunity to choose a career. Most of the world's population does not have such an opportunity. Having a career choice means that you are able to pursue your specific tastes, framing a life plan to suit your own character. Norman Care's classic article on the nature of careers suggests that people in this privileged position choose between two basic types of careers: those with a *shared fate* orientation and those oriented to *self-realization*. The former focuses on service to society, the latter solely on self-satisfaction.[1] Health (and other) professionals fall within both categories to some extent, but primarily within the shared fate category, with its straightforward service ethic. You have had an opportunity to think about this aspect of your role as a *professional* in several previous chapters.

The *right to work*, whatever the job, is seen as a basic right in democratic societies. Work as a professional, however, is not a basic right for everyone. Depending on your profession, society will give you a license, which certifies you or registers you in the state where you work. Your right to work (as a professional) comes about only after you have completed rigorous training, passed qualifying examinations, and promised to adhere to the code of ethics of your chosen profession. All these hurdles are society's reassurance that you are competent to do what you "profess" to do—namely, to be of service.

SUMMARY

Health professionals have chosen a career line that folds the opportunity for service into what will bring self-satisfaction in one's work. Society views this career choice as having special privileges and responsibilities that go beyond the more general privilege of a right to work and carry out one's duties as prescribed by a particular work site.

Of course, although this distinction is useful as a basic orientation to Michael's and the physician's place in society, it does not tell us definitively about how they should respond to Michael's discovery of trichloroethylene in the stream, or what he can reasonably expect from society in terms of support for any activity he undertakes to expose this environmental hazard.

Steps 1 and 2: Gather Relevant Information and Identify the Type of Ethical Problem

Perhaps some insight about what Michael should do can be gleaned from another look at the information he already has. He knows there is a deadly toxin in the stream near his home and other homes in their neighborhood. Every action he has taken so far suggests that he knows this is not a benign situation, rather it is a problem that should arrest the attention of others. He surmises, though does not have certainty, that something more is going on, perhaps an attempt by other leaders in the community to cover up any wrongdoing by the ExRad corporation that has brought needed jobs. His suspicion is shared by the physician who has offered to link arms with him in pursuing the issue. They are concerned just as any other good members of the community would be concerned.

However, these two individuals also are not like many other citizens in the community. This doctor and pharmacist are in a position to be heard if they choose to speak up because their roles carry a certain amount of status and weight in relation to most citizens. To at least a limited, and maybe a great, degree, they can be viewed as moral agents in this situation by virtue of their status and role, an issue we will take up in more detail as this chapter unfolds. They know that they are viewed accordingly, and they are conflicted, not because they are ignorant of their power but because they understandably are hesitant to get into the messy business of pursuing this issue. Michael knows he still is viewed as an "outsider," and therefore may more quickly be dismissed (and discriminated against) as a "troublemaker." He may become ostracized, even if proven to be right. He also knows he may be able to prove nothing.

We know he has had a discussion with his wife about the problems that might arise if they tackle this problem, and he admits to having some fear.

In summary, they are facing an ethical problem in the form of *ethical distress*. They know they should not let this matter drop until they are sure someone is taking care of it. But Michael dreads what is ahead.

Reflection

Using the diagram below, sketch out some details of their distress. Recall that Michael and his colleague are moral agents *(A)*, who must take a course of action *(C)* that has barriers that must be overcome to arrive at what they know is the correct outcome *(O)*. Name some barriers you imagine they have and also what you would consider a "correct outcome," ethically speaking.

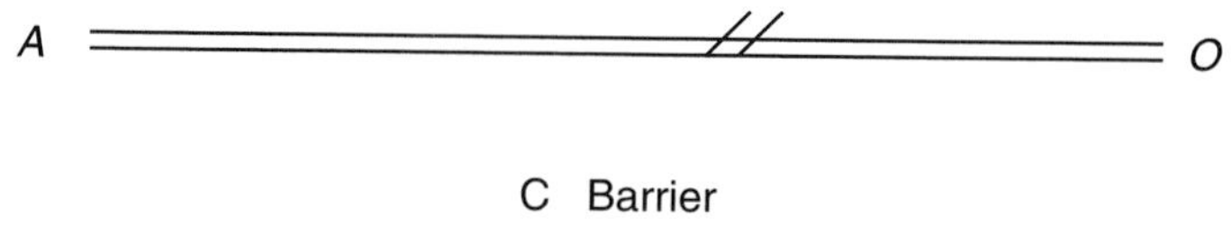

A ══════════//══════════ *O*

C Barrier

Ethical Distress

This type of ethical distress may include some uncertainties, but it can be best characterized as ethical distress type A, where known interior (e.g., fear) and exterior (resistance from at least one sector of leadership in the community) barriers are keeping them from pursuing what is right.

Step 3: Use Ethics Theories or Approaches to Analyze the Problem

Having identified their problem as one of ethical distress, let us look more closely at these two moral agents in a predicament they do not welcome.

Moral Courage as a Virtue

The caring response, the goal being the larger community, will require moral courage:

> Moral courage is a readiness of voluntary, purposive action in situations that engender realistic fear and anxiety in order to uphold something of great moral value.... A common term to describe courage is "bravery," but when the term "moral" is added to it, the ensuing action must always be with the goal of protecting a moral value that appears threatened.[2]

It is not surprising that one barrier to Michael's and his colleague's action is fear, and the reason they need courage is apparent. There is no body of ethical literature that makes courage a requirement of professional life, although on many occasions its cultivation will help the health professional do what is right. The current situation is one good example of that.

Often, courage can be built up by preparation for such action. In 1999, I had the privilege to conduct a series of interviews with exemplars of courageous action by professionals and others who fought the injustices of the apartheid system in South Africa. Several common themes emerged, among them the following:

1. Name the seriousness of the situation. Do not pretend that what is happening, or not happening, is acceptable and that it will go away. It is not and it will not.
2. Believe that good will prevail over wrongdoing. (One might call this the optimism of courage, or "hoping courage.")
3. Take the opportunity to nurture and be nurtured by essential sources of support. Everyone emphasized this, no matter their individual circumstances in other regards. In this chapter we see Michael, the physician, and Michael's family as one "support coalition" that already is in place, and others will surely follow as the word gets out.
4. Become fully invested in the outcome. As one interviewee said, "The cause I started out to embrace eventually embraced me."[3]

There were other themes, but these four seem to fit the situation facing Michael and the physician as they begin to stake out their strategies. Even if they find that their inquiries and probing reveal no wrongdoing, they will have prepared well and will benefit from the experience of having done so. In fact, in a report on their studies of moral development and moral agency in professionals, Bebeau, Rest, and Narvaez[4] attribute to Rest the idea of defining moral character as "having the strength of your convictions, having courage, persisting, overcoming distractions and obstacles, having implementing skills, [and] having ego strength." He singles out moral courage as the attribute needed to turn disposition into moral action.

SUMMARY

Moral courage is a virtue that, when cultivated, will prod one to the right action, even in the face of fear or other difficulties.

Another related moral resource of purposeful action is to understand fully the moral obligations supporting the idea that one must act on behalf of the well-being of the larger society, not just that of an identified patient.

Professional Responsibilities and Good Citizenship

The traditional oaths and codes of professional ethics say little about the health professional's obligations to society at large, except that direct patient care can be viewed as having a positive impact on the health of the larger society. But modern codes and ethical guidelines almost always include such a focus.

Reflection

Check the code of your particular profession to see how this focus is worded and jot it down. Professional codes often are worded broadly to allow for further interpretation in more specific circumstances. Is this true of the statement you just wrote from your code? If you were using the statement as your guide, what would you do if you were Michael?

You should now be aware that to guide your behavior you need to use some of the principles you learned earlier in this text rather than to rely solely on the code as a guide. Nonmaleficence will apply, as well as beneficence. Now the focus is society in general, not just an identified patient or client. Jennings and colleagues[5] distinguish two types of public service, each of which could be seen as meeting the criteria of nonmaleficence and beneficence. The first is service that seeks to promote the *public interest,* and the second is that which promotes the *common good.*

Public service that promotes the public interest includes the professions' contribution of *technical* expertise to public policy analysis and community problems, and indirect service to society as a byproduct of service to individual members of society. The sphere of influence is governed by your technical expertise.

Public service that promotes the common good includes the *distinctive and critical perspective* the various professions have to offer on basic human values and on facets of the human good and the good life. It also includes the profession's contribution to what may be called civic discourse—that ongoing conversation in a democratic society about our shared goals, our common purposes, and the nature of the good life in a just social order. Your influence partially is determined by your relatively high social standing in the community.

This thought about the two types of public service can be summarized as your professional responsibility to participate in the development of policies and solutions at the larger community level and to pay attention to those larger social issues by which you may help to create a better society. As Jennings and colleagues stated, there is a responsibility to contribute to "the well-being of the community: its safety, the integrity of its basic institutions and practices, the preservation of its core values."[5]

SUMMARY

Professionals engage in two types of public service—that which promotes the basic interests of individuals and that which promotes the public good. The former relies primarily on one's technical skills, the latter on one's solid standing in the community.

Of these two types of service, Michael's and the physician's opportunity to pursue the problem of the toxic waste being dumped into the stream more fully falls into the category of common good service.

Reflection

Let's think about this more specifically. What are the important values that could be served by Michael's involvement in this problem?

You probably agree that among the most important values is the safety of all living beings—the people, animals, and plants in the area; in other words, the environmental health or general ecologic balance. In recent years we have become more aware of the fragility of ecosystems and of the direct effects of imbalances on human health. Environmental or ecologic illnesses are major sources of public health problems today.[6]

To think about how the health professions play a role in maintaining and restoring this type of health, health professionals should be seen as affirming a definition of health and well-being that goes beyond medical interventions strictly speaking. Michael's decision to enter the public arena to prevent or to remove harm to the whole community is as important as his interventions at the bedside. As noted at the outset of this part of the discussion, his clear understanding of this moral dimension of his professional status may help him act courageously.

Step 4: Explore the Practical Alternatives

Social responsibility involves all the ways in which you may feel that you should become involved in making the world a better place. To suggest that Michael is obligated equally by the broader public health and narrower clinical arenas raises the critical problem of setting priorities. In prioritizing the expenditure of your time and energies, fulfilling the professional obligations for which you are specifically trained takes precedence. After that you may choose to become involved in activities where you can be of assistance, even if you are not specifically qualified to do so. The least claim on you is made by activities in which you are less qualified than others to make a significant impact. This approach to setting priorities can be of great assistance when the tug of responsibility calls and you feel overwhelmed about choosing what to do and what to leave undone.

In considering Michael's opportunity, the first thing to decide is whether his pursuit of the toxic waste problem will deter him from performing his professional services, as these skills have the greatest claim on his time and energies.

Using priority setting as their general guide, Jonsen and Jameton[7] offer this now classic paradigm for deciding actual responsibility in specific cases. They divide professional and political responsibilities of health professionals into three general categories of suitability for an individual's involvement:

- The most binding responsibilities are those directly related to patient care.
- The second most binding are those related to the broader public health issues that all health professionals share.
- The least binding are other opportunities for involvement.[7]

The third category, however, and this is key, will vary according to the health professional's judgment about how much difference her or his involvement is likely to make on the basis of the health professional's "symbolic weight" in some types of issues. Sometimes a job is more likely to get done because someone of high status, respect, or visibility throws weight behind the issue. Therefore, if Michael's status as a pharmacist (or health professional in general) will lend credence to the gravity of the offense or need for correcting the problem, his responsibility to get involved increases on that basis alone. Jonsen and Jameton[7] also stress that although these are useful *general* guidelines, an urgent crisis may arise in which health professionals feel compelled to change the order of these responsibilities. An example is the physicians, nurses, and others who threw themselves into open resistance against the Nazi regime, placing the urgency of this social situation above all else.[8] The issue does not necessarily have to involve health care (although Michael's problem involves a potentially serious public health issue). In summary, if Michael is trying to set priorities, he will have to ask himself about the appropriateness of his involvement according to the three criteria of suitability.

SUMMARY

Even when the health professional has determined that a problem warranting attention exists, priorities must be set.

Steps 5 and 6: Complete the Action and Evaluate the Process and Outcome

For purposes of our discussion, assume that Michael and the physician have decided they will pursue the issue.

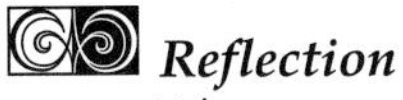

Reflection

What types of questions would you still need answers for to decide which of several practical strategies Michael (and his physician colleague) might follow will be the best one? Given what you know, what do you suggest?

In any challenge of the magnitude they may be facing, coalition building will become a major task in trying to assure success. Western cultures often believe that because we want to act responsibly, we must carry the moral weight of an issue on our individual shoulders. William May[9] points out that this is just one of the burdens we assume mistakenly because we fail to take into account the deep relationship of ourselves as individuals to others in the larger context in which we can indeed thrive. He reminds us that to cultivate "strong, nurturing, and self-restraining institutions [of society]. . . . we must cultivate the civic self." What does he mean by this term? He defines civic self as follows:

> The civic self, as opposed to the imperial self, understands and accepts itself as limited and amplified by others. The civic self recognizes that it enjoys an expansion of its life in and through its participation in community. The civic self . . . includes both a subjective and an objective element. Subjectively, the civic self requires the citizen and society to cultivate the ability to work in concert with others. Objectively, this working in concert with others must serve—at least in part—the common good.[9]

SUMMARY

Understanding our mutual interdependence as "civic selves" allows us not only to call on our colleagues and others to resolve problems they are more suited to handle, but also to count on their support when we are asked to share the larger societal burden.

The boundaries of professional responsibility as such do not have well-defined edges, therefore any of us could find ourselves involved in a great variety of societal issues during our professional careers. Working together with their colleagues and others, Michael and the physician can hope to have the energy, expertise, and wisdom needed to make a positive difference.

When they are engaged in reflection, the final step of ethical decision making, it would be appropriate for them to not only think about how they might have been more successful and why, but also to encourage themselves by reading from a great American novel, John Steinbeck's *The Grapes of Wrath*. It is a powerful literary statement about our interdependence and about the will to try to help fulfill high ethical goals such as they have undertaken. In this excerpt from the novel, Tom has decided to join the ranks of people struggling against the injustices being perpetrated on the migrant workers:

> They sat silent in the coal-black cave of vines. Ma said, "How'm I gonna know 'bout you? They might kill ya an' I wouldn' know. They might hurt ya. How'm I gonna know?"
>
> Tom laughed uneasily. "Well, maybe like Casy says, a fella ain't got a soul of his own, but on'y a piece of a big one: an' then:"
>
> "Then what, Tom?"
>
> "Then it don' matter. Then I'll be all aroun' in the dark. I'll be ever'where: wherever you look. Wherever they's a fight so hungry people can eat, I'll be there. Wherever they's a cop beatin' up a guy, I'll be there. I'll be in the way kids laugh when they're hungry an' they know supper's ready. An' when our folks eat the stuff they raise an' live in the houses they build: why, I'll be there. See?"[10]

Tom has made the decision to be where there is suffering and where he believes he is situated to make a difference. That commitment may indeed take you, too, into the heart of problem solving around issues that will not be resolved unless you "see" the difference your presence will make.

Summary

In this final chapter you have an opportunity to see yourself as a moral agent in regard to important social issues facing the larger human community. You will find a niche where your expertise, skills, high standing in the community, interests, and the urgency of the needs will help you set priorities. Your courage and professional responsibility to help prevent harm and promote the common good will seldom have to be exercised in issues as dramatic as the one discussed in this chapter; in fact, fortunately, that will be rare. At the same time, your readiness to be a positive force in society whatever the circumstances is a resource well worth cultivating as a part of the larger role you have a privilege to play. To echo William May's[9] words once again, "the civic self, understands and accepts itself as limited and amplified by others."

Questions for Thought and Discussion

1. Because you cannot become involved in every social issue that comes along, it is a good idea to choose the issues that hold some interest for you. If you were to become involved in trying to solve three social problems today, what would they be?

____

____

2. Your place of employment has been designated a first response site in case of the unthinkable—a bioterrorist attack. The administration has decided to identify key personnel on a volunteer basis, hoping to create a core group that will become the chief managers and caregivers in such an exigency. Each professional employee is asked to indicate his or her willingness to be a member of the core group and each is asked also to discuss the matter with loved ones before arriving at this decision. Some issues you are asked to consider are the heightened danger (in respect to the general population) you will be in either because the facility is hit directly or because exposed victims may quickly contaminate the facility, the likelihood that all communication will be cut off with the world outside your workplace, the likelihood that a triage network will be set up to include—and exclude—some victims for desperately needed attention, the likelihood that you will be "locked in" and not free to leave the site until such time as you are deemed not to be a biohazard to others. Will you volunteer? On what factors do you base your decision?

____

____

____

____

3. You have been invited to become a member of a state commission that will examine how to best use public space (parks, gardens, beaches, parking areas, and so on) for the welfare of the citizens. They have asked you because they think "your expertise as a health professional is needed." What, if anything, can you bring to such a commission from the point of view of your professional training and expertise?

____

____

____

____

4. Homelessness has reached momentous proportions. What can your profession do about meeting the health-related needs of people for whom the street is their "home," those who do not have so much as a roof over their heads? What can you personally do? What resources do your profession and you personally have to attend to their larger social, spiritual, and psychological needs? What benefits will such involvement offer you and your profession?

____

____

____

____

REFERENCES

1. Care, N. 1984. Career choice. *Ethics* 94(2):283–302.
2. Purtilo, R. 2000. Moral courage in times of change: Visions for the future. *Journal of Physical Therapy Education* 14(3):4–6.
3. Purtilo, R. 1999. Step up, speak out, stand firm! Moral courage lessons from South Africa. *Creighton Magazine* Fall:20–25.
4. Bebeau, M., Rest, T., Narvaez, D. 1999. Beyond the promise: A perspective on moral education. *Educational Researcher* 28(4):22.
5. Jennings, B., Callahan, D., Wolf, S. 1987. The professions: Public interest and the common good. *Hastings Center Report* (Suppl.):3–11.
6. Donnelley, S. 2002. Natural responsibilities. Philosophy, biology and ethics in Ernst Mayer and Hans Jonas. *Hastings Center Report* 32(4):36–43.
7. Jonsen, A., Jameton, A. 1977. Social and political responsibilities of physicians. *Journal of Medicine and Philosophy* 2(4):376–400.
8. O'Neill, O. 2002. *A Question of Trust: The BBC Reith Lectures 2002*. New York, Cambridge University Press.
9. May, W.F., 2001. Interlude: The shaping of public happiness. In *Beleaguered Rulers, The Public Obligation of the Professional*. Louisville, KY: Westminster John Knox Press, pp. 188–189.
10. Steinbeck, J. 1939. *The Grapes of Wrath*. New York: Penguin Books, p. 535.

Index

Page numbers followed by f refer to figures; page numbers followed by t refer to table